Intelligent Assistive Technologies
for Dementia

Intelligent Assistive Technologies for Dementia

Clinical, Ethical, Social, and Regulatory Implications

Edited by

FABRICE JOTTERAND

MARCELLO IENCA

TENZIN WANGMO

AND

BERNICE S. ELGER

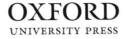

OXFORD
UNIVERSITY PRESS

Oxford University Press is a department of the University of Oxford. It furthers
the University's objective of excellence in research, scholarship, and education
by publishing worldwide. Oxford is a registered trade mark of Oxford University
Press in the UK and certain other countries.

Published in the United States of America by Oxford University Press
198 Madison Avenue, New York, NY 10016, United States of America.

CIP data is on file at the Library of Congress
ISBN 978–0–19–045980–2

This material is not intended to be, and should not be considered, a substitute for medical or other
professional advice. Treatment for the conditions described in this material is highly dependent on the
individual circumstances. And, while this material is designed to offer accurate information with respect
to the subject matter covered and to be current as of the time it was written, research and knowledge about
medical and health issues is constantly evolving and dose schedules for medications are being revised
continually, with new side effects recognized and accounted for regularly. Readers must therefore always
check the product information and clinical procedures with the most up- to- date published product
information and data sheets provided by the manufacturers and the most recent codes of conduct and
safety regulation. The publisher and the authors make no representations or warranties to readers, express
or implied, as to the accuracy or completeness of this material. Without limiting the foregoing, the
publisher and the authors make no representations or warranties as to the accuracy or efficacy of the drug
dosages mentioned in the material. The authors and the publisher do not accept, and expressly disclaim,
any responsibility for any liability, loss, or risk that may be claimed or incurred as a consequence of the use
and/ or application of any of the contents of this material.

1 3 5 7 9 8 6 4 2

Printed by Integrated Books International, United States of America

Contents

PART III ETHICAL AND REGULATORY IMPLICATIONS

A companion website with color versions of figures printed black and white in this text can be found at www.oup.com/us/intelligentassistivetechnologies

Contributor Biographies

Arlene Astell, PhD, is Professor of Neurocognitive Disorders at the University of Reading, Associate Scientist at the University Health Network and Associate Professor at the University of Toronto. She is a psychologist by training, and for the past 18 years, her research has explored the potential and application of technology to address challenges of later life, particularly enabling people to live well with dementia. Astell's work starts with understanding the context into which any innovation is to be introduced. This involves looking at physical, social, and psychological factors, to address challenges of adoption and facilitate cocreation with intended end-users. She has published across a wide range of fields and is the current Chair of the Alzheimer's Association Technology Professional Interest Area.

James Beauregard, PhD, is a Lecturer in the psychology doctoral program at Rivier University, Nashua, New Hampshire, where he teaches Neuropsychology, Biological Bases of Behavior, Health Care Ethics, and Aging. His research interests are in the fields of neuroethics and personalist philosophy including the intersection of these two areas as they impact our understandings of personhood.

Christophe J. Büla, MD, is the Head of the service of Geriatric Medicine and Geriatric Rehabilitation, Department of Medicine at the University of Lausanne Medical Center (CHUV), and full professor of Geriatric Medicine at the Faculty of Biology and Medicine at the University of Lausanne, Switzerland. His research interests focus on disability prevention in older persons. He conducted several projects aiming at improved detection and management of geriatric syndromes such as dementia, gait impairment, and falls; diseases such as depression; and infections that impact the frailty and disability pathway in different populations of older persons (community-dwelling; consulting the emergency department; hospitalized in acute, rehabilitation, and long-term care settings).

Cynthia Chen, PhD, MS, BA, is an independent postdoctoral researcher who continues to engage in bioethics research while pursuing a career in medical communications. She has conducted research for over a decade in centers of excellence, such as Imperial College London (UK), King's College London (UK), and Case Western Reserve University (US). Her research has included the genetics of complex traits such as cognitive abilities and psychiatric diseases, the effects of biological clocks on seasonal affective disorders and reproduction, and the ethical, legal, and social issues of direct-to-consumer genetic testing. She holds several degrees, including a PhD in neuroendocrinology from the University of Edinburgh (UK) and an Erasmus Mundus Masters of Bioethics from the consortium of KU Leuven (Belgium), Radboud University in Nijmegen (Netherlands), and the University of Padova (Italy). She has authored several publications in biomedical sciences and continues to publish in bioethics.

Gabriele Doblhammer, PhD, MSc, is a Full Professor for Empirical Methods and Demography at the University of Rostock (http://www.wiwi.uni-rostock.de/~esf/). She is head of the Demography Group at the German Center for Neurodegenerative Disease in Bonn (http://www.dzne.de/). In addition, she is a Distinguished Research Scholar at the Max Planck Institute for Demographic Research (http://www.demogr.mpg.de/). She completed her PhD in Demography and Statistics in 1997 at the University of Vienna. Her research focuses on patterns and trends in health, morbidity, and care needs at old age. She is particularly interested in life-course factors of cognitive and physical functioning and of neurodegenerative disease such as dementia and Parkinson disease.

Bernice S. Elger, MD, PhD, is head of the Institute for Biomedical Ethics at the University of Basel and associate professor at the Center for Legal Medicine at the University of Geneva, where she is head of the Unit for Health Law and Humanitarian Medicine. She studied medicine and theology in Germany, France, Switzerland, and the United States and obtained her specialty degree in internal medicine (FMH) in Switzerland. As part of her work at the Center for Legal Medicine at the University of Geneva, she has worked in prison medicine for 15 years. She has obtained several research awards: Arditi Award in Ethics (1997); Award of the Medical Faculty, University of Geneva (1999); Bizot Award (2005); and twice the Swiss Research Award in Primary Care (2010 and 2016). Her publications cover a wide range of fields including medical ethics in genetics, clinical ethics, research involving biobanks and human tissue, and ethical issues related to cutting-edge biotechnology.

Tanya E. Feng, BSc, completed her Bachelor's of Science in Psychology at the University of British Columbia and is currently studying in the MD undergraduate program at the university. Her research interests include patient engagement in dementia research and the impact of online information on health decision making. Her other areas of research include the role of dopamine in risky decision making and impulse control disorders in Parkinson's disease.

Anne Fink, PhD, has a PhD in Demography and is research associate at the German Center for Neurodegenerative Diseases (DZNE) in Bonn, Germany, and at the Rostock Center for the Study of Demographic Change in Rostock, Germany. Her research interests are the epidemiology of dementia in aging populations and modifiable risk factors of neurodegenerative diseases. Further, she is interested in data validation procedures. She has expertise in epidemiological methods for the research of dementia in health claims data and population-based surveys.

Thomas Fritze, PhD, has a PhD in Demography and is a research associate at the German Center for Neurodegenerative Diseases (DZNE) in Bonn, Germany, and at the Rostock Center for the Study of Demographic Change in Rostock, Germany. His research interests are the epidemiology of dementia in aging populations and the effect of risk factors over the life course on cognitive functioning and dementia late in life. He has expertise in demographic and epidemiological methods for the research of dementia in health claims data and population-based surveys.

Tsutomu Fujinami, PhD, is a Professor at the Japan Advanced Institute of Science and Technology (JAIST), Japan. His research interests include skill acquisition and dementia care. He studied philosophy at Waseda University and was engaged in the research of Artificial Intelligence at the Systems Development Laboratory, Hitachi Ltd. He studied Cognitive Science at the University of Edinburgh and was awarded his PhD.

Bert Gordijn, PhD, is professor of ethics and director of the Institute of Ethics at Dublin City University. Bert is Editor-in-Chief of two book series: *The International Library of Ethics, Law and Technology* and *Advances in Global Bioethics* as well as a peer-reviewed journal: *Medicine, Health Care and Philosophy*, all published by Springer Nature. Moreover, Bert is executive secretary of the European Society for Philosophy of Medicine and Healthcare, which was founded in 1987 with a view to the growing need for critical reflection on the role of medicine and healthcare in our present society. He is also President of the International Association of Education in Ethics. He has served on Advisory Panels and Expert Committees of the European Chemical Industry Council, the European Patent Organisation, the Irish Department of Health, and UNESCO. His research interests are in philosophical ethics, bioethics, and technoethics.

Elisabeth Hildt, PhD, is Professor of Philosophy and director of the Center for the Study of Ethics in the Professions at Illinois Institute of Technology, Chicago. After having completed her studies in biochemistry, she became a fellow of the postgraduate program Ethics in the Sciences and Humanities at the University of Tübingen. Then she spent several years as a postdoctoral student at the University of Tübingen and the University of Munich and was an assistant professor at the Chair for Ethics in the Life Sciences at the University of Tübingen (2002–2008). From 2008 to 2014, she was the head of the Research Group on Neuroethics/Neurophilosophy at the University of Mainz. Her research interests are bioethics, neuroethics, and science, technology, and society.

Marcello Ienca, PhD, MA, MSc, is a research fellow in the Health Ethics and Policy Lab, Department of Health Sciences & Technology at the Swiss Federal Institute of Technology (ETH Zurich). His research focuses on the convergence of natural and artificial intelligence in the digital age with particular emphasis on the ethical, legal, and social implications of neurotechnology, machine learning, big data, robotics, and other emerging socio-technical trends. Ienca has received several awards for social responsibility in science and technology such as the Vontobel Award for Aging Research and the European Association of Centres of Medical Ethics Schotsmans Prize. His research was featured in popular media such as *The Guardian, The Times, Die Welt*, and *Scientific American*. He has served on the Steering Committee on Neurotechnology of the Organisation for Economic Co-operation and Development (OECD).

Fabrice Jotterand, PhD, MA, is an Associate Professor and Director of the Graduate Program in Bioethics at the Center for Bioethics and Medical Humanities, Medical College of Wisconsin, Milwaukee, Wisconsin, and Senior Researcher at the Institute for Biomedical Ethics, University of Basel, Switzerland. He has published more than 50 articles and book chapters as well as reviews in leading academic journals, and has published four books. His scholarship and research interests focus on issues including moral enhancement, neurotechnologies and human identity, artificial intelligence, the use of neurotechnologies in psychiatry, medical professionalism, and moral and political philosophy.

Diane Feeney Mahoney, PhD, FGSA, FAAN, is Professor Emerita at the MGH Institute of Health Professions, Boston, Massachusetts, 02129, where from 2012 to 2017 she directed the Gerontechnology lab. Her program of research focused on developing interactive voice response (IVR) applications, home activity sensor monitoring, and cognitive orthotic family caregiver supports using new technologies to reduce their distress while simultaneously supporting persons with Alzheimer's disease to maintain their activities of daily living and well being. She is CEO of EDDEE Gerontechnology Consultants in Boston, Massachusetts. Considered one of the US female pioneers in the field of gerontechnology, she advises researchers, policymakers, and businesses. She has won numerous awards including the Cutting Edge Research Award for the Development of a Responsive Emotive Sensing System (DRESS) at the International Society of Gerontechnology 2015 competition in Taiwan. She has over 80 original research publications. She earned her PhD from the Heller Graduate School at Brandeis University, a master's degree as a Gerontological Nurse Practitioner from the University of Massachusetts Lowell, and a bachelor's degree in nursing from Boston College. She is a fellow in both the Gerontological Society of America and the American Academy of Nursing.

Osamu Moriyama, PhD, is a Professor at Kanazawa University. His research interests are in the field of social work and elderly care. Moriyama studied social welfare at Rissho University.

Andrew Y. C. Nee, DEng, PhD, is a Professor in the Mechanical Engineering Department, National University of Singapore. His research interests are in tool, die, and fixture design and virtual and augmented reality applications in manufacturing. He is a Fellow of the International Academy for Production Engineering (CIRP) and a Fellow of the Society of Manufacturing Engineers (SME). He received 13,935 citations and H-Index of 61.

Peter Novitzky, PhD, MA, MSc, is currently a post-doctoral researcher at the Philosophy Group of Wageningen University and Research. Peter's appointment follows research roles working on multiple European research projects, and at the National University of Singapore. Peter successfully completed his PhD in applied philosophy at Dublin City University (Ireland), where he specialised in the ethics of artificial intelligence for vulnerable populations. His research interests focus on the intersection of bioethics, ethics of technology, research integrity, and most recently, responsibility in research and innovation. Peter is a magna cum laude graduate of the Erasmus Mundus Master of Bioethics obtained at the consortium of Katholieke Universiteit Leuven (Belgium) – Radboud Universiteit Nijmegen (Netherlands) – Università degli Studi di Padova (Italy). He also studied and performed research at Pázmány Péter Catholic University (Hungary) and Charles University in Prague (Czechia).

S. K. Ong, PhD, is an Associate Professor in the Mechanical Engineering Department, National University of Singapore. Her research interests are in virtual and augmented reality applications in manufacturing and education, assistive technology, and rehabilitation engineering. She received 6,544 citations, H-Index 43 and over 350 international refereed journal and conference papers. She is a Fellow of the International Academy for Production Engineering (CIRP).

Julie M. Robillard, PhD, is an Assistant Professor of Neurology at the University of British Columbia, Scientist in Patient Experience at BC Children's and Women's Hospital and Health Centres, and Associate Director of Neuroethics Canada. Robillard brings her multidisciplinary background in neuroscience and biomedical ethics to the study of the intersection of aging, health, and technology. Her current work focuses on the development of tools for the evaluation of the quality, ethics, and experience of health intervention and health services, with a focus on brain health technology. She is also investigating the integration of artificial intelligence in technology for older adults with dementia and their caregivers as a means to ensure adherence to ethical norms.

James Semple, PhD, worked in the pharmaceutical industry for nearly 30 years developing, validating, and testing novel methodologies to be used in clinical trials of treatments for psychiatric and neurological disorders. He has published widely on using computers to test cognition in people with dementia, magnetic resonance imaging (MRI) to quantify brain changes as Alzheimer's disease progresses, and MRI and bedside electroencephalography to track and predict the development of infarction following stroke. He also coauthored a book on the neuropsychology of the dementias. Semple has also held visiting research fellowships at the Academic Department of Psychiatry; the University of Cambridge, UK; and the Institute for Artificial Intelligence, the University of Georgia, US.

Alan F. Smeaton, PhD, is Professor of Computing at Dublin City University where he is a Founding Director of the Insight Centre for Data Analytics. He is a member of the Board of the Irish Research Council and of the COST Scientific Committee. His research focuses on the development of theories and technologies to support all aspects of information discovery and human memory, allowing people to find the right information at the right time and in the right form. Alan has more than 600 peer-reviewed publications on Google SCHOLAR with over 14,000 citations and an H-index of 60. He is an elected member of the Royal Irish Academy and in 2016 was awarded the Academy's Gold Medal for Engineering Sciences. In 2017 he was elevated to Fellow of the Institute of Electrical and Electronic Engineers (IEEE) for contributions to multimedia indexing and retrieval and was also elected chair of ACM SIGMM.

Taro Sugihara, PhD, is an Assistant Professor at the Graduate School of Natural Science and Technology, Okayama University, Japan. His research interests are in the fields of users' behavior and workplaces for human–computer interaction, especially in the fields of caregiving for persons with dementia and university hospitals. He also conducts research in the area of technology management. Taro studied human–computer interaction at Kyoto Institute of Technology and was Doctor of Engineering.

Renaat Verbruggen, MMgt Sc, MMI, is a lecturer and researcher at the School of Computing at Dublin City University (Ireland). His research interests lie within software engineering and focus on the object-oriented construction of systems, the links between formal and informal methods in their approaches to software design, and higher-level process management issues. His current research focuses on testing and metrics approaches within the world of patterns and objects. Renaat has been engaged in numerous action research projects, involving Irish, European, and multinational companies (e.g., Microsoft, Bayer, Digital Galway, Ericsson, Verilog). Renaat's long-term interest is in the beneficence of software engineering and related ethical questions.

Eduard Fosch Villaronga, PhD, MA, LLM, LLB, is a Marie Skłodowska-Curie Postdoctoral Researcher at the eLaw Center for Law and Digital Technologies at Leiden University, the Netherlands. Eduard is the coleader of the Ethical, Legal, and Societal Aspects Working Group at the H2020 Cost Action 16116 on Wearable Robots. Eduard holds an Erasmus Mundus Joint Doctorate (EMJD) in Law, Science, and Technology. He has also held visiting PhD positions at the Center for Education Engineering and Outreach (CEEO) at Tufts University in the United States and the Laboratoire de Systèmes Robotiques (LSRO) at EPFL in Lausanne in Switzerland. Among receiving degrees from the University of Toulouse, the Autonomous University of Madrid, and the Autonomous University of Barcelona, he is also a qualified lawyer in Spain.

Tenzin Wangmo, PhD, is a gerontologist by training (PhD Gerontology, University of Kentucky) and holds a Senior Researcher position at the Institute for Biomedical Ethics, University of Basel. Her areas of expertise are rights of older persons, caregiving, intergenerational relationships, migration and aging, older prisoners, elder abuse, social justice, empirical methods, and research ethics. Her current research works focus on ethical issues related to the provision of mental health care to older prisoners, technology and aging, healthcare data sharing, and care relationships.

Mengyu Y. Zhao, PhD, received her BS in Biomedical and Information Engineering from Northeastern University, Shenyang, PRC, in 2010, specializing in lung segmentation in computed tomography images. She received her PhD in Mechanical Engineering, National University of Singapore, in 2016, specializing in augmented reality–assisted healthcare exercising systems for upper extremities.

1

Introduction

Fabrice Jotterand, Marcello Ienca, Tenzin Wangmo, and Bernice S. Elger

Dementia and especially Alzheimer disease (AD) are among the most expensive and burdensome diseases in Western societies. It is estimated that the number of older adults being diagnosed and living with dementia reached 35.6 million worldwide in 2010 and it is expected to increase up to 135.5 million in 2050 (Fritze et al., this volume). In the United States alone, 5.4 million individuals live with the condition, of which 5.2 million are 65 years old or older. This number could reach 13.8 million if no treatment becomes available (Alzheimer's Association, 2016). The increased incidence of the disease poses a major challenge for public health systems and health care services in terms of financial management and provision of specialized care to this patient population. The potential cost could reach up to $1.1 trillion by 2050 (Bharucha et al. 2009; Brookmeyer et al. 2007; Pollack 2005). Not surprisingly, the World Health Organization (WHO) and Alzheimer's Disease International published a report "to raise awareness of dementia as a public health priority" worldwide (WHO 2012).

In addition to issues surrounding financial considerations and the provision of specialized care, there are social and ethical considerations that require close scrutiny. The care of individuals with dementia demands an increased need for both formal and informal caregiving (Dall et al. 2013). Long-term care and the institutionalization of patients with dementia put additional constraints on public finances and the elders themselves. The coming Alzheimer's epidemic will require setting ethical guidelines concerning the allocation of healthcare resources as well as personnel. Family caregivers (spouses and children) of individuals with dementia are confronted with the task of caring for themselves or their own children in addition to caring for a family member with dementia. A fair decision-making process should occur as to which families taking care of a person suffering with AD should have access to healthcare professional help.

In light of these considerations, the development and implementation of smart assistive tools to compensate for the specific physical and cognitive deficits of older adults with dementia have been recognized by many as one of the most promising approaches to this emerging financial and caregiving burden (Newton and Robinson 2013; Peterson, Prasad, and Prasad 2012; Pollack 2005). In the past 15 years, advancements in artificial intelligence (AI), pervasive and ubiquitous computing (PUC), and other advanced trends in software and hardware technology have led to the development and design of a wide range of assistive technologies with their own computing capabilities and the capacity to mimic aspects of human intelligence, hence called intelligent assistive technologies (IATs). These technologies are expected to help older people compensate for the physical and sensory deficits that may accompany dementia and age-related cognitive decline. These technologies are designed to support impaired older adults in the completion of activities of daily living, assist them in the prevention or management of risk, and/or maintain their recreational and social environment (Bharucha et al. 2009; Singh et al. 2014). Examples of IATs for dementia and age-related cognitive decline include environmental sensors, biosensors, cognitive aids, audio and video technologies, advanced integrated systems, and social robots. The common denominator of these technologies lies in the fact that they are all aimed at helping dementia patients live independently at home or maintain a greater level of independence in assisted living or skilled nursing care facilities. The development and implementation of these technologies could provide a "triple-win" effect: (1) improving quality of life of people living with dementia and elders in general, (2) reducing the burden on caregivers and the health care system, and (3) being cost effective (Bharucha et al. 2009; Pollack 2005; Singh et al. 2014).

The widespread implementation and use of IATs is a very rapid process, which is reshaping dementia care and producing constantly changing strategies. This volume aims at providing an up-to-date overview of the current state of the art of IATs for dementia care, determining their current taxonomy, and defining their functionality, capability, and level of implementation. In addition, these technologies for dementia care raise several other important questions. First, there are implications at the medical level, including psychological and clinical issues. The evaluation of the possible psychological effects with the use of this type of technology is quintessential to avoid potential abuse and misuse. It is also crucial to identify how these technologies can enhance healthcare delivery, reduce psychological distress by improving social and family interactions, and promote important dimensions of human existence such as self-determination, independence, and dignity. Second, the implementation of IATs is not without its set of ethical and legal challenges such as problems related to their long-term effects (psychological and physiological), questions related to privacy, and the values and norms guiding the development of regulatory frameworks at the national and international stage. The overall goal of this book is to raise societal awareness on the use of IATs for dementia care and take a first step in developing an international regulatory and policy framework.

To optimize the analysis of the various dimensions outlined earlier, we structured the book into four main sections with a concerted effort aimed at bridging the interdisciplinary gap in current scholarship on the topic and producing a first comprehensive and multidisciplinary publication on IATs for dementia care and the ethical, psychological, clinical, social, and legal implications. To this end, we invited prominent scholars in the debate over assistive technologies for dementia care to discuss a broad set of issues within the four sections of the book.

Current Landscape of Assistive Technologies for Dementia Care

Part I delineates the current landscape of dementia in the aging world and the emergence of IATs for dementia care and age-related disability. In Chapter 2 ("Dementia in an Aging World"), Thomas Fritze, Anne Fink, and Gabriele Doblhammer present an overview of global demographic trends that contribute to worldwide population aging and to the increasing number of elderly people. The authors discuss the definition of dementia and its subtypes as well as mild cognitive impairment. They stress that "dementia is one of the most common diseases of old age" and include a discussion of potentially modifiable risk factors. The chapter describes the association important cardiovascular risk factors have with dementia and depicts recent and future trends in their prevalence. The authors also report estimates of current and future dementia prevalence and detail the costs and cost types showing how these differ between developing and developed countries. Indeed, both developed and developing countries are facing economic and social challenges posed by an aging population. The chapter presents dementia as one of the most common diseases in old age, which has major consequences for society. Given that in 2013 an estimated 44.4 million people worldwide suffered from dementia and that this number is expected to increase to 135.5 million by 2050, the authors report that the current worldwide costs of dementia have been estimated at $604 billion, primarily due to the high demand for care. It is underlined that "positive developments with respect to lifestyle and recognizing risk factors at young and middle ages might have positive long-term effects on the risk of dementia at old age" and that "prevention and adequate medical treatment of these risk factors might help postpone dementia into higher ages," which includes assistive technologies that "may help to mitigate the family and caregiver burden."

In Chapter 3 ("Dementia and Neurocognitive Disability"), Christophe J. Büla provides an overview of the clinical aspects of dementia, "a clinical syndrome characterized by—usually—progressive deficits in several cognitive domains such as memory, language, and impairments in a person's daily functional abilities as well as behavior." He underlines the extent to which dementia places considerable strain on patients and their relatives, who provide a large share of the required care and support. This chapter offers valuable information about the group of patients for which many IATs examined in this book are designed and addresses definitions and diagnostic criteria; prevalence and incidence; burden and costs; clinical course, from symptoms to disability; dementia management (including promises and limitations), in particular nonpharmacological and pharmacological interventions; and end-of-life care. It puts the clinical information in the context of global population ageing. Indeed, the burden of dementia has become a worldwide concern and will be further increasing over the next two decades. After discussing existing treatments, Büla concludes that "new pharmacological as well as nonpharmacological interventions are urgently needed to address this huge challenge."

Developing new methods of intervention to alleviate the burden of dementia faces challenges, as Arlene Astell outlines in her contribution. In Chapter 4 ("Can Robots, Apps, and Other Technologies Meet the Future Global Demands of Dementia?"), Astell provides a detailed summary of the major technological advances for supporting older people living with dementia. Her analysis shows that virtually all IAT families are hampered by a lack of research investment. However, some IAT types might benefit from increasing private-sector investment and hold a promising scalability potential. Among these, mobile health (m-Health) applications might be critical. M-health apps can support cognitive assessment, disease progression monitoring, and intervention delivery, and can even act as cognitive prostheses. As they can run on daily hardware technology such as smartphones and tablets, these applications can be of great benefit in developing countries. Astell's focus on low-income and developing countries is fundamental to address the question about IATs for dementia in the context of global health and distributive justice. In addition, she argues that it is important to correct the common misconception that the need to develop IATs for dementia is primarily a first world problem. Data show that the greater cost increases of dementia are occurring in low- and middle-income countries (Prince 2015), where the national healthcare budgets are already affected by structural financial limitations. Therefore, developing smart, pervasively deliverable, and low-cost technological solutions is a major public health challenge and moral obligation.

One example of a cutting-edge technology that could reduce the workload of caregivers and improve the quality of life of patients suffering from dementia is augmented reality (AR). Mengyu Y. Zhao, Soh K. Ong, and Andrew Y. C. Nee, in Chapter 5 ("Augmented Reality–Assisted Dementia Care"), describe the basic features and main applications of this technology and discuss how it can assist patients with their motor skills and cognitive abilities. They point out that AR has already been used in domains such as education, manufacturing, military, and the medical field, although there are only a few AR-based approaches being reported for dementia care. Based on a survey of current AR systems, they provide a "generic architecture of AR-assisted dementia care applications." This system structure, the authors contend, allows for the development of strategies for users to transfer what they learned in the virtual world into reality. The technology has many advantages such as a "highly controllable environment, intuitive interface, and real-time feedback" and represents the type of innovation that could provide venues to help improve the quality of life of individuals with AD. However, the authors of the chapter point out that AR in dementia care is quite new and therefore further studies are needed to test their efficacy and safety.

Psychosocial Implications

In Part II, contributions are aimed at addressing and analyzing the major psychosocial implications linked to the use of IATs in dementia care. In Chapter 6 ("Caring for Older Adults with Dementia: The Potential of Assisted Technology in Reducing Caregiving Burden"), Tenzin Wangmo examines the issue of caregiving burden for family members of persons with dementia. The focus of this chapter is on the caregivers and, in particular, on the discussion of whether, how, and to what extent IATs could help in supporting them. Wangmo reviews the literature delineating who are the informal caregivers of persons with dementia, the type of burden they face, and the consequences of such caregiving roles and responsibilities on their health. Thereafter, the chapter presents evidence concerning the potential of IATs in addressing the caregiving burden for these informal caregivers. Building on this twofold premise, the chapter seeks to make a justice-oriented case that equal access to IATs for older persons with dementia and IATs designed to reduce caregiving burden must be guaranteed by the state.

In the next contribution, Taro Sugihara, Tsutomu Fujinami, and Osamu Moriyama present an original case study involving qualitative interviews with formal caregivers from institutional care homes in Japan. While population aging is a global phenomenon, different world regions are affected by demographic trends in different magnitudes. With over 7.7 million people over the age of 65—of which over 2 million are aged 90 or older—Japan is particularly exposed to the consequences of population aging. Authors have called this accelerated and unprecedented aging trend "super-aging" (Muramatsu and Akiyama 2011). In Chapter 7 ("The Predestined Nature of Assistive Technologies for Dementia"), Sugihara et al. show a complex mosaic of psychological, physical, and logistic hardships that are currently affecting the caregivers of older adults with dementia. This analysis is an important exploration of the phenomenon of caregiving burden. In addition, the chapter explores a number of barriers that are currently limiting or delaying the successful introduction of IATs into standard institutional care. These barriers are presented at various levels of the caregiving continuum including at the micro, meso, and macro level.

In Chapter 8 ("Shaping the Development and Use of Intelligent Assistive Technologies in Dementia: Some Thoughts"), Elisabeth Hildt offers critical insights concerning the development and use of IATs in dementia care. In particular, she argues that these technologies must be designed, developed, and assessed according to the particular needs of end-users and "should not lead to a decrease in human-delivered care and services or a reduction in interpersonal contact, communication, and contact time." While other considerations are important, such as safety, security, and privacy, the users' goals and abilities ought to be the crucial concerns. According to Hildt, the improvement of quality of life and the quality of relationships should shape the design of these technologies, with particular attention to customization. Such a user-oriented approach not only would be morally preferable but also might increase technology acceptance and adoption. As she points out, "a user-centered approach that better takes user abilities and perspectives into consideration may also help to strengthen the practicability and attractiveness of IATs and may finally lead to an increase in user adoption." Based on these considerations, Hildt urges producers to adopt a user-centered approach to technology design and development.

Ethical and Regulatory Implications

The last section of the book, Part III, addresses and analyzes the major ethical and regulatory implications arising from the use of IATs in dementia care. In Chapter 9 ("Ethical Concerns About the Use of Assistive Technologies: How to Balance Beneficence and Respect for Autonomy in the Care of Dementia Patients"), Bernice S. Elger examines ethical issues that have been responsible for the slow uptake of potentially beneficial IATs. The aim of this contribution is to examine the ethical issues raised by distinct types of existing IATs in more detail, to obtain a nuanced judgment about "whether public health authorities and health care personnel should . . . offer patients and their informal caregivers more choice, or even actively recommend some of them [IATs]." This chapter focuses on four examples of IATs that, despite having been available for some time and being relatively simple to use, are not widely implemented: memory aid technology, "smart dresser" devices designed to help dementia patients with getting dressed, GPS tracking devices, and sensors to monitor patients in their private homes such as an intelligent wireless sensor system for the rapid detection of health issues. The first two technologies are chosen as examples for "aid technology," where the risk of harm is very low and compensated by significant benefits for patients, caregivers, and society. The second two are chosen because of their ethically relevant capacity to control, surveil, and monitor patient behavior. For each technology, the chapter discusses some major ethical issues associated with their use and draws normative conclusions on how to appropriately balance beneficence and respect for patient autonomy. The author claims that for an appropriate ethical judgment, it is important to clearly distinguish distinct types of technologies and to avoid unethical barriers, which may be the result of "ethical contamination" of one type of technology by the controversies related to others. She evaluates the first two types of technologies to represent a low-harm–potential benefit type about which more systematic information should be provided to all stakeholders, and she is more critical toward the other two discussed types. She argues that there is no justification to recommend use of the two latter technologies routinely but that there is equally no justification not to inform patients and caregivers about their existence as this information will expand their spectrum of choices on how to organize care.

The question of informing patients is further examined by Peter Novitzky, Cynthia Chen, Alan F. Smeaton, Renaat Verbruggen, and Bert Gordijn. In Chapter 10 ("Issues of Informed Consent from Persons with Dementia When Employing Assistive Technologies"), Novitzky et al. examine issues related to informed consent, which should be provided by persons suffering from dementia when employing assistive technologies. While on the one hand the use of IATs in the provision of healthcare promises to provide novel opportunities to protect, empower, and extend the autonomy of persons with dementia, on the other hand, it also poses autonomy-related challenges, especially regarding the traditional procedure of obtaining informed consent. Traditional consent procedures are aimed at the protection of the autonomy of research participants and patients undergoing treatment. They are not readily applicable to persons suffering from dementia when it comes to deciding about IATs. The authors analyze the ethical challenges of obtaining informed consent from dementia patients for research and development and the use of IATs. Their analysis reviews both traditional informed consent procedures and more innovative ones. Based on the findings of the ethical analysis, they provide the following recommendations: informed consent "interpreted solely on the basis of legal requirements should be avoided" in this context as the diagnosis of dementia does not automatically imply lack of competence to provide informed consent. However, they underline that research should be conducted wherever possible with healthy, or at least competent, volunteers instead of vulnerable populations, such as persons suffering from dementia. This research should be carried out in accordance with the UNESCO Universal Declaration on Bioethics and Human Rights. Research with persons who lack the capacity to consent should only be allowed if there is a direct health benefit to those participants and if no comparable study can be undertaken with participants who are able to consent. They also recommend using combinations of rolling informed consent, advanced directives, and alternative methods such as delayed informed consent and dynamic informed consent to obtain informed consent from persons with dementia because combined methods "are more likely to reflect the special conditions and needs of persons with dementia and may also improve the validity of the informed consent obtained."

In Chapter 11 ("Personal Identity, Neuroprosthetics, and Alzheimer's Disease"), Fabrice Jotterand focuses on the question of how the use of prosthetics in patients suffering from AD challenges our understanding of personal identity. This chapter explores two possible conceptualizations of personal identity, based on psychological continuity alone (memory) or on psychological continuity and embodiment. Jotterand argues that the latter should be favored and that the use of neuroprosthetics, such as an artificial hippocampus, should consider the intended goals of interventions in the brain of people with AD. Since the disease, in its early stages, impacts short-term memory, interventions can either restore and preserve identity integrity or allow the emergence of a new identity regardless of past memories. Jotterand argues that to capture the fullness of human experience and enhance the quality of life of this patient population, the implementation of neuroprosthetics should aim at restoring the identity of patients according to past and present psychological continuity and embodied identity.

In Chapter 12 ("Developing Assistive Technologies for Persons with Alzheimer's Disease and Their Carers: The Ethics of Doing Good, Not Harm"), Diane Mahoney examines the ethical principles applicable to gerontechnology and the development of in-home monitoring of persons with AD. This chapter brings forth the significance of gaining the opinions of IAT end-users prior to their testing to ensure that all important features are understood by the developers and incorporated appropriately. Her analysis of the ethical principles such as autonomy, do no harm, beneficence, and justice is well grounded on her long-standing experience as a professor in geriatric nursing research and as the director of gerontechnology at the MGH Institute in Boston, Massachusetts. She discusses critical issues, including the principles of respect for the person, do no harm, and beneficence. Her positive outlook on the potential of IATs for older persons with AD and their carers is partly rooted in the idea that technological use should be not only sensitive and useful for its users but also ethically sound. Mahoney notes that protectionist attitudes that view technology as inherently bad not only are paternalistic toward the end-users but also impede innovation, which may result in harming the population that they seek to protect rather than being benevolent. The author concludes that "technology is neither inherently harmful nor beneficial. Humans maintain the responsibility for developing applications that respect the personhood and dignity of those experiencing cognitive declines."

When it comes to medical technology, in particular technologies capable of accessing and transmitting sensitive information about their users, privacy and data security issues are paramount. This is of particular importance in the context of vulnerable individuals such as older adults with dementia. In Chapter 13 ("Privacy and Security Issues in Assistive Technologies for Dementia: The Case of Ambient Assisted Living, Wearables, and Service Robotics"), Marcello Ienca and Eduard Fosch Villaronga provide a detailed overview of privacy and security issues associated with three types of IATs: ambient assisted living (AAL), wearable computing, and service robotics. While some of these issues appear inherent to the entire IAT spectrum, specific privacy and security vulnerabilities appear associated with each of these three IAT families. After exploring a number of both category-specific and general ethical and legal implications, the authors propose a list of policy recommendations. These recommendations are aimed at informing calibrated policy interventions that can maximize the uptake of IATs while minimizing the risk of data insecurity and privacy erosion.

In Chapter 14 ("Developing Ethical Web- and Mobile-Based Technologies for Dementia: Challenges and Opportunities"), Julie M. Robillard and Tanya E. Feng examine another subtype of IAT, m-Health and web-based technologies, and provide in-depth ethical assessment. They explore the current capabilities of m-Health and web-based tools for people with dementia, including the promise of self-diagnostics, self-assessment, lifestyle monitoring, and cognitive engagement. At the same time, they identify critical ethical challenges including issues of privacy, data quality, reliability, and technology access. The scientific and ethical assessment offered by this chapter is an unavoidable resource to guide future technological innovation in the fields of m-Health and online health and to inform any risk-benefit assessment associated with the use of these technologies among older adults with dementia.

The final contribution to this volume, by James Beauregard (Chapter 15, "Dementia and the Regulation of Gerontechnology"), carefully assesses the regulation of gerontechnology in the United States. Underpinning that the deployment of technology to the public is regulated both at the federal and the state level in the United States, it highlights the complex regulatory framework that is in place to assess the utility of a technology before coming to the market. The chapter briefly presents the five types of gerontechnologies that are available: medical, monitoring, mobility, communication, and robotics. It brings forth an important point that not all dementias are equal and therefore special consideration should be given to technology development based on the specificity of the end-user population of interest. Thereafter, it delves into different federal regulatory bodies that oversee technology deployment such as the Department of Health and Human Services, the Food and Drug Administration, the Federal Trade Commission, and the General Accounting Office. The chapter provides a wealth of information related to what constitutes technology according to the federal guidelines, when and which type of technology requires prior approval from a federal agency, which agency regulates what technology, and what happens in the case of false marketing of technology to the general population. It further discusses the influence of the Veterans Administration and other healthcare providers (Medicare, Medicaid, and private insurance) in the adoption of technology for use by older persons with dementia. The chapter ends with detailed recommendations, for example, who should be informed about gerontechnology and what the stakeholders should know at the basic levels, and how different stakeholders can be educated about different concerns related to the issue of regulation of gerontechnology.

This volume provides a comprehensive, multidisciplinary, and international perspective on IATs for dementia care. This collection features contributions from highly respected researchers in the fields of public health, geriatric medicine, gerontology, computer science, engineering, psychology, neuroscience, sociology, anthropology, bioethics, law, and philosophy. As such, it provides a multifaceted overview of the promises and challenges associated with deploying IATs for people with dementia in the aging world. We believe this volume will benefit not only the academic community but also developers, designers, clinicians, and relevant policymakers working on IATs by offering a wide-ranging, easily accessible resource for comparative research on the topic. Furthermore, this volume enriches the ongoing public debate on the implementation of IATs for dementia care and provides a valid information source for informal caregivers, healthcare professionals, and patients themselves.

Acknowledgment

This collection of essays is the result of a collaborative effort between many individuals whom we would like to thank for their interest, enthusiasm, and encouragement. First, we are grateful for our contributors for their scholarship and commitment to deliver high-quality manuscripts. Without their contributions and insights this book could not have become a reality. Second, we would like to thank Oxford University Press for the opportunity to publish this volume. Special thanks go to Lucy Randall for her support and guidance throughout the whole process of bringing this volume together. Her guidance and prompt feedback made the completion of this project much easier. We also want to recognize the support of our respective academic institutions for allowing us to have the freedom and the privilege to work on this book. Financial support from the Swiss Academy of Medical Sciences under award Käthe-Zingg-Schwichtenberg-Fonds (KZS) 20/17 is gratefully acknowledged. In addition, we thank the following persons for reviewing some of the manuscripts: Pamela Teaster, Manya Hendriks, and Ralf Jox. Finally, we are thankful to our families for their support and patience while we were working on the book.

References

Alzheimer's Association. (2016). Alzheimer's disease facts and figures. *Alzheimer's & Dementia, 12*, 459–509.

Bharucha, A. J., Anand, V., Forlizzi, J., Dew, M. A., Reynolds III, C. F., Stevens, S., & Wactlar, H. (2009). Intelligent assistive technology applications to dementia care: current capabilities, limitations, and future challenges. *American Journal of Geriatric Psychiatry, 17*(2), 88–104.

Brookmeyer, R., Johnson, E., Ziegler-Graham, K., & Arrighi, H. M. (2007). Forecasting the global burden of Alzheimer's disease. *Alzheimer's & Dementia, 3*(3), 186–91.

Dall, T. M., Gallo, P. D., Chakrabarti, R., West, T., Semilla, A. P., & Storm, M. V. (2013). An aging population and growing disease burden will require a large and specialized health care workforce by 2025. *Health Affairs, 32*(11), 2013–2020.

Muramatsu, N., & Akiyama, H. (2011). Japan: Super-aging society preparing for the future. *The Gerontologist, 51*(4), 425–32.

Newton, L., & Robinson, L. (2013). Assistive technologies to maximise independence in people with dementia. *InnovAiT: Education and Inspiration for General Practice, 6*(12), 763–71. 1755738013504320.

Peterson, C. B., Prasad, N. R., & Prasad, R. (2012). *The Future of Assistive Technologies for Dementia*. Paper presented at the Workshop ISG-ISARC.

Pollack, M. E. (2005). Intelligent technology for an aging population: the use of AI to assist elders with cognitive impairment. *AI Magazine, 26*(2), 9.

Prince, M. J. (2015). World Alzheimer Report 2015: the global impact of dementia: An analysis of prevalence, incidence, cost and trends. London: Alzheimer's Disease International.

Singh, N. N., Lancioni, G. E., Sigafoos, J., O'Reilly, M. F., & Winton, A. S. (2014). Assistive technology for people with Alzheimer's disease. In *Assistive Technologies for People with Diverse Abilities* (pp. 219–50). Springer.

World Health Organization. (2012). *Dementia: A public health priority*. Geneva: WHO Press.

PART I

CURRENT LANDSCAPE
OF ASSISTIVE TECHNOLOGIES
FOR DEMENTIA CARE

2

Dementia in an Aging World

Thomas Fritze, Anne Fink, and Gabriele Doblhammer

Introduction

The world's population continues to grow, albeit at a slower pace than in the last century, and it will experience unprecedented population aging, particularly in the first half of the 21st century (Lutz, Sanderson, and Scherbov 2008). Population aging, defined as the shift to a larger proportion of the population at older ages, is a significant global trend that poses major challenges for the well-being of individuals and for the social and economic development of populations. Increasing life expectancy is both a major societal achievement and the driving force behind population aging and the growing number of old people. People are not only living longer but also appear to be healthier in terms of reduced disability (Christensen et al. 2009). Noncommunicable diseases (NCDs) tend to be associated with old age and make up a growing share of the disease burden. NCDs include not only cancer and chronic respiratory diseases (such as chronic obstructed pulmonary disease or asthma) but also dementia and cardiovascular diseases, diabetes, hearing and vision loss, and depression. It is particularly these latter diseases that are the major risk factors of dementia, which has become the fourth leading cause of death (Bickel 2003) and is a major predictor of death (Baldereschi et al. 1999). Vallin and Meslé (2004) postulate that the next steps in the epidemiological transition will depend on the ability of societies to fight cognitive impairment and dementia. At present, dementia is one of the most common diseases of old age and it is still incurable (Prince et al. 2013). In the future, there will be an increasing demand for preventing and treating dementia as well as mitigating its effect on patients and their families. It has been pointed out that assistive technologies may improve quality of life, extend the length of community residence, improve physical and mental health status, delay the onset of health problems, and reduce family and caregiver burdens (Blaschke, Freddolino, and Mullen 2009).

The present work provides an overview of global demographic trends that contribute to worldwide population aging and to the increasing number of elderly people. We discuss the definition of dementia and its subtypes as well as mild cognitive impairment. Because dementia is one of the most common diseases of old age, potentially modifiable risk factors are a major focus of this research. We describe the association that important cardiovascular risk factors have with dementia and depict recent and future trends in their prevalence. In the next section, we report estimates of current and future dementia prevalence. Finally, we detail the costs and cost types and describe how these differ between developing and developed countries.

Demographic Trends

World Population

According to United Nations estimates (United Nations 2015), in the middle of 2015 the world population reached 7.3 billion. Sixty percent of the global population (4.4 billion people) lives in Asia, followed by 16% in Africa (1.2 billion). Ten percent live in Europe (738 million), 9% in Latin America and the Caribbean (634 million), and 5% in North America (358 million) and Oceania (39 million).

Although current global population growth is slower than it was in the past, the world population is still projected to increase by more than 1 billion people by the year 2030. There will be 9.7 billion people by 2050 and 11.2 billion by 2100 (Figure 2.1). However, this development pattern varies according to region. Africa is the fastest-growing area, with more than half of all expected global population growth taking place there between 2015 and 2050. Asia is projected to add 0.9 billion people by 2050, while North America, Latin America, and the Caribbean and Oceania will experience much smaller population growth. Europe's population will take a very different turn, declining by 2050 due to low fertility levels (United Nations 2015).

The actual population development rates will depend heavily on future fertility levels. Current projections are based on the assumption that a substantial reduction in fertility levels of high-fertility countries will take place in the coming decades. However, there is significant uncertainty about projected fertility, particularly in countries with high fertility. A slower decline than expected would result in much higher population numbers in the future (United Nations 2015). While long-term low fertility below the replacement level of 2.1 children per woman does contribute to population aging, because there are fewer young people, increasing life expectancy is the true driving force behind population aging as it results in more old people (Christensen et al. 2009).

Trends in Life Expectancy

Life expectancy is the second major component of population development; its trend largely determines the number of elderly and the extent of population

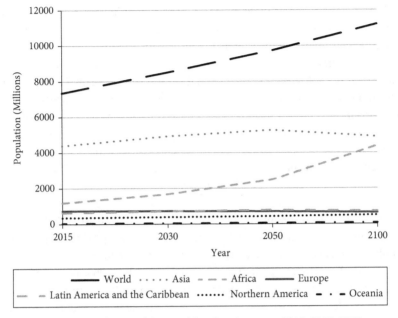

Figure 2.1 Total population of the World and major areas, 2015, 2030, 2050, and 2100, according to the medium-variant projection of the United Nations. Reproduced by permission from: United Nations, Department of Economic and Social Affairs, Population Division (2015). World Population Prospects: The 2015 Revision, DVD Edition. New York 2015. Downloaded: February 1, 2016.

aging. In industrialized countries, the 20th century yielded unprecedented and continuous mortality declines, resulting in ever-increasing life expectancy. Whereas in 1840 Swedish women had the highest life expectancy worldwide, about 45 years, by 2008 Japanese women were experiencing the highest life expectancy, 86.04 years. In 2015, the life expectancy of Japanese women had grown even more, to 87.05 years. Thus, since 1840, life expectancy has increased by an average of three months per year among the record-holding countries (Christensen et al. 2009; Ministry of Health 2015; Oeppen and Vaupel 2002; Shkolnikov et al. 2011), that is, those countries with the worldwide highest life expectancy at a specific time. This increase was similar also in those industrialized countries that did not have record life expectancy themselves (Rau et al. 2008). This upward trend was only interrupted by the two world wars and by the Spanish influenza pandemic in 1918, which, however, did not alter the pace of the steady increase. Even now, it does not appear that life expectancy is approaching a limit. There is no apparent deceleration in the increase; the rise has remained steady and is almost linear (Oeppen and Vaupel 2002).

These findings are based on the measure of period life expectancy, which is life expectancy estimated for a particular year combining the mortality regime of a newborn up to the oldest person. The underlying assumption is that this mortality regime will remain unchanged in the future. Because it is plausible to expect that mortality will also decline in the future, this measure is likely an underestimation of true life expectancy. In contrast to period life expectancy, the measure of cohort life expectancy follows the mortality regime of a birth cohort over time. Recent findings using cohort life expectancy show an even greater increase in record life expectancy of more than five months per year (Shkolnikov et al. 2011). To conclude, both cohort and period life expectancy indicate a further increase for both the best-practice countries and all other industrialized countries.

In general, determinants of this mortality decline consist of better living conditions; higher education and income; changes in lifestyle factors such as smoking, diet, and physical activity; and advances in medical technology (Meslé and Vallin 2002; Robine, Le Roy, and Jagger 2005; Vallin 2005; Vallin and Meslé 2001). The contribution of such factors to improved health, lower mortality, and increasing life expectancy has varied over time. In the first half of the 20th century the increase in life expectancy was due to the reduction of infant and child mortality as well as the successful fight against infectious disease. The latter is closely linked to the first epidemiological transition (Omran 1971), including advances in terms of nutrition, sanitation, and public health measures. During the second phase of the epidemiological transition, which began in the second half of the 20th century, a new pattern of mortality decline evolved. Advances in medical technology as well as changing lifestyle factors contributed significantly to the gains in life expectancy, which primarily stemmed from ages 60 and above, with a large fraction contributed by the old and oldest old (Christensen et al. 2009). All major groups of causes of death, with the exception of lung cancer among women, contributed to this mortality decline (Janssen, Kunst, and Netherlands Epidemiology and Demography Compression of Morbidity Research 2005; Janssen et al. 2004). A future third phase in the mortality development might be related to smoking patterns among women. Countries with high female smoking prevalence rates, such as the Netherlands, Denmark, and the United States, fared worse in terms of mortality than, for example, France or Japan (Janssen et al. 2004; Nusselder and Mackenbach 2000) and could benefit from a lower smoking prevalence among women. Particularly in aging societies, trends in neurodegenerative diseases such as dementia might be important for future gains in life expectancy.

Global life expectancy increased from 67 to 70 years between 2000–2005 and 2010–2015. During this period Africa's life expectancy increased by 6 years, up to 60 years in 2010–2015, which was the largest growth in the world. However, Africa still has the lowest life expectancy, followed by Asia (72 years), Latin America and the Caribbean (75 years), Europe and Oceania (77 years), and North America (79 years). While the decline in infant mortality had been the primary reason for increasing life expectancy in developed countries in the first half of the 20th century (Christensen et al. 2009), there is currently a similar trend in developing countries, particularly in Sub-Saharan Africa and in the least developed countries (United Nations 2015). According to United Nations forecasts, life expectancy will rise from 70 years in 2010–2015 to 77 years by 2045–2050 and to 83 years by 2095–2100. Again, Africa will have the largest gain, reaching 70 years by 2045–2050 and 78 years by 2095–2100. Such projections depend on future prevention and treatment of HIV and infectious diseases as well as NCDs, particularly in Africa. By end of this century Asia and Latin America and the Caribbean will have gained 13 to 14 years of life expectancy, and Europe, North America, and Oceania between 10 and 11 years.

World Population Aging

Europe was the first region to enter a demographic regime that combined low fertility with increasing life expectancy, resulting in population aging. Today, 24% of the population is aged 60 years or older. In the coming decades Europe will remain the most aged region in the world, followed by North America, Latin America and the Caribbean, Asia, Oceania, and finally Africa. United Nations population projections (United Nations 2015) estimate that in Africa the number of those aged 60 and above, which was barely over 5% in 2015, will have almost doubled by 2030. Globally, the 12% aged 60 and above today will rise to 21% by 2050. Thus, in the coming decades population aging will accelerate worldwide (Figure 2.2).

Unlike in the past, however, most of the projected increase in the number of elderly will occur in the global South. By 2050 the number of older persons is expected to double to 2 billion, reflecting a rapid growth of the elderly population in Africa, Latin America and the Caribbean, and Asia. The number will more than triple to 220 million in Africa, nearly triple to 200 million in Latin America and the Caribbean, and more than double to 1.3 billion in Asia. In comparison, the increase in Europe will be 38%, resulting in 242 million, and in North America will be 27%, reaching 123 million. Thus, the speed of population aging will be much faster in developing countries than in developed countries. It took France 114 years to double their proportion of people aged 65 years and over, from 7% to 14%, and it took the United Kingdom

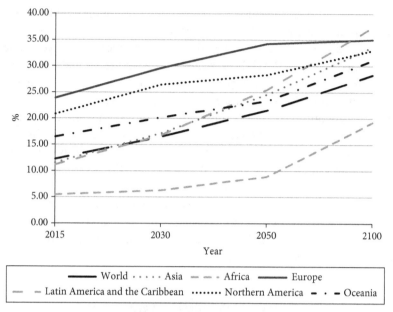

Figure 2.2 Percentage of the population aged 60 years or older for the World and major areas, 2015, 2030, 2050, and 2100, according to the medium-variant projection of the United Nations. Reproduced by permission from: United Nations, Department of Economic and Social Affairs, Population Division (2015). World Population Prospects: The 2015 Revision, DVD Edition. New York 2015. Downloaded: February 1, 2016.

45 years; in contrast, China will experience such a doubling within 25 years (Pison 2009).

The older population is itself aging, with ever more people reaching oldest old age. In 2015, 14% of those in the age group "60 and above" were 80 or older, and by 2050 this will be a full 20%. In 2015, most of the elderly were female, as women worldwide generally have higher a life expectancy than men, and this will hold true for the coming decades. Women account for 54% of those aged 60 and above, and for 61% of those aged 80 years and above. As the life expectancy of men is expected to slowly approach that of women by 2050, the proportion of women among the elderly will be reduced to 53%, and 58% among the oldest old.

Because dementia is a disease of old age, the number of dementia patients is closely linked with life expectancy. We now turn to the different types of dementia, which is a syndrome rather than a single disease.

Types of Dementia and Mild Cognitive Impairment

The term "dementia" describes a syndrome marked by cerebral changes that lead to cognitive declines and personality changes (World Health Organization 2015). According to the classification system of the 10th revision of the International Statistical Classification of Diseases and Related Health Problems (ICD-10), dementia

> is a syndrome due to disease of the brain, usually of a chronic or progressive nature, in which there is disturbance of multiple higher cortical functions, including memory, thinking, orientation, comprehension, calculation, learning capacity, language, and judgement. Consciousness is not clouded. The impairments of cognitive function are commonly accompanied, and occasionally preceded, by deterioration in emotional control, social behavior, or motivation. (World Health Organization 2010)

This syndrome can be caused by several diseases (Figure 2.3). Alzheimer disease (AD) is the most common cause of dementia. About 60% to 80% of all dementia cases are attributable to AD (Alzheimer's Association 2015; Ott et al. 1995; Schneider et al. 2007; Weyerer 2005), which is a slowly progressive brain disorder. Neuropathological changes may be detected 15 to 25 years prior to the occurrence of first clinical symptoms. All cognitive domains are affected over the course of the disease, resulting in an increasing need for care and assistance (Alzheimer's Association 2015; Kilimann and Teipel 2013). The second most common cause of dementia is vascular dementia (VaD), which usually results from strokes or bleeding in the brain due to cerebrovascular or cardiovascular pathologies (Alzheimer's Association 2015; Román 2003). VaD accounts for only 10% to 20% of all dementia cases; however, with increasing age, up to 50% of dementia cases show pathologies of VaD (Alzheimer's Association 2015; Ott et al. 1995; Román 2003; Weyerer 2005). Other causes of dementia are dementia with Lewy bodies, frontotemporal lobar degeneration, Parkinson disease dementia, depression, infectious diseases such as Creutzfeldt-Jakob disease, normal pressure hydrocephalus, nutritive-toxic factors, and metabolic diseases (Alzheimer's Association 2015; Doblhammer et al. 2012; Weyerer and Bickel 2007).

The term "mild cognitive impairment" (MCI) describes the intermediate stage between normal and pathological cognitive aging (Petersen et al. 2014). People with MCI are cognitively declined but not demented, which basically means that they experience no impairments in their activities of daily living (Petersen et al. 2014; Winblad et al. 2004). Annual progression rates to dementia vary between 6% and 15% (Petersen et al. 2009).

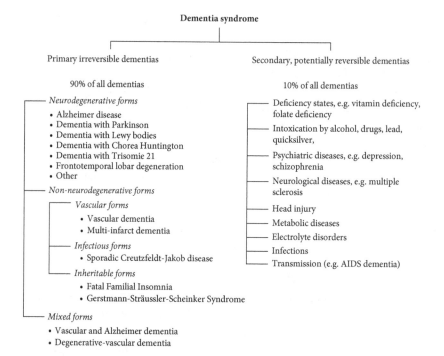

Figure 2.3 Types of dementia. Reproduced by permission from: Doblhammer, G., Schulz, A., Steinberg, J., Ziegler, U. (2012). Demografie der Demenz. Verlag Hans Huber, Hogrefe AG: Bern. Following: Gutzmann H., Zank S. (2005). Demenzielle Erkrankungen: Medizinische und psychosoziale Interventionen, Grundriss Gerontologie. Stuttgart: W. Kohlhammer. Kastner U., Löbach R. (2007). Handbuch Demenz. München, Jena: Urban & Fischer Verlag/ Elsevier GmbH. Kurz A. (2002). Demenzerkrankungen - Ursachen, Symptome und Verlauf. In: J. F. Hallauer, A. Kurz (Eds.). Weißbuch Demenz: Versorgungssituation relevanter Demenzerkrankungen in Deutschland. Stuttgart: Thieme-Verlag.

A Global Perspective on Occurrence and Trends in Major Dementia Risk Factors

A review by Kalaria et al. (2008) underlines the importance of several risk factors of dementia in both developed and developing countries. International evidence suggests that improvements in education and economic well-being subsequently lead to increasing life expectancy and reductions of late-life dementia risk in people who survive to old age. Both aspects also benefit from advances in the prevention and treatment of vascular diseases and other risk factors during midlife and early old age (Larson, Yaffe, and Langa 2013). This chapter presents information on the role of important vascular risk factors as well as mobility limitations and their occurrence worldwide.

Diabetes

Type 2 diabetes, the most common form of diabetes (Oputa and Chinenye 2012), is known to increase the risk of cognitive impairment (Fontbonne et al. 2001), dementia (Craft 2009; Luchsinger et al. 2004), and AD (Kopf and Frölich 2009; Weuve, McQueen, and Blacker 2008). In 2015, 415 million people worldwide suffered from diabetes (International Diabetes Federation 2015), more than 90% of whom were classified as type 2. The number of cases of type 2 diabetes is expected to increase in almost all countries (Oputa and Chinenye 2012). In 2040, the projected number of people aged 20 to 79 who suffer from diabetes will be about 642 million. The global age-standardized prevalence (a measure that allows for comparison of populations independent of the age profile of each population) (Naing 2000) will increase from 8.8% in 2015 to 10.4% by 2040. Europe has a comparatively low age-standardized prevalence, which will increase from 7.3% (59.8 million people) in 2015 to 7.6% (71.1 million) by 2040. In contrast, the age-standardized prevalence in North America and the Caribbean is high and it will increase from 11.5% in 2015 (44.3 million) to 12.0% by 2040 (60.5 million) (International Diabetes Federation 2015). Although diabetes is already highly prevalent, there are still many undiagnosed cases as well. Estimates suggest that globally almost 50% of people suffering from diabetes do not receive any diagnosis from a physician, meaning an estimated 193 million diabetics might not know of their illness. This could be due to unawareness or misdiagnosis of symptoms, but also because they are asymptomatic. The proportion of undiagnosed cases is particularly high in Sub-Saharan Africa (66.7%), South-East Asia (52.1%), and the Western Pacific (52.1%), but even in Europe (39.3%) and North America and the Caribbean (29.9%) a sizeable proportion of cases remains undiagnosed (International Diabetes Federation 2015).

Obesity

Being overweight or obese poses a significant burden to clinical and public health sectors. Globally the number of people with a high body mass index (BMI ≥ 25), which indicates being overweight or obese, has increased from 857 million in 1980 to 2.1 billion in 2013, and forecasts suggest continuing global increases (Basu 2010; Kelly et al. 2008; Sassi et al. 2009). Excessive weight is the leading global risk factor of disease burden, especially in Australasia and southern Latin America. It also ranks high in other high-income regions, such as North Africa and the Middle East, as well as Oceania. In 2010, having a high BMI was estimated to cause 3.4 million deaths, 4% of years of life lost, and 4% of disability-adjusted life-years (DALYs) worldwide (Lim et al. 2012). In combination with metabolic diseases (see section "Hypertension"), this increasing obesity prevalence poses a challenge for reducing dementia in the future, particularly in low- and middle-income countries (Anstey and Dixon 2014).

Hypertension

Hypertension is the most important cause of morbidity and mortality globally (Chow et al. 2013). While untreated hypertension increases the risk of dementia (Khachaturian et al. 2006; Lindsay, Hébert, and Rockwood 1997; Skoog 2004; Skoog et al. 1996; Wu et al. 2003), appropriate treatment of hypertension has been proven to decrease the risk of stroke (Garraway and Whisnant 1987) and dementia (Hajjar et al. 2005; Qui et al. 2003). Contrary to these findings, some cross-sectional studies have shown that dementia or lower cognitive performance was associated with lower blood pressure (Kontula et al. 1995; Lee 1994). Among others, Breteler (2000) has argued that while hypertension could increase the risk of dementia, blood pressure might have already declined prior to the onset of the disease and might continue to decrease as dementia progresses (Qiu, Winblad, and Fratiglioni 2005; Skoog and Gustafson 2006). The global age-standardized prevalence of hypertension in adults aged 18 years and over was around 22.2% in 2014. Prevalence was highest in Africa (30%) and lowest in North and South America (18.2%). In Europe prevalence was 23.3%, whereas the regions of South-East Asia (24.7%) and the Eastern Mediterranean (26.9%) had a prevalence above average (World Health Organization 2014). These numbers are likely an underestimation, especially in developing regions such as Africa. Hypertension is often poorly controlled and individuals are unaware of symptoms (Adeloye and Basquill 2014; Kayima et al. 2013). A meta-analysis (Adeloye and Basquill 2014) suggests that in Africa alone the numbers of 54.6 million cases (age >20) of hypertension in 1990 (prevalence: 19.1%), 92.3 million cases in 2000 (24.3%), and 130.2 million cases in 2010 (25.9%) will increase to 216.8 million cases (25.3%) by 2030. Another estimation (Kearney et al. 2005) listed the number of adults worldwide with hypertension in 2000 as being 972 million. This figure comprises 333 million in economically developed countries and 639 million in economically developing countries. The number of adults with hypertension is predicted to increase by about 60%, to a total of 1.56 billion, by 2025.

Hypertension is one of the essential components of the metabolic syndrome. The other components are visceral obesity, dyslipidemia, and glucose intolerance (Levesque and Lamarche 2008), although international definitions differ in their criteria and threshold values. This metabolic syndrome increases the risk of cardiovascular disease, type 2 diabetes mellitus, and all-cause mortality (Kaur 2014), and it is associated with AD (Vanhanen et al. 2006) as well as VaD (Solfrizzi et al. 2010). Depending on the region (urban or rural), demographic composition, and definition, the global prevalence of hypertension ranges from <10% to 84% (Kaur 2014). According to the International Diabetes Federation, one-quarter of the world's adult population suffer from this metabolic syndrome (International Diabetes Federation 2006).

Stroke

Stroke is a well-known risk factor of dementia (Desmond et al. 2002; Ivan et al. 2004; Patterson et al. 2007; Pendelbury and Rothwell 2009; Tatemichi et al. 1992; Zhu et al. 2000). The reason for dementia is either the stroke itself, which causes VaD (Pendelbury and Rothwell 2009), or a combination of degenerative and vascular pathologies, which may lead to the development of dementia after stroke (Ivan et al. 2004). A meta-regression analysis of 119 studies (Feigin et al. 2014) revealed a 12% decrease in the incidence of stroke in high-income countries and a 12% increase in low- and middle-income countries between 1990 and 2010. This global pattern was driven by the development in low- and middle-income countries. In 2010, the absolute number of people worldwide who had a first stroke was 16.9 million, and the number of stroke survivors was 33 million, both indicating a significant increase (68% and 84%, respectively) since 1990. In terms of distribution, 68.6% of all cases of first stroke and 52.2% of all stroke survivors live in low- and middle-income countries. Stroke also had an impact on DALYs. The 102 million DALYs lost in 2010 implicated an increase of roughly 12% since 1990. Strong, Mathers, and Bonita (2007) projected that in the absence of essential population-wide interventions, by 2030 the expected numbers of first-ever strokes and stroke-related deaths will be 23 million and 7.8 million, respectively.

Mobility Limitations

Mobility limitations have serious consequences on health. They limit social participation and reduce both psychosocial and physical activity. Mobility limitations are associated with depression as well as delirium, which is a common complication among elderly hospitalized patients, for example, after hip (Krogseth et al. 2014) or femoral neck fractures (Lundstrom et al. 2003). All such factors subsequently increase the risk of dementia (Bentler et al. 2009; Dal Bello-Haas et al. 2012; Krogseth et al. 2014; Lo et al. 2014; Lundstrom et al. 2003; Matheny et al. 2011; Zhou, Putter, and Doblhammer 2016). The prevention of falls and extremity injuries might help postpone dementia further into higher ages (Zhou, Putter, and Doblhammer 2016). Comparing the prevalence rates of mobility limitations is difficult because of varying operational measures in studies, particularly on a global level. The "World Report on Disability" published by the World Health Organization analyzed estimates based on the WHO World Health Survey 2002–2004, including 59 countries and representing 64% of the world population. It presented prevalence rates of a multidomain functioning indicator including domains of affect, cognition, interpersonal relationships, mobility, pain, sleep and energy, self-care, and vision. The total age- and sex-standardized prevalence rate of significant functioning difficulties in the everyday lives of adults aged 18 and older in 2004 was 15.6%, ranging from 11.8% in higher-income countries to 18.0% in lower-income countries. The prevalence for the age group 60 or older was 38.1%, with the higher prevalence in lower-income countries (43.4%) compared to higher-income countries (29.5%) (World Health Organization 2011). With regard to global population aging, the number of people with mobility limitations is likely to increase in the future.

Estimates of Current and Future Dementia Prevalence

In 2010, an estimated 36.6 million people worldwide suffered from dementia. This number is expected to double every 20 years, resulting in 65.7 million individuals with dementia by 2030 and 115.4 million by 2050 (Prince et al. 2013). An updated and less optimistic estimation posited that the number of people with dementia in 2013 was as high as 44.35 million, and it could reach 75.62 million by 2030 and 135.46 million by 2050 (Alzheimer's Disease International 2013). A recent meta-analysis (Prince et al. 2013) suggests that in most world regions the age-standardized prevalence of dementia at ages 60 and older is between 5% and 7%, with estimates for Latin America the highest (8.5%) and those for Sub-Saharan Africa the lowest (2% to 4%). Particularly in developing countries, dementia prevalence estimates vary widely due to differences in population age structure, genetics, lifestyles, difficulties in standardizing dementia assessment, and reduced survival after diagnosis (Brayne 2007). The most common subtypes of age-related dementia, both in developed and developing countries, are late-onset AD and VaD (Qiu, Kivipelto, and von Strauss 2009).

Dementia projections in general depend on assumptions about future life expectancy increases and trends in dementia prevalence. While dementia remains incurable and life expectancy will continue to increase, positive developments with respect to medical, lifestyle, and societal risk factors of dementia in young and middle age groups might have positive long-term effects, that is, decrease the risk of dementia in old age. Recent analyses also give some cause for hope. A review by Larson, Yaffe, and Langa (2013) presents results from five studies of higher-income countries (United States, Netherlands, Sweden, and England), all of which point toward a decline in dementia and severe cognitive impairment. A study by Doblhammer, Fink, and Fritze (2015) used German health claims data based on millions of observations up through the highest ages to explore short-term trends in the prevalence of dementia. Results revealed a significant yearly reduction of between 1% and 2% in dementia prevalence among women aged 75 to 84 years between 2007 and 2009. Further success in the reduction of vascular risk factors (Jacqmin-Gadda et al. 2013), changes in dietary habits (Barberger-Gateau et al. 2007), and increased physical activity (Jedrziewski, Lee, and Trojanowski 2007) may contribute to such trends and may also lead to a further delay in or even the prevention of dementia. Interventional and prevention programs, however, should not only target such single risk factors, as recent research has shown that overall health status is a major or contributing risk factor of dementia (Song, Mitnitski, and Rockwood 2014).

Cost Estimates and Projections

Dementia is a chronic disease and the leading cause of disability and care need in the elderly population; it imposes huge economic burdens on families, governments, and health and social care systems. The costs of dementia include direct, indirect, and intangible costs (Moise et al. 2004). Direct costs are primarily generated by professional health and nursing care, but also include costs of prevention, medical diagnosis, rehabilitation, research, or professional training. Indirect or informal costs are related to caring responsibilities by family or friends, as well as to the loss of added value to the national economy (Leicht et al. 2011; Wimo et al. 2013). Intangible costs are nonmonetary: they refer to the pain and suffering endured by patients and families, as well as the deterioration in the quality of life of patients and caregivers. Because it is difficult to evaluate intangible costs, estimations generally focus on direct and indirect costs (Zhu and Sano 2006). Estimations of total costs and costs per person vary between studies, due to different coverage of direct and indirect costs.

In 2010, the total estimated worldwide direct and indirect costs of dementia were $604 billion, with an uneven distribution across regions. Of all people with dementia, less than half (46%) lived in high-income countries, but this is where 89% of the total costs worldwide were incurred. Middle-income countries bore 10% of the costs, even though roughly 40% of all people with dementia lived there. Roughly 14% of all people with dementia lived in low-income countries, but they accounted for less than 1% of total costs (Wimo et al. 2013). The proportion of people with dementia living in care homes is higher in developed countries, which is the main expense. In developing countries, however, informal care at home has been dominant thus far, generating more indirect than direct costs (Kalaria et al. 2008; Wimo et al. 2013). It seems likely that this pattern will change due to new demographic, social, and economic developments. The need for institutionalized care will grow, thereby increasing the direct costs (Wimo et al. 2013).

In the EU27 states, estimated costs per person amounted to €21,045 in 2005 (Wimo, Jönsson, and Gustavsson 2008). In other studies the values in Western industrial nations range from €25,000 to €50,000 per person (Bickel 2001) or from $6,000 to $75,000 per person (Leung et al. 2003). Expenditures increase with the severity of the disease, as shown by a meta-analysis (Quentin et al. 2010) that revealed a wide range of results. The costs per persons were €10,500 to €29,100 for mild dementia, €18,300 to €43,900 for moderate cases, and €20,700 to €68,000 for severe cases of dementia.

Conclusion

Dementia is currently posing major challenges for societies with aging populations, and the number of people suffering from dementia will continue to increase. At present, dementia is mainly present in the developed world, but due to accelerated population aging in developing countries, dementia will also be an essential burden in these regions. Coping with the high demand for care and meeting the incurring costs are already key challenges and will continue to be so. In early and later stages of dementia, assistive technologies may help reduce the burden on the family and caregivers and postpone entrance into nursing homes, allowing individuals to remain in their communities longer.

References

1. Lutz W, Sanderson W, Scherbov S. The coming acceleration of global population ageing. Nature 2008;451:716–19.
2. Christensen K, Doblhammer G, Rau R, Vaupel JW. Ageing populations: the challenges ahead. Lancet 2009;374:1196–208.

3. Bickel H. Epidemiologie psychischer Erkrankungen im Alter. In: G. Förstl, editor. Lehrbuch der Gerontopsychiatrie und -psychotherapie. Stuttgart: Thieme Verlag; 2003, 11–26.

4. Baldereschi M, Di Carlo A, Maggi S, Grigoletto F, Scarlato G, Amaducci L, et al. Dementia is a major predictor of death among the Italian elderly. ILSA Working Group. Italian Longitudinal Study on Aging. Neurology 1999 Mar 10;52:709–13.

5. Vallin J, Meslé F. Convergences and divergences in mortality: a new approach of health transition. Demographic Research 2004;S2:11–44.

6. Prince M, Bryce R, Albanese E, Wimo A, Ribeiro W, Ferri CP. The global prevalence of dementia: a systematic review and metaanalysis. Alzheimer's & Dementia: Journal of the Alzheimer's Association 2013 Jan;9:63–75 e2.

7. Blaschke CM, Freddolino PP, Mullen EE. Ageing and technology: a review of the research literature. British Journal of Social Work 2009 Jun 1;39:641–56.

8. United Nations. Department of Economic and Social Affairs, Population Division (2015). World Population Prospects: The 2015 Revision, Key Findings and Advance Tables. ESA/P/WP.241.

9. Oeppen J, Vaupel JW. Broken limits to life expectancy. Science 2002 May 10;296:1029–31.

10. Shkolnikov VM, Jdanov DA, Andreev EM, Vaupel JW. Steep increase in best-practice cohort life expectancy. Population and Development Review 2011;37:419–34.

11. Abridged Life Tables for Japan 2015 [Internet]. Ministry of Health, Labour, and Welfare, Japan. 2015 [cited October 10, 2016]. Available from: http://www.mhlw.go.jp/english/database/db-hw/vs02.html.

12. Rau R, Soroko E, Jasilionis D, Vaupel JW. Continued reductions in mortality at advanced ages. Population and Development Review 2008;34:747–68.

13. Meslé F, Vallin J. Mortality in Europe: the divergence between East and West. Population and Development Review 2002;57:157–97.

14. Vallin J. Disease, death, and life expectancy. Genus 2005;61:279–96.

15. Vallin J, Meslé F. Trends in mortality in Europe since 1950: age-, sex- and cause-specific mortality. In: J. Vallin, F. Meslé, & T. Valkonen, editors, Trends in mortality and differential mortality. Strasbourg: Council of Europe Publishing (Population Studies No. 36); 2001, 31–186.

16. Robine JM, Le Roy S, Jagger C. Changes in life expectancy in the European Union since 1995: similarities and differences between the 25 EU countries. In: Institut des sciences de la santé, editor. Europe blanche XXVI. Budapest, Hungary: Institut des sciences de la santé; 2005, 9–48.

17. Omran AR. The epidemiologic transition. A theory of the epidemiology of population change. Milbank Memorial Fund Quarterly Health and Society 1971 Oct;49:509–38.

18. Janssen F, Kunst AE, Netherlands Epidemiology and Demography Compression of Morbidity Research Group. Cohort patterns in mortality trends among the elderly in seven European countries, 1950–99. International Journal of Epidemiology 2005 Oct;34:1149–59.

19. Janssen F, Mackenbach JP, Kunst AE, Nedcom. Trends in old-age mortality in seven European countries, 1950–1999. Journal of Clinical Epidemiology 2004 Feb;57:203–16.

20. Nusselder WJ, Mackenbach JP. Lack of improvement of life expectancy at advanced ages in the Netherlands. International Journal of Epidemiology 2000 Feb;29:140–48.

21. Pison G. Population ageing will be faster in the South than in the North. Population and Societies 2009;457:1–4.
22. World Health Organization. Dementia 2015 [cited August 5, 2015]. Available from: http://www.who.int/mediacentre/factsheets/fs362/en/.
23. World Health Organization. ICD-10 Version: 2010 [cited August 5, 2015]. Available from: http://apps.who.int/classifications/icd10/browse/2010/en#/F00-F09.
24. Weyerer S. Altersdemenz. Berlin: Robert Koch-Institut; 2005.
25. Ott A, Breteler MMB, Van Harskamp F, Claus JJ, Van der Cammen TJM, Grobbee DE, et al. Prevalence of Alzheimer's disease and vascular dementia: association with education. The Rotterdam study. British Medical Journal 1995;310:970–73.
26. Alzheimer's Association. 2015 Alzheimer's disease facts and figures. Alzheimer's & Dementia 2015;11:332–84.
27. Schneider JA, Arvanitakis Z, Bang W, Bennett DA. Mixed brain pathologies account for most dementia cases in community-dwelling older persons. Neurology 2007;69:2197–204.
28. Kilimann I, Teipel S. Alzheimer-Krankheit. Gedächtnisstörungen—Diagnostik und Rehabilitation. Berlin, Heidelberg: Springer; 2013, 239–63.
29. Román GC. Vascular dementia: distinguishing characteristics, treatment, and prevention. Journal of the American Geriatrics Society 2003;51:S296–304.
30. Doblhammer G, Schulz A, Steinberg J, Ziegler U. Demografie der Demenz. Bern: Verlag Hans Huber, Hofgrefe AG; 2012.
31. Weyerer S, Bickel H. Epidemiologie psychischer Erkrankungen im höheren Lebensalter. Tesch-Römer C, Wahl H-W, Weyerer S, Zank S, editors. Stuttgart: Verlag W. Kohlhammer; 2007.
32. Petersen RC, Caracciolo B, Brayne C, Gauthier S, Jelic V, Fratiglioni L. Mild cognitive impairment: a concept in evolution. Journal of Internal Medicine 2014;275:214–28.
33. Winblad B, Palmer K, Kivipelto M, Jelic V, Fratiglioni L, Wahlund LO. Mild cognitive impairment: beyond controversies, towards a consensus-report of the international working group on mild cognitive impairment. Journal of Internal Medicine 2004;256:240–46.
34. Petersen RC, Roberts RO, Knopman DS, Boeve BF, Geda YE, Ivnik RJ, et al. Mild cognitive impairment: ten years later. Archives of Neurology 2009;66:1447–55.
35. Kalaria RN, Maestre GE, Arizaga R, Friedland RP, Galasko D, Hall K, et al. Alzheimer's disease and vascular dementia in developing countries: prevalence, management, and risk factors. Lancet Neurology 2008 Sep;7:812–26.
36. Larson EB, Yaffe K, Langa KM. New insights into the dementia epidemic. New England Journal of Medicine 2013 Dec 12;369:2275–77.
37. Oputa RN, Chinenye S. Diabetes mellitus: a global epidemic with potential solutions. African Journal of Diabetes Medicine 2012;457:33–35.
38. Fontbonne A, Berr C, Ducimetiere P, Alperovitch A. Changes in cognitive abilities over a 4-year period are unfavorably affected in elderly diabetic subjects: results of the epidemiology of vascular aging study. Diabetes Care 2001;24:366–70.
39. Craft S. The role of metabolic disorders in Alzheimer disease and vascular dementia. Two roads converged. Archives of Neurology 2009;66:300–5.
40. Luchsinger JA, Tang M-X, Shea S, Mayeux R. Hyperinsulinemia and risk of Alzheimer disease. Neurology 2004;63:1187–92.
41. Kopf D, Frölich L. Risk of incident Alzheimer's disease in diabetic patients: a systematic review of prospective trials. Journal of Alzheimer's Disease 2009;16:677–85.

42. Weuve J, McQueen MB, Blacker D. The AlzRisk database. Alzheimer Research Forum. 2008 [cited June 1, 2016]. Available from: http://www.alzforum.org.
43. International Diabetes Federation. IDF Diabetes Atlas. 7th ed. Brussels, Belgium: International Diabetes Federation; 2015.
44. Naing NN. Easy way to learn standardization: direct and indirect methods. Malaysian Journal of Medical Sciences: MJMS 2000;7:10–15.
45. Kelly T, Yang W, Chen CS, Reynolds K, He J. Global burden of obesity in 2005 and projections to 2030. International Journal of Obesity 2008 Sep;32:1431–37.
46. Basu A. Forecasting distribution of body mass index in the United States: is there more room for growth? Medical Decision Making: International Journal of the Society for Medical Decision Making 2010 May-Jun;30:E1–11.
47. Sassi F, Marion D, Cecchini M, Rusticelli E. The Obesity Epidemic: Analysis of Past Trends and Projected Future Trends in Selected OECD Countries. 2009 Contract No.: 45.
48. Lim SS, Vos T, Flaxman AD, Danaei G, Shibuya K, Adair-Rohani H, et al. A comparative risk assessment of burden of disease and injury attributable to 67 risk factors and risk factor clusters in 21 regions, 1990-2010: a systematic analysis for the Global Burden of Disease Study 2010. Lancet 2012 Dec 15;380:2224–60.
49. Anstey KJ, Dixon RA. Applying a cumulative deficit model of frailty to dementia: progress and future challenges. Alzheimer's Research & Therapy 2014;6:84.
50. Chow CK, Teo KK, Rangarajan S, Islam S, Gupta R, Avezum A, et al. Prevalence, awareness, treatment, and control of hypertension in rural and urban communities in high-, middle-, and low-income countries. JAMA 2013 Sep 4;310:959–68.
51. Lindsay J, Hébert R, Rockwood K. The Canadian Study of Health and Aging. Risk factors for vascular dementia. Stroke 1997;28:526–30.
52. Khachaturian AS, Zandi PP, Lyketsos CG, Hayden KM, Skoog I, Norton MC, et al. Antihypertensive medication use and incident Alzheimer disease. Archives of Neurology 2006;3:686–92.
53. Skoog I. Psychiatric epidemiology of old age: the H70 study—the NAPE Lecture 2003. Acta Psychiatrica Scandinavica 2004;109:4–18.
54. Skoog I, Lernfelt B, Landahl S, Palmertz B, Andreasson LA, Nilsson L, et al. 15-year longitudinal study of blood pressure and dementia. Lancet 1996;347:1141–45.
55. Wu C, Zhou D, Wen C, Zhang L, Como P, Qiao Y. Relationship between blood pressure and Alzheimer's disease in Linxian County, China. Life Sciences 2003;72:1125–33.
56. Garraway WM, Whisnant JP. The changing pattern of hypertension and the declining incidence of stroke. Journal of the American Medical Association 1987;258:214–17.
57. Hajjar I, Catoe H, Sixta S, Boland R, Johnson D, Hirth V, et al. Cross-sectional and longitudinal association between antihypertensive medications and cognitive impairment in an elderly population. Journals of Gerontology Series A—Biological Sciences and Medical Sciences 2005;60:67–73.
58. Qui C, Winblad B, Fastbom J, Fratiglioni L. Combined effects of APOE genotype, blood pressure, and antihypertensive drug use on incident AD. Neurology 2003;61:655–60.
59. Kontula K, Ylikorkala A, Miettinen H, Vuorio A, Kauppinen-Mäkelin R, Hämäläinen L, et al. Arg506Gln factor V mutation (factor V Leiden) in patients with ischaemic cerebrovascular disease and survivors of myocardial infarction. Thrombosis and Haemostasis 1995;73:558–60.
60. Lee PN. Smoking and Alzheimer's disease: a review of the epidemiological evidence. Neuroepidemiology 1994;13:131–44.

61. Breteler M. Vascular risk factors for Alzheimer's disease: an epidemiologic perspective. Neurobiology of Aging 2000;21:153–60.
62. Qiu C, Winblad B, Fratiglioni L. The age-dependent relation of blood pressure to cognitive function and dementia. Lancet Neurology 2005;4:487–99.
63. Skoog I, Gustafson D. Update on hypertension and Alzheimer's disease. Neurology Research 2006;28:605–11.
64. World Health Organization. Global Status Report on Noncommunicable Diseases 2014. Geneva, Switzerland: World Health Organization; 2014.
65. Adeloye D, Basquill C. Estimating the prevalence and awareness rates of hypertension in Africa: a systematic analysis. PLoS One 2014;9:e104300.
66. Kayima J, Wanyenze RK, Katamba A, Leontsini E, Nuwaha F. Hypertension awareness, treatment and control in Africa: a systematic review. BMC Cardiovascular Disorders 2013;13:54.
67. Kearney PM, Whelton M, Reynolds K, Muntner P, Whelton PK, He J. Global burden of hypertension: analysis of worldwide data. Lancet 2005 Jan 15–21;365:217–23.
68. Levesque J, Lamarche B. The metabolic syndrome: definitions, prevalence and management. Journal of Nutrigenetics and Nutrigenomics 2008;1:100–8.
69. Kaur J. A comprehensive review on metabolic syndrome. Cardiology Research and Practice 2014;2014:943162.
70. Vanhanen M, Koivisto K, Moilanen L, Helkala EL, Hänninen T, Soininen H, et al. Association of metabolic syndrome with Alzheimer disease. Neurology 2006;67:843–47.
71. Solfrizzi V, Scafato E, Capurso C, D'Introno A, Colacicco AM, Frisardi V, et al. Metabolic syndrome and the risk of vascular dementia: the Italian Longitudinal Study on Ageing. Journal of Neurology, Neurosurgery, and Psychiatry 2010 Apr;81:433–40.
72. International Diabetes Federation. The IDF consensus worldwide definition of the metabolic syndrome. 2006 [cited June 1, 2016]. Available from: http://www.idf.org/metabolic-syndrome.
73. Desmond DW, Moroney JT, Sano M, Stern Y. Incidence of dementia after ischemic stroke: results of a longitudinal study. Stroke 2002;33:2254–60.
74. Ivan CS, Seshadri S, Beiser A, Au R, Kase CS, Kelly-Hayes M, et al. Dementia after stroke. The Framingham Study. Stroke 2004;35:1264–69.
75. Patterson C, Feightner J, Garcia A, MacKnight C. General risk factors for dementia: a systematic evidence review. Alzheimer's & Dementia 2007;3:341–47.
76. Pendelbury ST, Rothwell PM. Prevalence, incidence, and factors associated with pre-stroke and post-stroke dementia: a systematic review and meta-analysis. Lancet Neurology 2009;8:1006–18.
77. Tatemichi TK, Desmond DW, Mayeux R, Paik M, Stern Y, Sano M, et al. Dementia after stroke. Baseline frequency, risks, and clinical features in a hospitalized cohort. Neurology 1992;42:1185–93.
78. Zhu L, Fratiglioni L, Guo Z, Basun H, Hedlund Corder E, Winblad B, et al. Incidence of dementia in relation to stroke and the apolipoprotein E4 allele in the very old. Findings from a population-based longitudinal study. Stroke 2000;31:53–60.
79. Feigin VL, Forouzanfar MH, Krishnamurthi R, Mensah GA, Connor M, Bennett DA, et al. Global and regional burden of stroke during 1990-2010: findings from the Global Burden of Disease Study 2010. Lancet 2014 Jan 18;383:245–54.
80. Strong K, Mathers C, Bonita R. Preventing stroke: saving lives around the world. Lancet Neurology 2007 Feb;6:182–87.

81. Krogseth M, Wyller TB, Engedal K, Juliebo V. Delirium is a risk factor for institutionalization and functional decline in older hip fracture patients. Journal of Psychosomatic Research 2014 Jan;76:68–74.
82. Lundstrom M, Edlund A, Bucht G, Karlsson S, Gustafson Y. Dementia after delirium in patients with femoral neck fractures. Journal of the American Geriatrics Society 2003 Jul;51:1002–6.
83. Matheny ME, Miller RR, Shardell MD, Hawkes WG, Lenze EJ, Magaziner J, et al. Inflammatory cytokine levels and depressive symptoms in older women in the year after hip fracture: findings from the Baltimore Hip Studies. Journal of the American Geriatrics Society 2011 Dec;59:2249–55.
84. Dal Bello-Haas VP, Thorpe LU, Lix LM, Scudds R, Hadjistavropoulos T. The effects of a long-term care walking program on balance, falls and well-being. BMC Geriatrics 2012;12:76.
85. Lo AX, Brown CJ, Sawyer P, Kennedy RE, Allman RM. Life-space mobility declines associated with incident falls and fractures. Journal of the American Geriatrics Society 2014 May;62:919–23.
86. Bentler SE, Liu L, Obrizan M, Cook EA, Wright KB, Geweke JF, et al. The aftermath of hip fracture: discharge placement, functional status change, and mortality. American Journal of Epidemiology 2009 Nov 15;170:1290–99.
87. Zhou Y, Putter H, Doblhammer G. Years of life lost due to lower extremity injury in association with dementia, and care need: a 6-year follow-up population-based study using a multi-state approach among German elderly. BMC Geriatrics 2016;16:9.
88. World Health Organization. World Report on Disability. Geneva, Switzerland: World Health Organization; 2011.
89. Alzheimer's Disease International. Policy Brief: The Global Impact of Dementia 2013-2050. London: Alzheimer's Disease International (ADI); 2013.
90. Brayne C. The elephant in the room—healthy brains in later life, epidemiology and public health. Nature Reviews Neuroscience 2007 Mar;8:233–39.
91. Qiu C, Kivipelto M, von Strauss E. Epidemiology of Alzheimer's disease: occurrence, determinants, and strategies toward intervention. Dialogues in Clinical Neuroscience 2009;11:111–28.
92. Doblhammer G, Fink A, Fritze T. Short-term trends in dementia prevalence in Germany between the years 2007 and 2009. Alzheimer's & Dementia: Journal of the Alzheimer's Association 2015 Mar;11:291–99.
93. Jacqmin-Gadda H, Alperovitch A, Montlahuc C, Commenges D, Leffondre K, Dufouil C, et al. 20-Year prevalence projections for dementia and impact of preventive policy about risk factors. European Journal of Epidemiology 2013 Jun;28:493–502.
94. Barberger-Gateau P, Raffaitin C, Letenneur L, Berr C, Tzourio C, Dartigues JF, et al. Dietary patterns and risk of dementia: the three-city cohort study. Neurology 2007 Nov 13;69:1921–30.
95. Jedrziewski MK, Lee VM, Trojanowski JQ. Physical activity and cognitive health. Alzheimer's & Dementia: Journal of the Alzheimer's Association 2007 Apr;3:98–108.
96. Song X, Mitnitski A, Rockwood K. Age-related deficit accumulation and the risk of late-life dementia. Alzheimer's Research & Therapy 2014;6:54.
97. Moise P, Schwarzinger M, Um MY, Dementia Experts Group. Dementia care in 9 OECD countries: a comparative analysis. OECD Health Working Papers 2004;13.

98. Wimo A, Jonsson L, Bond J, Prince M, Winblad B, Alzheimer disease I. The world-wide economic impact of dementia 2010. Alzheimer's & Dementia: Journal of the Alzheimer's Association 2013 Jan;9:1–11 e3.
99. Leicht H, Heinrich S, Heider D, Bachmann C, Bickel H, van den Bussche H, et al. Net costs of dementia by disease stage. Acta Psychiatrica Scandinavica 2011;124:384–95.
100. Zhu CW, Sano M. Economic considerations in the management of Alzheimer's disease. Clinical Interventions in Aging 2006;1:143–54.
101. Wimo A, Jönsson L, Gustavsson A. The cost of illness and burden of dementia in Europe. In: Alzheimer Europe, editor. Dementia in Europe Yearbook 2008. Luxembourg: Alzheimer Europe; 2008, 67–70.
102. Bickel H. Demenzen im höheren Lebensalter. Schätzungen des Vorkommens und der Versorgungskosten. Zeitschrift Fur Gerontologie Und Geriatrie 2001;34:108–15.
103. Leung GM, Yeung RYT, Chi I, Chu LW. The economics of Alzheimer disease. Dementia and Geriatric Cognitive Disorders 2003;15:34–43.
104. Quentin W, Riedel-Heller S, Luppa M, Rudolph A, König H-H. Cost-of-illness studies of dementia: a systematic review focusing on stage dependency of costs. Acta Psychiatrica Scandinavica 2010;121:243–59.

3

Dementia and Neurocognitive Disability

Christophe J. Büla

Definitions and Diagnostic Criteria

Dementia can be broadly defined as a decline in cognitive abilities in comparison with a previous level of performance that interferes with a person's function in daily activities. Until recently, the most widely used criteria defined dementia as a clinical syndrome (i.e., a constellation of clinical symptoms and signs) characterized by the—usually—progressive development of multiple cognitive deficits including memory impairments and disturbances in at least one other cognitive domain (e.g., praxis, language, gnosis, executive functions, etc.). The diagnosis of dementia requires that these cognitive deficits are severe enough to cause impairments in social and/or occupational functioning. In addition, the deficits must not occur exclusively during a delirium and must not be attributable to a major psychiatric disorder, such as depression or schizophrenia.

A difficulty in diagnosing dementia relates to the observation that cognitive performance varies among older persons. The limit between usual, age-related decline and abnormal impairment remains fuzzy. Furthermore, recent data from autopsy studies showed that whereas some cognitively well-functioning individuals had extensive signs of neurodegenerative cellular pathologies, others with significant cognitive decline had only few of these cellular abnormalities (Boyle et al. 2013). The term "mild cognitive impairment" (MCI) was proposed to describe an intermediate stage between normal cognition and dementia (Langa and Levine 2014; Petersen 2011). The concept of MCI defines situations where cognitive complaints and/or concerns are associated with objective modest impairments in memory (amnestic MCI) or other nonmemory (nonamnestic MCI) cognitive domains, but in the absence of functional repercussion and dementia. Impairment may affect only one (single-domain MCI) or multiple (multidomain MCI) cognitive domains. Persons with MCI, especially those with amnestic MCI, are at increased risk of progressing to dementia, about 10% to 15% per year, with extremes ranging from an annual conversion rate of less than 5% to 20% depending on the population studied (Petersen 2011).

More recently, the fifth edition of the *Diagnostic and Statistical Manual of Mental Disorders* (DSM-5) proposed to replace the terms "dementia" and "MCI" with the concepts of "major" and "minor" neurocognitive disorder, respectively (Association D-AP 2013). Until this revision, the presence of memory impairment was required for the diagnosis of all dementia syndromes, indiscriminate of their etiology. The new DSM-5 definition recognized that memory is not the first impaired cognitive domain in several dementias from etiologies other than Alzheimer's disease (AD), such as frontotemporal dementias, where language can be affected first. DSM-5 criteria for diagnosing a major and a minor neurocognitive disorder are presented in Table 3.1.

Once the presence of a dementia syndrome (i.e., of a major neurocognitive disorder) has been established, healthcare professionals need to determine its underlying etiology (Table 3.1).

In older persons, AD is the most common etiology of dementia (about 60% to 75% of cases), followed by vascular dementia (VaD, about 10% to 25% of cases), mixed dementia (AD and VaD, about 25% included AD and VaD), and dementia with Lewy bodies (about 15% of cases). Other types of dementia (e.g., frontotemporal dementia, Parkinson's disease, Huntington's disease, Creutzfeldt-Jakob disease, etc.) are much less frequent in older persons (about 5% of cases).

The specific description of the set of diagnostic criteria as well as of the clinical course of each of these entities is beyond the scope of this chapter. For the interested reader, a detailed description of diagnostic criteria for AD (Dubois et al. 2007) and frontotemporal (Bang, Spina, and Miller 2015), Lewy body (Walker et al. 2015), and VaDs (O'Brien and Thomas 2015) can be found elsewhere.

Epidemiology: Dementia as a Global Challenge

Prevalence and Incidence

In high-income countries, the prevalence of dementia is about 5% to 10% in older persons aged 65 and over. However, dementia prevalence varies within this older population and increases exponentially with increasing age, from 2% to 5% among those aged 65 to 74 years up to 30% to 45% among those aged 85 years or more. As life expectancy continues to extend in most countries, the prevalence of dementia is expected to further increase worldwide. In 2013, it was estimated that about 47.5 million people worldwide suffered from dementia and that a new case appeared every 5 to 10 seconds (Alzheimer's Disease International 2013; Ferri et al. 2005; Prince et al. 2013). Thus, the worldwide prevalence of dementia is expected to amount to about 75.6 million by 2030 and 135.5 million by 2050. Currently, about 58% of people with dementia live in low- and middle-income countries, a proportion expected to increase to about 71% by 2050 because of the population aging in countries such as China and India (Figure 3.1).

Table 3.1 Diagnostic Criteria for Major and Minor Neurocognitive Disorders

Major Neurocognitive Disorder (Dementia)	Mild Neurocognitive Disorder (Mild Cognitive Impairment [MCI])
A. Evidence of significant cognitive decline from a previous level of performance in one or more cognitive domains (complex attention, executive function, learning and memory, language, perceptual motor, or social cognition) based on: 1. Concern of the individual, a knowledgeable informant, or the clinician that there has been a significant decline in cognitive function; and 2. A substantial impairment in cognitive performance, preferably documented by standardized neuropsychological testing (test performance in the range of two or more standard deviations below appropriate norms, i.e., below the third percentile) or, in its absence, another quantified clinical assessment. B. The cognitive deficits interfere with capacity for independence in everyday activities (i.e., complex instrumental activities of daily living such as paying bills or managing medications are impaired).	A. Evidence of modest cognitive decline from a previous level of performance in one or more cognitive domains (complex attention, executive function, learning and memory, language, perceptual motor, or social cognition) based on: 1. Concern of the individual, a knowledgeable informant, or the clinician that there has been a mild decline in cognitive function; and 2. A modest impairment in cognitive performance, preferably documented by standardized neuropsychological testing (test performance in the range of one and two standard deviations below appropriate norms, i.e., between the 3rd and 16th percentiles) or, in its absence, another quantified clinical assessment. B. The cognitive deficits do not interfere with capacity for independence in everyday activities (i.e., complex instrumental activities of daily living such as paying bills or managing medications are preserved, but greater effort, more time, compensatory strategies, or accommodation may be required).

C. Deficits do not occur exclusively during delirium.

D. Deficits are not better explained by another mental disorder (e.g., major depressive disorder, schizophrenia).

E. Specify one or more causal subtypes caused by:
- ☐ Alzheimer's disease
- ☐ Cerebrovascular disease (vascular cognitive disorder)
- ☐ Frontotemporal lobar degeneration (frontotemporal cognitive disorder)
- ☐ Dementia with Lewy bodies (neurocognitive disorder with Lewy bodies)
- ☐ Parkinson's disease
- ☐ Huntington disease
- ☐ Traumatic brain injury
- ☐ Human immunodeficiency virus infection
- ☐ Prion disease
- ☐ Another medical condition
- ☐ Multiple causes

Adapted from Association D-AP. Diagnostic and statistical manual of mental disorders. Arlington: American Psychiatric Publishing; 2013.

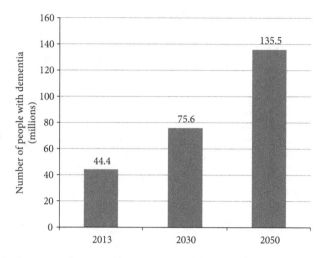

Figure 3.1 Current and projected estimations of the number of people with dementia worldwide.

Adapted from Alzheimer's Disease International. Policy brief for G8 heads of government. The Global Impact of Dementia 2013–2050. Alzheimer's Disease International; 2013, London.

Recent data on dementia incidence, however, suggests that these projections might be somewhat modified. Older studies all observed steady increases in dementia incidence until age 90 to 95 years, with age-specific incidence rates ranging from 0.1% to 0.3% at age 60 to 64 years up to 8.6% to 17.5% at age 95 years (Gao et al. 1998; Jorm and Jolley 1998). However, several more recent studies from Europe as well as from the United States strongly suggest that the age-specific incidence of dementia might actually be declining (Matthews et al. 2013; Qiu et al. 2013; Satizabal et al. 2016). For instance, over a 20-year period in the Framingham study, the age- and gender-adjusted hazard rates of dementia decreased steadily from 3.6 per 100 persons in 1970–1980 to 2.8 in 1980–1990, 2.2 in 1990–2000, and 2.0 in 2000–2010, representing a 44% decline in incidence rate (Satizabal et al. 2016). Moreover, this study observed that the age at diagnosis increased from about 80 years in 1970–1980 to about 85 years in 2000–2010. Similarly, a recent UK study found that among men aged 85 or over, dementia incidence fell from about 70 to about 40 cases per 1000 person-years in just two decades (Matthews et al. 2016). Better control of risk factors, especially cardiovascular; increased wealth; and better education likely explains some of this decrease. Overall, these studies suggest that the expected massive increase in dementia prevalence might be somewhat buffered by this favorable trend, even though the overall public health burden will likely remain enormous.

Burden and Costs

Dementias have important consequences for affected individuals, their families, and the whole healthcare system. In 2010, total worldwide yearly costs of dementia care were estimated to amount to €548 billion (US $604 billion), an amount about equivalent to 1% of the world's gross domestic product (Prince, Prina, and Guerchet 2013; Wimo et al. 2013). These costs are related mainly to *informal* care (up to 65% of total care costs) in low-income countries, whereas *social* care (professional in-home and long-term care) is the main driver of costs in high-income countries (about 45% of total care costs) (Prince, Prina, and Guerchet 2013). The share of healthcare (ambulatory, hospital)–related costs vary between about 15% (high-income countries) and 32% (upper-middle-income countries).

In 2010, dementia ranked 10th on the worldwide list of the 15 most burdensome disorders in people aged 60 years and over. Dementia accounted for 10.0 million disability-adjusted life years (DALYs), a 112.8% increase compared to 1990 (Prince et al. 2015). Specific studies in populations from low- and middle-income countries have shown that, in these countries, dementia was the leading contributor to disability (Sousa et al. 2009). Previous estimations reported that dementia accounted for 11.2% of disability years among persons aged 60 years and over, a share larger than stroke (9.5%), musculoskeletal disorders (8.9%), cardiovascular diseases (5.0%), or cancers (2.4%) (Ferri et al. 2005).

But the burden of dementia is not limited to these figures. For each patient affected by the disease, it is usually estimated that about two to three relatives (i.e., family members or friends) are involved in their care. As will be discussed later in this chapter, these informal caregivers face tremendous strain over the course of the disease. Early on, caregiving tasks relate to instrumental activities of daily living (ADLs), such as preparing meals, doing the laundry, providing transportation, and managing finances and legal affairs. Later on, caregivers are involved in assistance in basic ADLs such as bathing, dressing, grooming, and helping the person to walk. Eventually, caregivers face difficulties managing behavioral symptoms such as aggressive behavior, wandering, agitation, or anxiety. They also frequently have to face intensely painful care decisions, such as decisions about the need for institutionalization in a long-term care facility.

Caregivers provide a large amount of care, and as such, they need to be recognized as a partner by health professionals caring for a demented patient. Caregivers are more likely to experience depressive episodes and anxiety and have worse general health than informal caregivers of similarly old patients suffering from other types of chronic diseases (Brodaty, Green, and Koschera 2003; Cooper, Balamurali, and Livingston 2007; Grasel 2002; Mahoney et al. 2005). Supporting caregivers can be difficult as they are frequently reluctant to request professional support (Brodaty et al. 2005), but this appears essential as burnout and depression are major determinants in the decision to institutionalize a person with dementia (Downs and Bowers 2008). Still, caregivers sometimes also report more satisfaction with their lives even though they experience more burden (Cohen, Colantonio, and Vernich 2002), and some interventions supporting their role could provide important benefits for both patients and caregivers, as will be discussed later in this chapter.

Clinical Course: From Symptoms to Disability

This section will focus on AD, the main type of dementia that represents between 60% and 75% of dementia cases. Clinical manifestations in other types of dementia will not be discussed in detail here. In early stages, these manifestations can be very similar to those in AD, as in dementia with Lewy bodies, where dementia occurs before or concurrently with parkinsonism. In addition, dementia with Lewy bodies is associated with early sleep behavior disorders and with predominant deficits in attention, executive function, and visuospatial ability (Walker et al. 2015). Indeed, visual hallucinations appearing in early dementia seem very specific to differentiate dementia with Lewy bodies from AD (Tiraboschi et al. 2006). In contrast, frontotemporal dementias are characterized by relatively earlier onset (i.e., before age 65) than AD and predominant deficits in behavior, executive functions, or language (Bang, Spina, and Miller 2015). Finally, manifestations in VaDs vary according to type and location of the vascular lesions (O'Brien and Thomas 2015). Mean duration of survival also differs across dementia types but is highly variable according to the age of onset as well as the stage at the time of diagnosis. Durations of survival range from several months in rapidly progressive dementias such as Creutzfeldt-Jakob disease, to 8 to 12 years in AD, to 6 to 8 years in dementia with Lewy bodies and frontotemporal dementias (Todd et al. 2013).

AD itself is also heterogeneous in its presentation and clinical course. Its main clinical manifestations combine cognitive, behavioral, psychological, and functional impairments (Knopman et al. 2001). Despite this heterogeneity, a common pattern of clinical manifestations can be broadly identified over the course of the disease in most patients, as shown in Figure 3.2.

Usually, patients do not seek medical advice on their own and are referred by a relative who noticed some alarming symptoms. Most frequently, decline in memory (reflected by difficulties in remembering recent events, recent conversations, and the name of familiar persons, or repeating self) is one of the initial symptoms reported by relatives of a patient with AD. The gradual onset of these symptoms, however, makes it difficult to differentiate from normal aging,

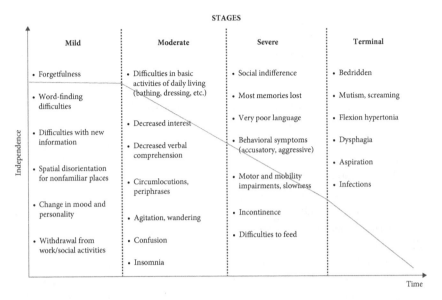

STAGES

Mild	Moderate	Severe	Terminal
• Forgetfulness	• Difficulties in basic activities of daily living (bathing, dressing, etc.)	• Social indifference	• Bedridden
• Word-finding difficulties		• Most memories lost	• Mutism, screaming
	• Decreased interest	• Very poor language	• Flexion hypertonia
• Difficulties with new information	• Decreased verbal comprehension	• Behavioral symptoms (accusatory, aggressive)	• Dysphagia
• Spatial disorientation for nonfamiliar places	• Circumlocutions, periphrases	• Motor and mobility impairments, slowness	• Aspiration
			• Infections
• Change in mood and personality	• Agitation, wandering	• Incontinence	
• Withdrawal from work/social activities	• Confusion	• Difficulties to feed	
	• Insomnia		

Figure 3.2 Schematic description of the most frequent clinical manifestations of Alzheimer's disease over its evolution.

and patients frequently minimize their difficulties. Even though patients are usually not aware of some difficulties such as repeating themselves, they frequently develop strategies such as taking notes for grocery shopping or referring to their spouse or relative to answer specific questions that challenge their memory. Progressive difficulty in word finding is another early observation commonly reported by relatives, whereas changes in mood and/or personality are early symptoms that are less frequently spontaneously reported. Although rarer, an episode of disorientation in a nonfamiliar place may also be mentioned and appears highly significant. Withdrawal from hobbies or social activities usually happens when these difficulties interfere with these activities.

As the disease progresses from mild to moderate to severe stages (Figure 3.2), additional difficulties are observed in memory (difficulties recalling names of relatives or familiar addresses or phone numbers), orientation (disorientation in familiar places, driving problems), comprehension, daily activities (e.g., misplacing things, decreased interest for hygiene, apathy, inability to dress), and behavior (social indifference, aggressivity, wandering, sleep problems). Patients are progressively unable to stay alone and are becoming fully dependent in all basic ADLs, including feeding. Behavioral problems are distressing for both the patient and his or her relatives and, with the need for full care, are major drivers in the decision to institutionalize a patient.

In the terminal stage, patients cannot walk anymore and become mute and unable to feed themselves. Eating and swallowing problems frequently result in aspiration pneumonia, one of the most frequent modes of death (Mitchell 2015).

Dementia Management: Promises and Limitations

To date, there is no curative treatment for dementia, indiscriminate of its etiology. Thus, primary goals of care are to maximize the patient's remaining functional performance and to maintain or improve his or her quality of life, as well as his or her caregivers' well-being. To achieve these goals, dementia management requires, at each evolutionary stage, combining pharmacological and nonpharmacological interventions to enhance cognition, to treat comorbid illnesses such as diabetes or hypertension, and to prevent further decline in daily function and mobility. As the disease progresses, patients' and caregivers' needs adapt and evolve. Advance care planning is a critical component of the management of dementia patients, and hospice care is still underused in advanced dementia (Mitchell et al. 2012).

Nonpharmacological Interventions
Mild to Moderate Stages

When dementia is diagnosed, the first intervention is to communicate this diagnosis to the patient and his or her relatives. When diagnosed early enough, patients can complete advanced directives and design a surrogate decision maker to anticipate when the disease will progress and the patient becomes incompetent. Arranging for legal matters (living will) and deciding about driving privileges are also important decisions that can still be made by the patient when dementia is diagnosed early enough.

The patient and family can be advised about potential sources of support such as the Alzheimer's Disease Association or other caregiver support groups. Caregivers can benefit from specific advice about appropriate level of assistance to provide to the patient as well as about communication approaches. They usually also have important information needs about the disease's prognosis, course, treatment, and overall management. Although evidence is still scarce, providing early support to caregivers appears to be a rewarding strategy to prevent their burnout and extend the duration of patients' remaining at home (Livingston et al. 2014). Indeed, community-based interventions delivered through caregivers have been shown to reduce behavioral symptoms in the patients and to improve caregivers' reactions to these behaviors (Brodaty and Arasaratnam 2012). Environmental interventions have also been shown to help in preventing or reducing disturbing wandering and agitation, but evidence is only of moderate methodological quality (Gitlin, Liebman, and Winter 2003). Similarly, evidence supporting nonpharmacological interventions directed to the patients, such as validation therapy, aromatherapy, Snoezelen, or light therapy, is still limited (Kales, Gitlin, and Lyketsos 2015). Additional support from respite care services and day hospitals are provided in most high-income countries.

Moderate to Severe Stages

Similar interventions aiming at training caregivers to enhance communication and better manage specific behavioral and psychological symptoms of dementia are proposed (Kales, Gitlin, and Lyketsos 2015). These programs typically provide caregiver education and support, and to train them in stress reduction as well as in the management of specific behavioral problems to prevent burnout and potential situations of abuse.

Several disease management interventions that combined nonpharmacological and pharmacological interventions according to guidelines have shown significant improvements in patients' outcomes and health-related quality of life and caregivers' burden and distress, resulting in prolonged home survival (Callahan et al. 2006; Mittelman et al. 2006; Vickrey et al. 2006).

Pharmacological Interventions

Mild to Moderate Stages

The first pharmacological intervention consists in reviewing all current medications and stopping those potentially deleterious to cognition such as anticholinergic drugs and hypnosedatives (Risacher et al. 2016).

Management of other diseases (hypertension, diabetes, etc.) that could be deleterious in these patients is mandatory. Among those diseases, about a third of patients with dementia develop an episode of major depression that can be effectively treated with antidepressants. Selective serotonin reuptake inhibitors are preferred because of their favorable side-effect profile (Kales, Gitlin, and Lyketsos 2015).

Unfortunately, there is currently no cure for dementias and only symptomatic treatments are available. Cholinesterase inhibitors (donepezil, galantamine, and rivastigmine) are used to treat AD, dementia with Lewy bodies, and Parkinson's disease dementia (Birks 2006; Rolinski et al. 2012). Cholinesterase inhibitors had similar efficacy and side-effect profile (mostly digestive) for mild to moderate AD. Overall, these drugs have limited, albeit clinically significant, effects on cognition and, to a lesser extent, function that correspond to a 6-month delay in cognitive symptom progression.

Huge efforts are being made to develop disease-modifying drugs that target amyloid production, deposition, or clearance (inhibitors of cleavage enzymes beta- and gamma-secretase, passive immunization), but currently all have failed clinical trials.

Moderate to Severe Stages

Memantine, a glutamatergic partial agonist, is used in moderate to severe stages of AD and has modest but significant benefits on cognition and function (McShane et al. 2006).

As dementia progresses, other pharmacological interventions are usually needed to address the behavioral and psychological symptoms of dementia. Antipsychotics, antidepressants, mood stabilizers, cholinesterase inhibitors, and memantine have all been used when nonpharmacological approaches have failed (Kales, Gitlin, and Lyketsos 2015). Among these, antipsychotics have shown the strongest evidence of efficacy, although increased mortality risk is a serious concern.

End-of-Life Care

Despite all the interventions described previously, a substantial proportion of demented patients will still need to be institutionalized in long-term care. This decision is never easy to make for involved caregivers. Caregivers' stress is a strong predictor of nursing home placement and, although institutionalization certainly relieves some strain for them, the frequent additional financial burden adds to frequent feelings of guilt, anger, or anxiety.

The quality of end-of-life care in residents suffering from dementia remains heterogeneous. Decisions regarding eating problems and treatment of infections are the most frequent that relatives face. Studies have shown that management of these frequent complications frequently results in potentially deleterious interventions, such as tube feeding or unnecessary transfers to the hospital (Mitchell et al. 2012).

Better use of advance care planning, improved counseling of relatives to antic-ipate complex end-of-life decisions, and easier access to palliative care services to better manage terminal symptoms are some examples of interventions likely to enhance the quality of end-of-life care in patients with advanced dementia.

Conclusions

Dementia is characterized by multiple cognitive deficits that result in signifi-cant impairments in social and daily functioning. Indeed, dementia is a leading cause of dependence and disability in older people. Its incidence and prevalence are closely associated with increasing age, and as life expectancy increases in the population throughout the world, the overall burden will likely further increase over the next two decades. Thus, dementia has become a global challenge in high- as well as in middle- and low-income countries worldwide.

Most types of dementia are not curable, and hearing this diagnosis is distressing for both the patient and his or her relatives. As the disease progresses, caring for affected patients can become more and more burdensome so that informal caregivers can become overwhelmed if they do not receive formal help early enough. Indeed, dementia places considerable strain on patients and their relatives, who provide a large share of the required care and support over the course of the disease. Dementia also places a heavy burden on the healthcare system because of this need for long-term care. However, despite the lack of cure, tailored pharmacological and nonpharmacological interventions can be proposed to optimize medical treatment for general medical conditions, control behavioral and psychiatric manifestations of dementia, and support caregivers. Overall, these interventions have been shown to improve the patients' quality of life and their caregivers' well-being, thus easing their burden and extending the time spent at home. However, new preventative as well as curative interventions remain dreadfully needed to address dementia's huge challenge.

References

1. Boyle PA, Wilson RS, Yu L, Barr AM, Honer WG, Schneider JA, et al. Much of late life cognitive decline is not due to common neurodegenerative pathologies. Ann Neurol. 2013;74(3):478–89.
2. Petersen RC. Clinical practice. Mild cognitive impairment. N Engl J Med. 2011;364(23):2227–234.
3. Langa KM, Levine DA. The diagnosis and management of mild cognitive impairment: a clinical review. JAMA. 2014;312(23):2551–61.
4. Association D-AP. Diagnostic and statistical manual of mental disorders. Arlington: American Psychiatric Publishing; 2013.
5. Dubois B, Feldman HH, Jacova C, Dekosky ST, Barberger-Gateau P, Cummings J, et al. Research criteria for the diagnosis of Alzheimer's disease: revising the NINCDS-ADRDA criteria. Lancet Neurol. 2007;6(8):734–46.
6. Bang J, Spina S, Miller BL. Frontotemporal dementia. Lancet. 2015;386(10004):1672–82.
7. Walker Z, Possin KL, Boeve BF, Aarsland D. Lewy body dementias. Lancet. 2015;386(10004):1683–97.
8. O'Brien JT, Thomas A. Vascular dementia. Lancet. 2015;386(10004):1698–706.
9. Ferri CP, Prince M, Brayne C, Brodaty H, Fratiglioni L, Ganguli M, et al. Global prevalence of dementia: a Delphi consensus study. Lancet. 2005;366(9503):2112–217.
10. Prince M, Bryce R, Albanese E, Wimo A, Ribeiro W, Ferri CP. The global prevalence of dementia: a systematic review and metaanalysis. Alzheimers Dement. 2013;9(1):63–75.e2.

11. Alzheimer's Disease International. Policy brief for G8 heads of government. The Global Impact of Dementia 2013–2050. Alzheimer's Disease International, London; 2013.

12. Jorm AF, Jolley D. The incidence of dementia: a meta-analysis. Neurology. 1998;51(3):728–33.

13. Gao S, Hendrie HC, Hall KS, Hui S. The relationships between age, sex, and the incidence of dementia and Alzheimer disease: a meta-analysis. Arch Gen Psychiatry. 1998;55(9):809–15.

14. Satizabal CL, Beiser AS, Chouraki V, Chene G, Dufouil C, Seshadri S. Incidence of dementia over three decades in the Framingham Heart Study. N Engl J Med. 2016;374(6):523–32.

15. Matthews FE, Arthur A, Barnes LE, Bond J, Jagger C, Robinson L, et al. A two-decade comparison of prevalence of dementia in individuals aged 65 years and older from three geographical areas of England: results of the Cognitive Function and Ageing Study I and II. Lancet. 2013;382(9902):1405–12.

16. Qiu C, von Strauss E, Backman L, Winblad B, Fratiglioni L. Twenty-year changes in dementia occurrence suggest decreasing incidence in central Stockholm, Sweden. Neurology. 2013;80(20):1888–94.

17. Matthews FE, Stephan BC, Robinson L, Jagger C, Barnes LE, Arthur A, et al. A two decade dementia incidence comparison from the Cognitive Function and Ageing Studies I and II. Nat Commun. 2016;7:11398.

18. Wimo A, Jonsson L, Bond J, Prince M, Winblad B, Alzheimer disease I. The worldwide economic impact of dementia 2010. Alzheimers Dement. 2013;9(1):1–11.e3.

19. Prince M, Prina M, Guerchet M. World Alzheimer Report 2013. Journey of caring: an analysis of long-term care for dementia. Alzheimer's Disease International, London; 2013.

20. Prince MJ, Wu F, Guo Y, Gutierrez Robledo LM, O'Donnell M, Sullivan R, et al. The burden of disease in older people and implications for health policy and practice. Lancet. 2015;385(9967):549–62.

21. Sousa RM, Ferri CP, Acosta D, Albanese E, Guerra M, Huang Y, et al. Contribution of chronic diseases to disability in elderly people in countries with low and middle incomes: a 10/66 Dementia Research Group population-based survey. Lancet. 2009;374(9704):1821–30.

22. Grasel E. When home care ends—changes in the physical health of informal caregivers caring for dementia patients: a longitudinal study. J Am Geriatr Soc. 2002;50(5):843–49.

23. Cooper C, Balamurali TB, Livingston G. A systematic review of the prevalence and covariates of anxiety in caregivers of people with dementia. Int Psychogeriatr. 2007;19(2):175–95.

24. Mahoney R, Regan C, Katona C, Livingston G. Anxiety and depression in family caregivers of people with Alzheimer disease: the LASER-AD study. Am J Geriatr Psychiatry. 2005;13(9):795–801.

25. Brodaty H, Green A, Koschera A. Meta-analysis of psychosocial interventions for caregivers of people with dementia. J Am Geriatr Soc. 2003;51(5):657–64.

26. Brodaty H, Thomson C, Thompson C, Fine M. Why caregivers of people with dementia and memory loss don't use services. Int J Geriatr Psychiatry. 2005;20(6):537–46.

27. Downs M, Bowers B. Caring for people with dementia. BMJ. 2008;336(7638):225–26.

28. Cohen CA, Colantonio A, Vernich L. Positive aspects of caregiving: rounding out the caregiver experience. Int J Geriatr Psychiatry. 2002;17(2):184–88.

29. Tiraboschi P, Salmon DP, Hansen LA, Hofstetter RC, Thal LJ, Corey-Bloom J. What best differentiates Lewy body from Alzheimer's disease in early-stage dementia? Brain. 2006;129(Pt 3):729–35.

30. Todd S, Barr S, Roberts M, Passmore AP. Survival in dementia and predictors of mortality: a review. Int J Geriatr Psychiatry. 2013;28(11):1109–24.

31. Knopman DS, DeKosky ST, Cummings JL, Chui H, Corey-Bloom J, Relkin N, et al. Practice parameter: diagnosis of dementia (an evidence-based review). Report of the Quality Standards Subcommittee of the American Academy of Neurology. Neurology. 2001;56(9):1143–53.

32. Mitchell SL. Advanced dementia. N Engl J Med. 2015;373(13):1276–77.

33. Mitchell SL, Black BS, Ersek M, Hanson LC, Miller SC, Sachs GA, et al. Advanced dementia: state of the art and priorities for the next decade. Ann Intern Med. 2012;156(1 Pt 1):45–51.

34. Livingston G, Barber J, Rapaport P, Knapp M, Griffin M, King D, et al. Long-term clinical and cost-effectiveness of psychological intervention for family carers of people with dementia: a single-blind, randomised, controlled trial. Lancet Psychiatry. 2014;1(7):539–48.

35. Brodaty H, Arasaratnam C. Meta-analysis of nonpharmacological interventions for neuropsychiatric symptoms of dementia. Am J Psychiatry. 2012;169(9):946–53.

36. Gitlin LN, Liebman J, Winter L. Are environmental interventions effective in the management of Alzheimer's disease and related disorders? A synthesis of the evidence. Alzheimer's Care Today. 2003;4(2):85–107.

37. Kales HC, Gitlin LN, Lyketsos CG. Assessment and management of behavioral and psychological symptoms of dementia. BMJ. 2015;350:h369.

38. Vickrey BG, Mittman BS, Connor KI, Pearson ML, Della Penna RD, Ganiats TG, et al. The effect of a disease management intervention on quality and outcomes of dementia care: a randomized, controlled trial. Ann Intern Med. 2006;145(10):713–26.

39. Callahan CM, Boustani MA, Unverzagt FW, Austrom MG, Damush TM, Perkins AJ, et al. Effectiveness of collaborative care for older adults with Alzheimer disease in primary care: a randomized controlled trial. JAMA. 2006;295(18):2148–57.

40. Mittelman MS, Haley WE, Clay OJ, Roth DL. Improving caregiver well-being delays nursing home placement of patients with Alzheimer disease. Neurology. 2006;67(9):1592–99.

41. Risacher SL, McDonald BC, Tallman EF, West JD, Farlow MR, Unverzagt FW, et al. Association between anticholinergic medication use and cognition, brain metabolism, and brain atrophy in cognitively normal older adults. JAMA Neurol. 2016;73(6):721–32.

42. Birks J. Cholinesterase inhibitors for Alzheimer's disease. Cochrane Database Syst Rev. 2006;(1):CD005593.

43. Rolinski M, Fox C, Maidment I, McShane R. Cholinesterase inhibitors for dementia with Lewy bodies, Parkinson's disease dementia and cognitive impairment in Parkinson's disease. Cochrane Database Syst Rev. 2012;3:CD006504.

44. McShane R, Areosa Sastre A, Minakaran N. Memantine for dementia. Cochrane Database Syst Rev. 2006;(2):CD003154.

4

Can Robots, Apps, and Other Technologies Meet the Future Global Demands of Dementia?

Arlene Astell and James Semple

The Rising Challenge of Dementia

"Dementia" is an umbrella term for an acquired syndrome that affects cognitive function and associated behavior. Dementia has many causes, the most common being Alzheimer's disease (AD), a progressive degenerative neurological disease that destroys brain cells. Age is the biggest risk factor for developing AD, and as dementia develops, cognitive capacity declines. This ultimately leads to an inability to carry out daily activities and growing dependency on other people. Currently pharmacological treatments to enhance cognition produce comparatively modest improvements, while disease modification remains a much-sought-after but still distant goal (1). Even if there were to be significant improvements in pharmacotherapy, the need for care provision will remain and indeed may increase.

At this time, fewer than half of the people in the world with dementia actually have a diagnosis, highlighting the global lack of resources (2). Most people with dementia, with and without a diagnosis, live at home, cared for by family and community resources. Caring for a family member with dementia is challenging and time-consuming and commonly has a detrimental impact on the primary caregiver's own mental and physical well-being (3). In countries that have institutional care for older adults, the transition from home frequently occurs late in the disease progression and is triggered by caregiver exhaustion and/or ill health.

The biggest impact of increasing life span will be felt in lower income and low-to-middle income (LMI) countries, where the numbers of older adults are predicted to increase by 239% and 185%, respectively, in the next 35 years, versus 56% in higher-income countries (2). Set against this massive disparity, "poorer" countries have fewer economic and human professional resources to meet the health and social care needs of their rapidly growing older populations. Many of these countries face the challenge of a " "double burden" of persistently high rates of maternal, childhood, and infectious diseases combined with a growing epidemic of chronic noncommunicable diseases." ((2), page 8).

The World Health Organization (WHO) dementia survey in 2012 (4) showed that, compared to high-income countries, awareness of dementia was lower in LMI countries, specifically highlighting that symptoms were viewed as a normal part of aging and that the causes were more likely to be perceived as having a metaphysical origin involving the supernatural and interventions from the spirit world. Studies in Nigeria (5); South Africa (6); Bangui, Central African Republic; and Brazzaville, Republic of Congo (7), all commented on the need for public education and raising awareness before any forms of screening or assessment are considered. One approach is to combine education with outreach, as employed by Nair et al. (8) in establishing a community-based memory clinic in Mumbai. Additionally, linguistically and culturally appropriate screening tests of cognitive function are needed, such as the Mandarin and Cantonese versions of the Montreal Cognitive Assessment (9). Modified or new screening and assessment tools for use in non-Western countries must also take account of differences in perceptions about dementia across countries and cultures (10).

This chapter examines research that has taken place in higher-income countries over the past 25 years into the potential of technology for meeting the needs of people living with dementia, and possible application of this work to lower-income countries. The information is structured as follows: a brief review of the areas of technology research focus, an evaluation of the potential of technology for dementia caregiving, and consideration of the practical applications for LMI countries. We do this because these nations are facing the greatest demographic and epidemiological changes with the least developed health and social care infrastructures. Moreover, their problems are compounded by additional social and economic factors. Low- and middle-income countries have witnessed massive internal migration from rural to urban communities, primarily involving younger population cohorts. This is maximally disruptive to the capacities of traditional family networks that hitherto provided the most support (11, 12). For example, in China, many rural areas are dominated by large numbers of isolated elderly individuals (13). These problems have been further exacerbated by the significant restructuring of the age pyramid by the now-abandoned one-child policy (14). However, it must be remembered that while today there are major problems in caring for those left behind in rural environments, the next generation of individuals with dementia will be dominated by those living in poorly resourced cities. Another factor has been the increasing education of women. While improving women's education is a long overdue human rights achievement, it has had the effect of diverting women from traditional caregiving roles into other more economically advantageous careers (15). Finally, many healthcare professionals trained in LMI countries migrate to high-income countries, tempted by the lure of better and more lucrative working conditions, educational advancement, and so forth for them and their families (16).

Technology for Dementia

The potential of technology to address the gap between the growing need for dementia care and the declining numbers of people to meet this need is increasingly being explored. Solutions vary from robots, fully equipped smart homes, and remote control of devices to automated systems and wearables that include GPS. In this section, we summarize the main directions of technological developments at the time of writing (February 2016) and examine their potential for improving the lives of people with dementia and those caring for them (Table 4.1). The aim is to identify what this research can offer to address the dementia care challenges that LMI countries are beginning to face.

Robotics

Robots are increasingly being promoted as solutions to the huge need for caregivers for older adults. Potential roles include robots as (a) direct caregivers, (b) household assistants, and (c) facilitators of social interaction.

Attempts to create robot replacements for human caregivers began in the 1990s (e.g., NurseBot (17)), and more recent examples include the Robear (18), which attracted a lot of media attention as a potential provider of physical care for frail, older adults. To date, robotic nurses have been deployed in some acute hospital settings, for example, in Japan as a solution to their shortage of nurses (19). However, creating a replacement human to provide care to people living with dementia, which combines physical, cognitive, emotional, social, and relationship elements, is much more complex and is still in its infancy.

More progress has been made with robotic assistance in the domestic or institutional environment. For example, Care-o-bot (20) is a service device that can be purchased to "be used for a variety of household tasks, for example to deliver food and drinks, to assist with cooking or for cleaning." However, it is unclear whether it has been utilized in care settings or to support people living with dementia. "Brian" (21), on the other hand, a prototype humanoid robot, was developed specifically to provide support to people with dementia at mealtimes in long-term care facilities. This robot was created to take the place of a human caregiver, not to physically do care but instead to prompt and support, and utilizes the Kinect motion controller to recognize emotion in the person it is interacting with to provide personalized interaction (22). The same research

Table 4.1 Potential of Main Categories of Technology Innovation for Dementia Care

Technology Type	Functionality	Intended User(s)	Impact	Global Applicability	Comment
Robot caregiver	Deliver physical care in place of a human	Institution, care services, family caregivers	Minimal	Minimal	Expensive, needs high-tech support base
Robot assistant	Support daily activity in place of a human	Institution, care services, family caregivers	Minimal	Minimal	Expensive, needs high-tech support base
Robot facilitator of social interaction	Support social participation in place of or with a human	Institution, care services, family caregivers	Minimal	Minimal	Current examples simplistic Culturally inappropriate?
Smart environment	Monitoring and support to augment human care	Institution, care services, family caregivers	Moderate to high	Moderate	Depends on complexity and cost reductions Requires stable energy supply
PCs, laptops, and tablets	Assessment and cognitive testing	Institution, care services, family caregivers	High	High	Need validated assessments in the culture of use
	Access to education and support	Institution, care services, family caregivers, people with a dementia diagnosis	High	High	Internet access widespread and growing
	Interventions	Services, people with a dementia diagnosis	Moderate to high	High	Efficacy of many interventions unproven
Wearable devices	Monitoring and assessment in and out of home	Institution, care services, family caregivers	Moderate	Moderate	Early stages of development Smart watches expensive but in the future less so
Mobile and smartphones	Reminders, navigation, contacts	Family caregivers, people with a dementia diagnosis	High	High	Mobile phones widely available

group is also working on "Casper," a robot to prompt and support older people in meal preparation that at this stage is still in development (23). One other study has demonstrated the feasibility of a robot to assist older adults with dementia in daily activities, but it was within the controlled environment of a simulated (laboratory) home setting with only five people (24). These developments highlight the future potential of robotic support but are primarily all still prototypes that have yet to be tested in the real world or at scale.

Somewhat more developed are robots for social interaction, or "telepresence" robots. These basically consist of a video conferencing system navigated and controlled by a remote operator, so-called "Skype on wheels." Currently a range of telepresence robots are available to purchase including Giraff, Anybots QB, Beampro, VGO, Double Robotics, and MantaroBot (25). Of these, Giraff has been developed and used in a number of European research projects focused on supporting older adults at home. Giraff is promoted as supporting "virtual" visits from caregivers (26) and as part of the Giraffplus system is being tested in 15 people's homes combined with a network of sensors to monitor their activities within the domestic environment.

Finally, "Tangy" is a robot being developed to promote participation in recreational activity in long-term care facilities (27). This nonhumanoid robot can act as a bingo caller, prompt players to mark their bingo cards, and check winning cards. Working with specially created digital bingo cards, Tangy can respond to four different scenarios that might occur in the game (28). However, this is yet another prototype that has so far only been tested for feasibility with a very small group of participants.

Despite the number of products available for purchase, particularly telepresence robots, evidence about the utility, acceptability, and benefit of robots for people living with dementia is lacking. This is due to the low number of research projects, especially large-scale projects, funded to date across the world specifically exploring the application of robots with people living with dementia.

Smart Environments

Another approach to addressing the growing demands for care and support for people living with dementia is smart environments. A smart home is a dwelling that has been augmented by sensors and actuators (29). Utilizing a variety of technologies including active and passive infrared, visible light, audible sound and infrasound, pressure, and temperature, they can be used to measure ambient environmental conditions including lighting and temperature and to detect smoke or gas, whether cookers have been left on, whether taps have been left running, and so forth. Sensors can also be used to detect motion, label objects and indicate their location, and monitor levels of activity in specific locations as well as actions by inhabitants such as entering and leaving rooms and opening and closing doors (front and back doors being particularly important as their use may signal leaving the premises or the entry of others). These can be supplemented by additional sensors affixed to the body or clothes of the participating individual (see also "Wearables Technologies" later). In summary, sensors can be used to detect environmental parameters, information about the occupant of the environment, and his or her interactions within it.

The data collected may be used in a number of ways, including general monitoring, issuing warnings to the occupier and to external agencies, and providing prompts to the occupier. For example, Ficocelli and Nejat (30) have described promising early trials of a prototype system to support activity in the kitchen using a voice recognition interface and automated cabinets to provide items of interest to support initiation, planning, and monitoring of kitchen tasks. Although this early work did not include people with dementia, the potential to prompt and support people living with cognitive impairment through daily tasks is clear.

It has been proposed that prompts delivered via computer systems can increase the capacity of people with dementia to maintain activities, but the supporting empirical literature is sparse, particularly beyond small feasibility or proof-of-concept studies. For example, Mihailidis et al. (31) conducted an efficacy study of the COACH system to prompt six older adults with dementia through handwashing using artificial intelligence. Another group "demonstrated proof of feasibility" of the concept of automated prompting to support people with dementia through dressing using a combination of audio and visual cues presented on a tablet built into a chest of drawers, context-aware/skeletal movement (using Kinect), and tags on clothing (32).

In principle, smart home–based systems offer the potential to record activities over a period of time, making it possible to collect sufficient data to model "normal" patterns of activity, thereby enabling the identification of anomalous behaviors and, ideally, prediction of their future occurrence (33). This could facilitate rapid responses to incidents and potentially prevent their occurrence. This is a very attractive line of research, but at this time extending it to take account of situations where more than one person is present (e.g., a carer, other family members or pets living with the person with dementia, or visitors) is still proving challenging. Such research is being carried out in a number of laboratories (e.g., Coradeschi et al. (26); Palumbo et al. (34)), but space limitations preclude a detailed examination of specific studies (see (35) for a relatively recent review).

Wearable Technologies

"Wearable technologies" encompasses a variety of platforms characterized by being attached to the body of the person using them on a temporary or more or less permanent basis. A looser definition would include attaching the technologies to clothing worn by individuals or in accessories carried by them such as key rings and mobile phones (see "Mobile Phones" later). Due to space constraints, we limit consideration to the example of wearables used to monitor people with dementia outside the home, rather than a broader consideration of general health-monitoring wearables applicable to the wider population.

The potential of wearables for people living with dementia was recognized in the 1990s with the first, and possibly most controversial, application of electronic tags. This ignited a polarized debate that rages on, with advocates arguing that people living with dementia can experience greater freedom, less use of locked doors, and reduced need for medication as a result of tagging (36). However, this is weighed against the perceived stigmatization of tagging, the ability of people with dementia to consent to being tagged (37), how often tagging is used to address caregiver concerns, and the ways in which the benefits of tagging to people with dementia are evaluated (38).

More recently GPS-enabled mobile devices have offered the potential to move from actual tags that are not removable by the individual with dementia to remote tracking of their location and movement. This is proposed as enabling vulnerable individuals to continue with their daily activities with the security that someone else is monitoring them. For example, Carr and McCullagh, (39) described the application of "geo-fencing," whereby certain areas of the environment are designated as "safe" and others as more dangerous, and leaving the safe area can trigger an alarm. Other proposed applications include the measuring of "life space," the geographical area a person covers in a day, to monitor progression of dementia (40), but more research is required to clarify this potential and how these data could be used.

Personal Computers, Laptops, and Tablets

Utilization of personal computers falls largely into three areas: (a) assessment, (b) education, and (c) interventions. Assessment is a key element in the care of people with dementia to identify cases, assist diagnosis, evaluate need, monitor disease progression, and measure the effectiveness of interventions. Early case identification will be vital if and when disease-modifying agents become available, and it allows for the advance planning of care packages.

There is a long history of using computer-based assessments, a process facilitated by the increased portability of laptops and tablets and the introduction of touchscreens (41). Computer-based tests offer a number of potential advantages over more traditional approaches, including standardized presentation of stimuli, response logging, and data processing and collating in a database, and may be more sensitive than existing measures (42). Moreover, response times can be recorded more accurately, offering the possibility of new outcome measures. Computer-based assessments may reduce the level of training required, thus potentially increasing capacity for diagnostic assessments, especially in countries with few trained diagnosticians. These data could be processed and interpreted at a central hub and returned with recommendations for treatments and interventions.

Regarding computerized education, (43) reported that an Internet-delivered training package significantly improved dementia care knowledge among nursing assistants and enhanced their self-perceptions of competency. Another study demonstrated that providing an observational scale on a handheld device increased care assistants' confidence and the quality of the data they passed on to nursing staff (44). However, working relationships worsened as the care assistants felt their increased contributions were not appreciated by the nurses. This highlights the need for a systematic approach to the rollout of technology at the organizational level to ensure all aspects of the impact are addressed.

Caregiving makes taxing demands on families, and people may turn to currently available technologies including voice and video communications for education and advice and to address feelings of isolation and abandonment. A recent review of Internet-based supportive interventions for informal caregivers concluded that while the limited number of studies to date reported largely positive outcomes, they were methodologically weak, with very few large-scale randomized controlled trials (45).

For people living with a dementia diagnosis, computer-delivered interventions may be classified into two broad and overlapping strategic categories. The first is an "internal" strategy aimed at boosting the existing cognitive resources of the person with dementia, and the second is "external," involving prostheses to circumvent lost functionality. The internal approach is exemplified by "brain training" interventions aimed at improving memory, attention, and so forth. Brain training straddles two clinical questions: "Can it enhance the cognitive processing power of people who have identified dementia?" and "Can training retard disease progression from preclinical to clinical states?"

Recent evidence has found some benefits of computerized cognitive training for "healthy" older adults (46), people who have been diagnosed with mild cognitive impairment (MCI) (47,48), and those already living with dementia (49). While training produces modest benefits in the trained tasks, there is no evidence regarding the durability of effects, generalizability to nontrained tasks, or altered risk of future morbidity. Regarding people already living with dementia, the number of studies since 1990 of technology-delivered interventions is very small ($n = 16$), with researchers tending to target people with MCI instead (49). In the few studies with people living with dementia, the computer-based training has focused on purely cognitive functions (e.g., memory or attention) (50), functional activities of daily life (e.g., shopping) (51), or a combination of both (52). From this small evidence base, a picture is emerging of promising interventions for supporting people with dementia to complete tasks, which has important implications for improving performance in daily life activities, but this is tempered by the understanding that task-specific training may not and indeed should not be expected to generalize to overall improvements of global cognitive status. Nor is there any evidence yet that undertaking such training slows disease progression.

Regarding external strategies, the notion of "cognitive prosthetics" has been proposed to utilize the functionality of computers to mitigate the loss of specific cognitive abilities experienced by people with dementia (53). This loss is progressive and variable across cognitive functions, with some being affected earlier in the disease process, providing the opportunity to leverage those that are relatively unaffected. For example, CIRCA (Computer Interaction Reminiscence and Conversation Aid) (54) has been shown to effectively mitigate the working memory problem common in people with AD that interferes with holding a conversation, to enable them to successfully interact with caregivers. Given the current cheapness and widespread availability of computing capacity, particularly through mobile devices, this line of research could easily be scaled up to develop direct support for people who receive a dementia diagnosis.

Mobile Phones

The revolution in communications technology brought about by the advent of mobile cellular phones is nothing less than remarkable. So-called smartphones, with increasing memory and processing capacity, blur the lines between phones and personal computers. Thus, it is little surprise that mobile phones have been used for many of the same purposes as personal computers (PCs), laptops, and computer tablets (55).

O'Connor et al. (56) compared the effectiveness of delivering a "dementia risk reduction" program via the Internet and as a phone app. Participants preferred the web-based programs, but it is not clear whether this was due to differences in content, familiarity with use of apps, or even physical limitations such as screen size of the phone. The potential of phones for assessment is also being explored (57)—for example, comparison of a battery of three commercially available computerized cognitive screening instruments implemented on a tablet and a smartphone, which were shown to have similar sensitivity and specificity to the Montreal Cognitive Assessment (58).

Mobile phones have also been used as tracking devices (e.g., (59)) with the exploration of the potential of GPS-based systems to enhance the autonomy of individuals. Frequently used routes to local amenities can be programmed into the device to provide continuous directions and warnings of deviations from the route (e.g., (60)). An example of what is possible using existing functionality is the commercially available app BlindSquare (MIPsoft) (61), developed for visually impaired people. This not only facilitates route following but also can provide warning information regarding upcoming hazards such as roads to cross. This system, or something similar, could be an empowering technology for people living with dementia.

Potential of Technological Developments

We now evaluate the potential of the developments discussed previously for improving the lives of people with dementia and their caregivers in high-income (HI) countries, where they have been developed, with specific consideration of the ethical issues raised. Table 4.1 summarizes the major areas of technological research, the intended end-users of the technology, impact thus far, and likely global applicability. It is important to note that at the present time the potential of technology is significantly underexplored, due to low funding and lack of prioritization by funders of dementia research across the world.

Technology in High-Income Countries

Coughlin (62) suggested that robots could potentially reduce the skyrocketing costs of long-term care (approximately $219.9 billion in the United States in 2012) and the $522 billion per annum of informal, unpaid caregiving provided by family or friends of the care recipient. In response, there is also a growing backlash against technology, with concerns voiced about the possibility of robots taking jobs away from humans (63). However, projections from current functionality suggest that any reduction in the workforce will be minimal and potentially outweighed by the numbers of engineers required to support a robot workforce—a redistribution of work rather than a reduction, something noted previously in healthcare innovations (64).

Current instantioations of humanoid robots to replace human caregivers seem far from being available at any scale or functional capacity to have an impact on the needs of people living with dementia in the near future. Robots operate best when required to perform repetitive, well-defined tasks in controlled and constant environments. Every act of a caregiver will be unique in many aspects and performed in a highly complex domestic environment. Additionally, safety issues and longer-term problems such as integrating progress made on specific challenges across different delivery platforms, the envirnonmental challenges for robot outside institutions, the level of technical support they need to operate, their cultural acceptability and their costs with regard to capital expenditure and recurring maintenance, and the availability of backups if they malfunction currently make robots an impractical solution in HI countries let alone middle- and low-income countries.

The development of smart homes has not been specifically motivated to provide for the care needs of vulnerable individuals. To date, smart environment research groups have pursued their own preferred approaches to problems and specific underlying technology platforms for arriving at these. Moreover, studies have involved relatively few participants, particularly with dementia, and of course the technology has been supported by the expertise residing in the research groups. While this is a necessary first step, if solutions are to be implemented more widely, they have to be tested and demonstrated in more "realistic" settings and involve much larger numbers of participants. Preferably field testing will be carried out by individuals who were not members of the original research groups and whose familiarity and expertise regarding the system realistically match that which could be expected when the systems are rolled out to potential users. Additionally, potential end-users of smart home technology need to be involved in the process from the start. Researchers are expert in understanding available technologies, their limitations, and how to circumvent these; their expertise is focused around what can be done. People with dementia are experts in the experience of being part of a specific population, while carers have first-hand experience of the challenges of trying to respond to these needs, plus experience of what works.

While the Internet is awash with personal recommendations from individual carers for a variety of electronic devices and aids, there is no empirical evidence to support adoption of these. Additionally, there is little evidence about what caregivers actually want from such aids, how available products match these needs, and how they are actually used in real life, beyond some pilot data (65). As such, there is a huge scope to engage with people with dementia, their families, and communities across the world to develop and share accessible resources to support people living with dementia in their own homes.

There is also an urgent need for empirically based research to support the use of computer-based training for people living with dementia. Brain training has emerged as a billion-dollar industry (66) that positions itself as offering more than recreational activities. However, there is a lack of evidence to (a) confirm that training actually enhances performance in clinical populations, (b) identify optimal training tasks and regimens, and (c) show that the training produces clinically meaningful benefits in terms of everyday functioning and/or alteration of disease progression. This deficiency has recently been highlighted by the payment of $2 million by Lumos Labs, the producer of an extremely widely used package of "brain training" games, to the Federal Trade Commission to settle a pending prosecution for making "false and/or unsubstantiated claims" in its advertising regarding the beneficial effects of using its products.

Ethical Issues Relating to Technology

A progress review in 2011 (19) suggested the need for a robot that can make complicated decisions and deal with a variety of situations, illustrated with the example of a human refusing to take medication. This scenario was generated to highlight the challenges for robotic nurses in acute care within the controlled hospital setting. For people living with dementia, the complexity of their cognitive challenges and their needs in everyday life, both in and out of the house, all present highly complex technical and ethical challenges for robotic caregivers to be able to replace humans.

Felzmann et al. (67) idetentified the following specific ethical issues regarding robotic care: identified the following ethical issues relating to the potential introduction of robots in dementia care: (a) privacy, with regard to data captured by the robot and also the individual's personal privacy in relation to the robot carrying out monitoring functions; (b) safety of the device during interactions with the human care recipient and in relation to the monitoring functions; and (c) replacing human care, with respect to the subjective experience of older people living with dementia and wider implications in society (67). These authors also highlighted the current "neglect of user perspectives regarding the development and use of those robots" ((67), page 1). This latter point can be addressed by engaging people with a dementia diagnosis as partners in all stages of the technology development process (68), a critical step to avoid excessively disablingpeople by taking away their autonomy and personhood through the inappropriate introduction of technology (69).

The smart environment paradigm also raises important ethical and security issues, some of which are shared by other technological applications (70). Monitoring of the position and activity of the occupier of a house on a potential real-time, 24-hour basis could be considered intrusive. The level of scrutiny occupiers will be under needs to be explained and consented to, to avoid gross violation of their privacy. For cultural reasons occupiers may consider that there are circumstances, times of the day, and so forth when they feel less comfortable about being monitored in detail. The level of monitoring should not exceed the requirements of the care program unless its purpose is to develop that program, and then only with the consent of the occupier.

Occupiers also need to be aware and consent to the fact that such detailed data about their lives may be open to individuals whom they have never met in a remote monitoring station. Data about patterns of daily activity should be treated with the same level of respect and confidentiality that we accord to medical records. It should be accessible only on a need-to-know basis and be subject to the same rules of nondisclosure. Moreover, if data are collected, stored, and/ or transferred to remote monitoring centers, it should be subject to best practice with respect to encryption and data protection, as with other medical information. Knowledge about patterns of behavior could be exploited by individuals with malevolent intent and must therefore be protected. If these issues can be adequately addressed, the reducing costs of sensor technology and energy requirements, together with cheap microcomputers, suggest that smart homes may have application for people living with dementia beyond high-income countries.

In reality, current instantiations are actually far from being available at any scale or functional capacity to have an impact on caregiving needs in the near future. Creating robots that can carry out everyday tasks is proving to be a difficult problem. For example, BRETT can now fold towels in a minute thanks to a neural network, but that took 7 years to perfect. Selecting and manipulating clothes is even more challenging, and it is difficult to see a robot being physically able to help a person dress in the near future. The limits of progress are highlighted by the fact that research on such fundamental issues as soft-touch lifting remains ongoing in the lab (71).

Finally, regarding wearable technologies, the move to tracking using mobile devices, as opposed to affixing tags, does not obviate ethical considerations with respect to whether and to what extent tracking violates the rights of the individual to privacy, who has access to the information and under what circumstances, how the data can be made secure and not accessible to individuals with malintent, its potential for covert unapproved monitoring, and who decides whether this technology should be employed (72, 73, 74, 75).

Is "Dementia" Technology Globally Applicable?

The 10/66 phenomenon (76) refers to the fact that only 10% of the research is being carried out in countries where 66% of individuals affected by dementia live. As such, there is a dearth of field studies in countries where the need is greatest, meaning that our current picture of the problems they face is at best a low-resolution one, particularly as diagnostic procedures and knowledge about dementia may be less advanced.

Based on what has been achieved to date, robots as a like-for-like replacement for human caregivers appear to be an unlikely solution for the growing numbers of people living with dementia across the world. At this time, there are many unanswered questions, ranging from whether robots need to be humanoid or not, how people feel about having them roaming their homes, and how acceptable people would find physical care delivered by a robot. To date, successful implementation of robots in healthcare has been in specific and highly focused activities, such as urological surgery, although even here opinion is strongly divided about the cost-effectiveness of this innovation (77, 78). However, this experience suggests that the potential of robotics in the care of people living with dementia must also be necessarily selective and focused on very specific activities. In this respect robots can do what they are good at, repetitive mechanical tasks, freeing up human caregivers to do what they are best at -social interaction and personal relationships.

Smart environments also have the potential for benefitting people living with dementia, but again currently available systems, including computational and artificial intelligence (AI) components and backup support, are very expensive and underinvestigated. Research to date has focused on the most sophisticated systems that are realizable by today's technology. There has been little effort to identify the minimum requirements for a system that could make a difference to the quality of life of people with dementia and their families. This brings us back to the need to involve people with dementia and their carers as key participants in the design loop (79). It is also vital that researchers explore how to achieve their goals with the minimum of resources. For example, researchers at the Eindhoven University of Technology have been able to manufacture tiny sensors that are powered by and report back by Wi-Fi for as little as 20 cents per unit (80), which could revolutionize capacity. Microcomputers such as Raspberry Pi could be used to collate data, execute local responses, or pass information to remote data centers. These processors and the necessary routers could be powered by the local main supply and backed up by rechargeable batteries or capacitors where this is unreliable, or even be powered by solar power or some other source of renewable energy to be usable in LMI countries.

Technologies that have the most immediate potential and applicability in LMI countries are wearables, PCs, and mobile devices, subject to ethical issues being addressed. In LMI countries smartwatches have great potential as their perception as desirable objects should lead to mass production and reduce production costs. This will help promote global penetration in a similar manner to mobile cellular phones; however, at this time there is a lack of research into exactly how smartwatches could be used to help people living with dementia.

There is some evidence that computer technologies can be used with people with dementia, but again, much still needs to be done to establish what can be achieved, with whom it can be achieved, and how best to achieve it. The use of personal computers and related technologies is most prevalent in developed countries, where 79 out of 100 people have a personal computer, compared with 28.3 in LMI countries (81). Nevertheless, these figures are not insubstantial and suggest that PCs in all their forms may be a viable route of transfer of expertise, which, with suitable adaptation to local need and culture, may improve the lives of people living with dementia and their families.

Meanwhile, there are nearly 7 billion subscriptions to mobile phones worldwide (82), with some 54% of all mobile phones sold described as smartphones and the greatest growth in sales of these expected to come from the developing world, where Internet access is primarily mediated via mobile devices (83). It seems obvious that of all the available technology platforms that could be used to support people with dementia and their carers, the mobile phone is by far the cheapest and the most accessible globally. However, there is a lack of empirical studies about how useful currently available apps actually are both in delivering what they claim and their acceptability to people with dementia and caregivers. A recent case study, coauthored by a gentleman living with dementia, highlighted how a smartphone supported him to undertake independent travel and retain social connectivity using Skype and email (84). However, to exploit this functionality, further work is needed to develop training materials for people with dementia and their families as well as services that might provide mobile devices and/or apps to enable them to make the most of these developments.

Moreover, in the continuously evolving world of mobile phone technology, nothing stands still for long and the "life span" of many devices and accompanying apps is ephemeral. This poses a problem for research which, because of the logistics of study design, participant recruitment, data analysis, and peer review, operates on a somewhat different timescale to commercial cycles. However, we suggest that to address this it is sufficient to select a few examples from the current state of the art and show their utility to establish proof of principle. LMI countries have demonstrated huge innovation in developing mobile apps to solve a broad spectrum of local problems—for example, the Mobile Alliance for Maternal Action (85), a mobile app to improve maternal health in South Africa, which includes daily tips and access to an interactive website (MAMA Mobi) (86). In addition, the potential barriers, opportunities, and research directions of mobile health in LMI countries are already being identified (87).

Conclusions

Across the world, the biggest limitation of technology for dementia is the lack of evidence. Although explorations started in the 1990s, the majority of projects to date have been small-scale pilot or feasibility studies, with many single case studies. This is a great pity as technology has huge potential to address the needs of growing numbers of people living with dementia across the world: first, through exploitation of expertise developed in HI countries to rapidly advance developments in LMI countries; second, through the cheapness and availability of mobile technology; and third, through the largely untapped functionality of existing smart devices as "cognitive prostheses" to mitigate the cognitive problems of people living with dementia.

The real heart of technology development for LMI countries should be exploitation of technologies that can make a difference such as expert systems and mobile apps building from a local, bottom-up process, not a top-down, imported one. Building on home-grown initiatives could also help to address the huge need for public education and raising awareness about dementia in most LMI countries by encouraging local development of apps and training materials.

As indicated earlier, the second area to focus on is mHealth, which has the biggest potential for LMI countries due to cheapness and accessibility. This platform could be used for supporting assessment, monitoring progression, and delivering interventions, advice, and education.

In addition, the potential for mobile technology to act as cognitive prostheses for people living with dementia is currently underdeveloped. This is the third area ripe for development and deployment at scale as existing and future functionality could be used to support individuals with a dementia diagnosis. Today, the majority of smartphone users in the world rely on their devices to store phone numbers and appointments, that is, to save their own cognitive function. However, this aspect of technology deployment in dementia has been underserved in HI countries where the bulk of technology developments have focused on caregivers, either supplementing or replacing them. Much less attention has been paid to how technology could enhance or maintain the functioning of individuals with a dementia diagnosis. Yet, supporting people in looking after themselves and maintaining their independence for as long as possible by adopting smart devices from the point of diagnosis should delay or reduce demand on families and services for direct caregiving.

In the absence of medication, these developments highlight the huge potential for a brand-new way of thinking about dementia as a condition that can be aided with carefully and sensitively designed technology that can supplement and respond to changes in their cognitive function. This would provide a global solution to dementia, revolutionizing the way the world approaches this rapidly growing, costly, and stressful condition, and could see LMI countries taking the lead ahead of the slow but steady advances in HI countries.

References

1. Burke M. Why Alzheimer's drugs keep failing. Sci Am [Internet]. July3rd, 2014 [cited 2016 Feb 9]. Available from: http://www.scientificamerican.com/article/why-alzheimer-s-drugs-keep-failing/

2. Prince M, Wimo A, Guerchet M, Gemma-Claire A, Wu Y-T, Prina M. World Alzheimer Report 2015: The Global Impact of Dementia—An analysis of prevalence, incidence, cost and trends. Alzheimer's Dis Int. 2015;84.

3. Jerrom B, Mian I, Rukanyake NG, Prothero D. Stress on relative caregivers of dementia sufferers, and predictors of the breakdown of community care. Int J Geriatr Psychiatry [Internet]. 1993;8(4):331–37. Available from: http://onlinelibrary.wiley.com/doi/10.1002/gps.930080409/abstract\nhttp://onlinelibrary.wiley.com/doi/10.1002/gps.930080409/abstract?systemMessage=Wiley+Online+Library+will+be+disrupted+on+15+December+from+10:00-12:00+GMT+(05:00-07:00+EST)+for

4. World Health Organization. Dementia: a public health priority. Dementia [Internet]. 2012;112. Available from: http://whqlibdoc.who.int/publications/2012/9789241564458_eng.pdf

5. Yusuf AJ, Baiyewu O. Beliefs and attitudes towards dementia among community leaders in northern Nigeria. West Afr J Med [Internet]. 2012;31(1):8–13. Available from: http://ovidsp.ovid.com/ovidweb.cgi?T=JS&PAGE=reference&D=medl&NEWS=N&AN=23115089

6. Khonje V, Milligan C, Yako Y, Mabelane M, Borochowitz KE, Jager CA De. Knowledge, attitudes and beliefs about dementia in an urban Xhosa-speaking community in South Africa. Adv Alzheimer's Dis. 2015;4:21–36.

7. Faure A, Guerchet M, Mbelesso P, Mouanga AM, Dalmay F, Dubreuil C-M, et al. Dementia and cognitive impairment: beliefs and attitudes towards elderly in Central Africa (edac survey). Alzheimer's Dement [Internet]. 2010 Jul [cited 2016 Aug 1];6(4):S95–96. Available from: http://linkinghub.elsevier.com/retrieve/pii/S1552526010004206

8. Nair G, Van Dyk K, Shah U, Purohit DP, Pinto C, Shah AB, et al. Characterizing cognitive deficits and dementia in an aging urban population in India. International Journal of Alzheimer's Disease, vol. 2012, Article ID 673849, 8 pages, 2012.

9. Zheng L, Teng EL, Varma R, MacK WJ, Mungas D, Lu PH, et al. Chinese-language Montreal cognitive assessment for Cantonese or Mandarin speakers: age, education, and gender effects. International Journal of Alzheimer's Disease, vol. 2012, Article ID 204623, 10 pages, 2012.

10. Faure-Delage A, Mouanga AM, M'Belesso P, Tabo A, Bandzouzi B, Dubreuil C-M, et al. Socio-cultural perceptions and representations of dementia in Brazzaville, Republic of Congo: the EDAC survey. Dement Geriatr Cogn Dis Extra [Internet]. 2012 [cited 2016 Aug 1];2(1):84–96. Available from: http://www.karger.com/doi/10.1159/000335626

11. He C, Ye J. Lonely sunsets: impacts of rural-urban migration on the left-behind elderly in rural china. Popul Space Place. 2014;20(4):352–69.

12. Nabalamba A, Chikoko AfDB M. Aging population challenges in Africa. Chief Econ Complex African Dev Bank. 2011. https://www.afdb.org/fileadmin/uploads/afdb/Documents/Publications/Aging%20Population%20Challenges%20in%20Africa-distribution.pdf. Accessed 3rd August 2016.

13. Ao X, Jiang D, Zhao Z. The impact of rural–urban migration on the health of the left-behind parents. China Econ Rev. 2016;37:126–39.

14. Powell TM. The negative impact of the one child policy on the Chinese society as it relates to the parental support of the aging population. A thesis submitted to Georgetown University for a Master of Arts. 2012. https://repository.library.georgetown.edu/bitstream/handle/10822/557704/Powell_georgetown_0076M_11971.pdf?sequence=1&isAllowed=y. accessed 1st August 2016.

15. Prince M, Prina M, Guerchet M. World Alzheimer Report 2013 Journey of Caring: an analysis of long-term care for dementia. Alzheimer's Dis Int. 2013;1–92.

16. Health at a Glance. Statistics/Health at a Glance/2015: OECD Indicators. http://apps.who.int/medicinedocs/documents/s22177en/s22177en.pdf. Accessed 31st July 2016.

17. Roy N, Baltus G, Fox D, Gemperle F, Goetz J, Hirsch T, et al. Towards personal service robots for the elderly. Work Interact Robot Entertain (WIRE 2000). 2000;25(2000):184.

18. Moon M. Robear is a robot bear that can care for the elderly. Engaget [Internet]. 2015 [cited 2016 Feb 13]. Available from: https://www.engadget.com/2015/02/26/robear-japan-caregiver/

19. Charova K, Schaeffer C, Garron L. Robotic nurses | computers and robots: decision-makers in an automated world [Internet]. 2011 [cited 2016 Jul 25]. Available from: https://cs.stanford.edu/people/eroberts/cs201/projects/2010-11/ComputersMakingDecisions/robotic-nurses/index.html

20. Schraft RD, Schaeffer C, May T. Care-O-bot™: the concept of a system for assisting elderly or disabled persons in home environments. IECON '98 Proc 24th Annu Conf IEEE Ind Electron Soc (Cat No98CH36200). 1998;4.

21. Derek M, Chan J, Nejat G. A socially assistive robot for meal-time cognitive interventions. J Med Device [Internet]. 2012 Mar 12 [cited 2016 Aug 1];6(1):17559. Available from: http://medicaldevices.asmedigitalcollection.asme.org/article.aspx?doi=10.1115/1.4026737

22. McColl D, Nejat G. A socially assistive robot that can monitor affect of the elderly during mealtime assistance. J Med Device [Internet]. 2014 Jul 21 [cited 2016 Aug 1];8(3):30941. Available from: http://medicaldevices.asmedigitalcollection.asme.org/article.aspx?doi=10.1115/1.4027109

23. Bovbel P, Nejat G. Casper: an assistive kitchen robot to promote aging in place. J Med Device [Internet]. 2014 Jul 21 [cited 2016 Aug 1];8(3):30945. Available from: http://medicaldevices.asmedigitalcollection.asme.org/article.aspx?doi=10.1115/1.4027113

24. Begum M, Wang R, Huq R, Mihailidis A. Performance of daily activities by older adults with dementia: the role of an assistive robot. In: IEEE International Conference on Rehabilitation Robotics; 2013.

25. Kristoffersson A, Coradeschi S, Loutfi A. A review of mobile robotic telepresence. Vol. 2013, Advances in Human-Computer Interaction. 2013.

26. Coradeschi S, Cesta A, Cortellessa G, Coraci L, Gonzalez J, Karlsson L, et al. GiraffPlus: Combining social interaction and long term monitoring for promoting independent living. In: 2013 6th International Conference on Human System Interactions (HSI 2013). 2013, pp. 578–85.

27. Louie W-Y, Han R, Nejat G. Did anyone say BINGO: a socially assistive robot to promote stimulating recreational activities at long-term care facilities. J Med Device [Internet]. 2013 Jul 3 [cited 2016 Aug 1];7(3):30944. Available from: http://medicaldevices.asmedigitalcollection.asme.org/article.aspx?doi=10.1115/1.4024511

28. Louie W-Y, Li J, Mohamed C, Despond F, Lee V, Nejat G. Tangy the Robot bingo facilitator: a performance review. J Med Device [Internet]. 2015 Mar 1 [cited 2016 Aug 1];9(2):20936. Available from: http://medicaldevices.asmedigitalcollection.asme.org/article.aspx?doi=10.1115/1.4030145

29. Rashidi P, Mihailidis A. A survey on ambient-assisted living tools for older adults. IEEE J Biomed Heal Informatics. 2013;17(3):579–90.

30. Ficocelli M, Nejat G. Cognitive and physical assistance for the elderly in kitchen environments. J Med Device [Internet]. 2012 Mar 12 [cited 2016 Aug 1];6(1):17561. Available from: http://medicaldevices.asmedigitalcollection.asme.org/article.aspx?doi=10.1115/1.4026739

31. Mihailidis A, Boger JN, Craig T, Hoey J. The COACH prompting system to assist older adults with dementia through handwashing: an efficacy study. BMC Geriatr [Internet]. 2008;8(1):28. Available from: http://www.biomedcentral.com/1471-2318/8/28

32. Mahoney DF, Burleson W, Lozano C, Ravishankar V, Mahoney EL. Prototype Development of a Responsive Emotive Sensing System (DRESS) to aid older persons with dementia to dress independently. Gerontechnology [Internet]. 2014 Dec 19 [cited 2016 Aug 1];13(3):345–58. Available from: http://gerontechnology.info/index.php/journal/article/view/2267

33. Lotfi A, Langensiepen C, Mahmoud SM, Akhlaghinia MJ. Smart homes for the elderly dementia sufferers: identification and prediction of abnormal behaviour. J Ambient Intell Humaniz Comput. 2012;3(3):205–18.

34. Palumbo F, Ullberg J, Stimec A, Furfari F, Karlsson L, Coradeschi S. Sensor network infrastructure for a home care monitoring system. Sensors (Basel) [Internet]. 2014;14(3):3833–60. Available from: http://www.scopus.com/inward/record.url?eid=2-s2.0-84927170280&partnerID=tZOtx3y1

35. Miller K, Ozanne E, Hansen R, Pearce AJ, Santamaria N, et al. Smart-home technologies to assist older people to live well at home. J Aging Sci [Internet]. 2013 [cited 2016 Aug 1];1(1). Available from: http://www.esciencecentral.org/journals/smart-home-technologies-to-assist-older-people-to-live-well-at-home-2329-8847.1000101.php?aid=12044

36. Bail KD. Electronic tagging of people with dementia. Devices may be preferable to locked doors. Br Med J. 2003;326(7383):281.

37. Hughes JC, Louw SJ. Electronic tagging of people with dementia who wander. BMJ. 2002;325:847–48.

38. Astell AJ. Technology and personhood in dementia care. Qual Ageing [Internet]. 2006;7(1):15. Available from: http://proquest.umi.com/pqdweb?did=1019254741&Fmt=7&clientId=16331&RQT=309&VName=PQD

39. Carr N, McCullagh P. GeoFencing on a mobile platform with alert escalation. Ambient Assist Living Dly Act [Internet]. 2014 [cited 2016 Aug 1];1–4. Available from: http://link.springer.com/10.1007/978-3-319-13105-4_38

40. Tung JY, Rose RV, Gammada E, Lam I, Roy EA, Black SE, et al. Measuring life space in older adults with mild-to-moderate Alzheimer's disease using mobile phone GPS. Gerontology. 2014;60(2):154–62.

41. Joddrell P, Astell AJ. The use of touchscreen technology with people living with dementia : A review of the literature. JMIR Rehabilitation and Assistive Technologies (JRAT). 2016;3(6):e10.
42. Wright DW, Nevárez H, Kilgo P, LaPlaca M, Robinson A, Fowler S, et al. A novel technology to screen for cognitive impairment in the elderly. Am J Alzheimers Dis Other Demen [Internet]. 2011;26(6):484–91. Available from: http://www.ncbi.nlm.nih.gov/pubmed/22110158
43. Hobday JV, Savik K, Smith S, Gaugler JE. Feasibility of Internet training for care staff of residents with dementia: The CARES program. J Gerontol Nurs. 2010;36(4):13–21.
44. Corazzini K, Rapp CG, McConnell ES, Anderson RA. Use of a handheld computer observational tool to improve communication for care planning and psychosocial well-being. J Nurses Staff Dev. 2009;25(1):E1–7.
45. Boots LMM, de Vugt ME, van Knippenberg RJM, Kempen GIJM, Verhey FRJ. A systematic review of Internet-based supportive interventions for caregivers of patients with dementia. Int J Geriatr Psychiatry [Internet]. 2014 Apr [cited 2016 Aug 2];29(4):331–44. Available from: http://doi.wiley.com/10.1002/gps.4016
46. Lampit A, Hallock H, Valenzuela M. Computerized cognitive training in cognitively healthy older adults: a systematic review and meta-analysis of effect modifiers. PLoS Med. 2014;11(11):e1001756. https://doi.org/10.1371/journal.pmed.1001756
47. Coyle H, Traynor V, Solowij N. Computerized and virtual reality cognitive training for individuals at high risk of cognitive decline: systematic review of the literature. Am J Geriatr Psychiatry [Internet]. 2014;23(4):335–59. Available from: http://www.ncbi.nlm.nih.gov/pubmed/24998488
48. Gates NJ, Sachdev PS, Fiatarone Singh MA, Valenzuela M. Cognitive and memory training in adults at risk of dementia: a systematic review. BMC Geriatr [Internet]. 2011;11:55. Available from: http://www.pubmedcentral.nih.gov/articlerender.fcgi?artid=3191477&tool=pmcentrez&rendertype=abstract
49. Mahendra N, Lange B, Harinath L, Jimison H, Astell A. Review of technology-based cognitive interventions for adults with mild cognitive impairment and dementia. in Prep. 2016;Contact Author.
50. Cipriani G, Bianchetti A, Trabucchi M. Outcomes of a computer-based cognitive rehabilitation program on Alzheimer's disease patients compared with those on patients affected by mild cognitive impairment. Arch Gerontol Geriatr. 2006;43(3):327–35.
51. Hofmann M, Hock C, Kühler A, Müller-Spahn F. Interactive computer-based cognitive training in patients with Alzheimer's disease. J Psychiatr Res. 1996;30(6):493–501.
52. Requena C, Maestú F, Campo P, Fernández A, Ortiz T. Effects of cholinergic drugs and cognitive training on dementia: 2-year follow-up. Dement Geriatr Cogn Disord. 2006;22(4):339–45.
52. Astell AJ, Alm N, Gowans G, Ellis MP, Dye R, Campbell J. CIRCA: a communication prosthesis for dementia. In: Mihailidas A, Normie L, Kautz H, Boger J, editors. Technology and Aging [Internet]. IOS Press; 2012, pp. 67–76. Available from: http://ebooks.iospress.nl/volumearticle/793
54. Astell AJ, Ellis MP, Bernardi L, Alm N, Dye R, Gowans G, et al. Using a touch screen computer to support relationships between people with dementia and caregivers. Interact Comput. 2010;22(4):267–75.
55. Ericsson Consumer Lab. Europe Ericsson Mobility Report Appendix. Ericsson Mobil Rep [Internet]. 2015;(June):1–8. Available from: http://www.ericsson.com/mobility-report

56. O'Connor E, Farrow M, Hatherly C. Randomized comparison of mobile and web-tools to provide dementia risk reduction education: use, engagement and participant satisfaction. JMIR Ment Heal. 2014;1(1):e4.
57. Brouillette RM, Foil H, Fontenot S, Correro A, Allen R, Martin CK, et al. Feasibility, reliability, and validity of a smartphone based application for the assessment of cognitive function in the elderly. PLoS One. 2013;8(6):e65925.
58. Scanlon L, O'Shea E, O'Caoimh R, Timmons S. Usability and validity of a battery of computerised cognitive screening tests for detecting cognitive impairment. Gerontology [Internet]. 2015 Jun 24 [cited 2016 Aug 2];62(2):247–52. Available from: http://www.karger.com/?doi=10.1159/000433432
59. Miskelly F. Electronic tracking of patients with dementia and wandering using mobile phone technology. Age Ageing. 2005;34:497–99.
60. Palmer M, Hancock J. Jurojin: Designing a GPS Device for People Living with Dementia. Springer International Publishing; 2015 [cited 2016 Aug 2], pp. 660–68. Available from: http://link.springer.com/10.1007/978-3-319-20684-4_63
61. MIPSoft. BlindSquare [Internet]. Available from: http://blindsquare.com/. Accessed 2016 Feb 9.
62. Coughlin, Joseph F. (2015). When robots begin to care [Internet]. Huffington Post. 2015 [cited 2016 Feb 9]. Available from: http://www.huffingtonpost.com/Joseph-f-coughing/when-robots-begin-to-care_b_6826022.html
63. Sherman E. 5 Jobs that robots already are taking [Internet]. Fortune. 2015 [cited 2016 Feb 9]. Available from: http://fortune.com/2015/02/25/5-jobs-that-robots-already-are-taking/
64. Oudshoorn N. Diagnosis at a distance: the invisible work of patients and healthcare professionals in cardiac telemonitoring technology. Sociol Heal Illn. 2008;30(2):272–88.
65. Boger J, Quraishi M, Turcotte N, Dunal L. The identification of assistive technologies being used to support the daily occupations of community-dwelling older adults with dementia: a cross-sectional pilot study. Disabil Rehabil Assist Technol [Internet]. 2014;9(1):17–30. Available from: http://www.ncbi.nlm.nih.gov/pubmed/23607569\nhttp://search.ebscohost.com/login.aspx?direct=true&db=c8h&AN=2012406479&site=ehost-live
66. Burch D. What could computerized brain training learn from evidence-based medicine? PLoS Med. 2014;11(11): e1001758.
67. Felzmann H, Murphy K, Casey D, Beyan O. Robot-assisted care for elderly with dementia: is there a potential for genuine end-user empowerment? Ind Robot An Int J [Internet]. 2013;40(5):433–40. Available from: http://www.emeraldinsight.com/doi/abs/10.1108/IR-12-2012-451
68. Astell A, Alm N, Gowans G, Ellis M, Dye R, Vaughan P. Involving older people with dementia and their carers in designing computer based support systems: Some methodological considerations. Univers Access Inf Soc. 2009;8(1):49–58.
69. Astell AJ. Supporting a Good Life with Dementia. In: Prendergast D, Garattini C, editors. Aging and the Digital Life Course. Berghahn Books; 2015, pp. 691–99.
70. Mahoney DF, Purtilo RB, Webbe FM, Alwan M, Bharucha AJ, Adlam TD, et al. In-home monitoring of persons with dementia: ethical guidelines for technology research and development. Alzheimer's Dement. 2007;3(3):217–26.
71. Robear. https://www.theverge.com/2015/4/28/8507049/robear-robot-bear-japan-elderly

72. Cragg H. GPS systems for people with dementia: the human rights issues. 2015 [cited 2016 Feb 9]. Available from: http://www.nash.co.uk/wp-content/uploads/2015/02/GPS-Systems-for-people-with-Dementia.pdf

73. Landau R, Auslander GK, Werner S, Shoval N, Heinik J. Who should make the decision on the use of GPS for people with dementia? Aging and Mental Health. 2011;15910:78–84.

74. Landau R, Werner S. Ethical aspects of using GPS for tracking people with dementia: recommendations for practice. Int Psychogeriatrics. 2012;24(3):358–66.

75. White EB, Montgomery P. Electronic tracking for people with dementia: an exploratory study of the ethical issues experienced by carers in making decisions about usage. Dementia [Internet]. 2014 Mar 1 [cited 2016 Aug 1];13(2):216–32. Available from: http://www.ncbi.nlm.nih.gov/pubmed/24599815

76. 10/66 Dementia Research Group. Alzheimer's Disease International [Internet]. [cited 2016 Feb 12]. Available from: http://www.alz.co.uk/10/66-group

77. Liberman D, Trinh Q-D, Jeldres C, Zorn KC. Is robotic surgery cost-effective: yes. Curr Opin Urol [Internet]. 2012;22(1):61–65. Available from: http://www.ncbi.nlm.nih.gov/pubmed/22037320

78. Seideman CA, Sleeper JP, Lotan Y. Cost comparison of robot-assisted and laparoscopic pyeloplasty. J Endourol [Internet]. 2012;26(8):1044–48. Available from: http://www.ncbi.nlm.nih.gov/pubmed/22494052

79. Martin S, Augusto J, McCullagh P, Carswell W, Zheng H, Wang H, et al. Participatory research to design a novel telehealth system to support the night-time needs of people with dementia: NOCTURNAL. Int J Environ Res Public Health [Internet]. 2013 Dec 4 [cited 2016 Aug 2];10(12):6764–82. Available from: http://www.mdpi.com/1660-4601/10/12/6764/

80. Gao H. Fully integrated ultra-low power mm-wave wireless sensor design methods [Internet]. Technische Universiteit Eindhoven; 2015 [cited 2016 Aug 2]. Available from: http://repository.tue.nl/800521

81. Islamic Development Bank. Key socio-economic statistics on IDB member countries 2015 [Internet]. Jeddah; 2015 [cited 2016 Aug 2]. Available from: http://www.isdb.org/irj/go/km/docs/documents/IDBDevelopments/Internet/English/IDB/CM/Publications/Statistical Monograph No. 35 Final.pdf

82. mobiThinking. Global mobile statistics 2014 part A: mobile subscribers; handset market share; mobile operators [Internet]. mobiForge. 2014 [cited 2016 Feb 9]. Available from: https://mobiforge.com/research-analysis/global-mobile-statistics-2014-part-a-mobile-subscribers-handset-market-share-mobile-operators

83. mobiThinking. Global mobile statistics 2014 part B: mobile web; mobile broadband penetration; 3G/4G subscribers and networks; mobile search [Internet]. mobiForge. 2014 [cited 2016 Feb 9]. Available from: https://mobiforge.com/research-analysis/global-mobile-statistics-2014-part-b-mobile-web-mobile-broadband-penetration-3g4g-subscribers-and-ne

84. Astell AJ, Malone B, Williams G, Hwang F, Ellis MP. Leveraging everyday technology for people living with dementia: a case study. J Assist Technol. 2014;8(4):164–76.

85. MAMA. MAMA—Mobile Alliance for Maternal Action—learn more [Internet]. [cited 2016 Feb 12]. Available from: http://askmama.co.za/learn_more.html

86. MAMA. MAMA—Mobile Alliance for Maternal Action—Mobi [Internet]. [cited 2016 Feb 12]. Available from: http://askmama.co.za/mobi.html

87. Aranda-Jan CB, Mohutsiwa-Dibe N, Loukanova S. Systematic review on what works, what does not work and why of implementation of mobile health (mHealth) projects in Africa. BMC Public Health [Internet]. 2014;14(1):188. Available from: http://www. pubmedcentral.nih.gov/articlerender.fcgi?artid=3942265&tool=pmcentrez&render type=abstract\nhttp://www.biomedcentral.com/1471-2458/14/188

5

Augmented Reality–Assisted Dementia Care

Mengyu Y. Zhao, S. K. Ong, and Andrew Y. C. Nee

Introduction

Nowadays, the number of people suffering from dementia is rising continuously. Hence there is an increasing demand for treatments and assistive devices to help people with dementia. However, current treatments only assist in decelerating the progress of the disease, instead of stopping or reversing it. New approaches need to be considered to prevent and diagnose dementia and relieve its symptoms. Augmented reality (AR) is a technology that evolves from virtual reality (VR). VR allows individuals to become "immersed" in a virtual environment that is built using computer-generated 3D objects as well as audio and haptic information (1). AR enables human-computer interaction via superimposing virtual elements on the real world instead of the virtual environment (2). These virtual elements, including visual, audio, and tactile information, are used to add supplementary information, enhance real objects, and provide aids for the execution of a task (3). In comparison with VR, AR is closer to the real environment, which allows AR to provide a more realistic interaction. Azuma (4) defined three characteristics of AR systems: combining real and virtual elements together in one application, allowing human-machine interaction in real time, and registering in 3D.

During the last 10 years, considerable progress in AR has been achieved. This technology has been utilized in numerous applications in education, military, manufacturing, and the medical field. On the other hand, it has been documented that environmental interventions are important in improving the quality of life of people suffering from cognitive impairments, including dementia (5). It is essential to create an ideal environment that neither underuses the patients' existing abilities nor puts too much pressure on them. As AR supports a highly controllable environment and real-time feedback (6), it is able to achieve a balance between individual capabilities and the demands of the environment. However, only few AR-based approaches for dementia have been reported.

This chapter discusses the application of AR in dementia care. The second section introduces the state of the art of AR-based assistive and rehabilitation applications for dementia care. A generic system structure for AR-assisted dementia care applications, as well as techniques and devices used in this structure, is provided in the third section. To provide more details about using AR in dementia care, an AR-assisted healthcare exercising system that aims to enhance the user's motor skills, cognition, and planning capability is presented in the fourth section. Finally, the last section summarizes the advantages and future directions of using AR in the field of dementia.

AR-Assisted Applications for Dementia

This section provides a succinct overview of AR-based assistive and rehabilitation applications for dementia. As dementia has various symptoms, these applications are categorized according to the focused symptom(s), including memory decline, spatial impairment, and so forth. Although some applications are designed for specific cognitive impairments other than dementia, they can also be utilized to help dementia patients. Table 5.1 summarizes most of the existing AR-assisted applications for dementia care.

AR-Based Assistive Systems

The objective of assistive applications is to enhance the user's capability for independent living. As the major symptom of dementia is memory loss (7), many AR-based assistive applications have been developed to aid patients to cope with frequent memory-related issues, such as recalling their relatives, friends, and daily tasks (Table 5.1). The Development Augmented Reality for Dementia (DARD) system (8) helps a dementia patient remember his or her family members and friends. While using this system, pictures and details about relatives and friends are rendered on the screen when the camera detects an AR marker. A case study demonstrated that in comparison with audio stimulation, the information provided by AR is more helpful in retaining memory. Thus far, this system only provides a simple scenario where only visual information is augmented on a registered AR marker. Al-Khafaji et al. (9) proposed a system that is similar to DARD for helping people with Alzheimer's disease (AD) remember relatives and happy moments. Instead of using AR markers, this system compares color pictures with images in a database and generates visual and audio information about these pictures. As compared with conventional healthcare interventions, AR systems can assist the user to retrieve memory without help from caregivers.

Table 5.1 AR-Based Assistive and Rehabilitation Applications for Dementia Care

Application	User Group	Objective	Characteristics	Limitations
DARD (Sahar, MatNasir, and Zainudin 2014)	Dementia patients	Help dementia patients remember their relatives	Visual information augmented	Simple scenario
Al-Khafaji et al. (Al-Khafaji et al. 2013)	People with AD	Help dementia patients remember their relatives and moments	Use color pictures as markers Augment visual and audio information	No assessment of the user's performance
Ambient aNnotation System (Quintana and Favela 2013)	Persons suffering from memory loss and their caregivers	Notify the user of everyday objects and daily tasks	Consists of two modules: one allows the caregiver to create tags and another one alerts the user of the presence of tags Portable	Can only be used in a prepared environment
Hervás et al. (Hervas, Bravo, and Fontecha 2014)	Cognitively impaired people	Supply spatial orientation	Plan a route based on familiar places Portable Allow caregivers to supervise the activities of the user	Only visual information is provided
Zhang et al. (Zhang, Ong, and Nee 2009)	Visually impaired persons	Provide orientation information to approach user-defined destinations	Map-less User-centric orientation information	Prepared environment
Wearable navigation system (Zhang et al. 2012)	Visually impaired persons	Provide orientation information	Guided by Google Maps API Provides audio and tactile feedbacks	Bulky device
TARDIS (Wood and McCrindle 2012)	People with memory loss	Assist users to perform daily activities	Guides a user to complete a task through audio hints and visual information	More scenarios are desired

(continued)

Table 5.1 Continued

Application	User Group	Objective	Characteristics	Limitations
dGames-VI memory game (Kirner, Cerqueira, and Kirner 2012)	Cognitively disabled people	Exercise cognitive skills, such as association and memory	Developed using blended tactile and audition sense	Therapist intervention is necessary
GenVirtual (Correa et al. 2007)	People with learning disability	Stimulate memory and concentration	Uses music to enhance memory	Therapist intervention is necessary
ARVe (Richard et al. 2007)	Cognitively impaired children	Aid the children in decision making	Mixed-scene is rendered on a large screen through a video projector Provides visual, olfactory, and auditory cues	Relatively complex setup
ARCoach (Chang, Kang, and Huang 2013)	People with cognitive impairments	Enhance job skills	Reduces the trainer's workloads Provides audio and visual information	No assessment of the user's performance
Artifact-AR (Kirner and Kirner 2011)	Cognitively disabled people	Enhance cognitive functions	Overlaps visual information on a three-plane model	Dependent on webcam quality
Frutos-Pascual et al. (Frutos-Pascual, García-Zapirain, and Méndez-Zorrilla 2012)	People with cognitive problems	Improve cognitive capacities	Trains users by tangram pieces	The VR goggle is uncomfortable to wear
Eldergames (Gamberini et al. 2009)	Elderly people	Preserve cognitive function	Remote communication Enables the user to play with other players	Relatively costly device
AR cube system (Boletsis and Mccallum 2014)	People in the initial stages of mild dementia	Prevent cognitive impairment	Portable Trains the user's capability of logical reasoning	Affected by the occlusion problem

However, systems with moderate involvement of caregivers can enhance the users' experience using these systems. The Ambient Annotation System (ANS) (10) assists persons with AD to notify tags or notes placed by their caregivers. This indoor application involves two subsystems. The first one allows a caregiver to create tags about daily tasks on certain objects. The second subsystem recognizes these objects and uses AR to augment visual, audio, and tactile feedbacks to alert the users of these tags. ANS is installed on a mobile phone, so that the tag recognition is automatic and in real time.

Navigation systems are another common type of assistive approaches for AD patients. Hervás et al. (11) proposed a mobile AR-based navigation system that generates user-friendly routes to a destination according to points of interest or well-known places. This system is developed for cognitively impaired users who often suffer from disorientation and relies on familiar places to find the way to a destination. AR is applied in this system to render important information entities (e.g., the user's home and the closest point of interest) on the road scene that is captured using an Android device. Currently, this system is the only navigation system that is developed specifically for cognitively impaired persons. Although some approaches are not designed for dementia, they are suitable for individuals who become disoriented, including dementia patients. Zhang et al. (12) proposed an AR-based map-less navigation system for visually impaired people (Figure 5.1). In this system, infrared emission markers are attached on specific locations to help detect the user's orientation and provide user-centric orientation information for approaching a destination. However, this system is only suitable in a

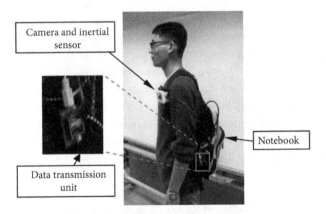

Figure 5.1 Navigation assistance system.

From Zhang J, Ong S, Nee AYC. Design and development of a navigation assistance system for visually impaired individuals. In: Proceedings of the 3rd International Convention on Rehabilitation Engineering & Assistive Technology (i-CREATe); 2009 Apr 22–26; Singapore.

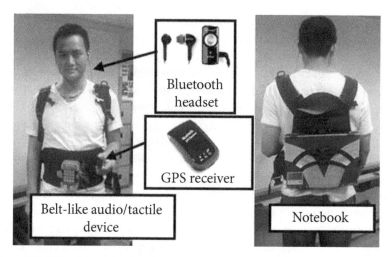

Figure 5.2 Wearable navigation system.
From Zhang J, Zhao MY, Ong SK, Nee AYC. A wearable navigation system for visually impaired users. In: Proceedings of the 6th International Convention on Rehabilitation Engineering & Assistive Technology (i-CREATe); 2012 Jul 24–26; Singapore.

prepared environment. To overcome this limitation, the research group has developed a wearable navigation system based on the information produced by the Google Maps API (Figure 5.2) (13). When a user wearing this system walks outdoor, Google Maps API as well as audio and tactile feedbacks are used to guide the user with respect to the heading direction adjustment and distance notification. However, the devices applied in this system are cumbersome and the accurate tracking needed requires high computational cost.

People who suffer from dementia may encounter difficulty with planning and organizing, which would affect their capability of undertaking everyday tasks. The Augmented Reality Discovery and Information System (TARDIS) (14) is an AR-based system that assists users with memory loss to perform daily activities, such as making a hot drink. TARDIS splits each task into several stages and guides a user through completing the task via augmented visual information and audio hints. Thus far, this system consists of only one exercise. More exercises are required to evaluate its applicability.

AR-Based Rehabilitation Systems

Rehabilitation systems concentrate on recovering the lost mental functions through training, such as repetitive training. It has been identified that multiple feedbacks are conducive to draw a user's attention even during a repetitive training (23). AR can stimulate users through multimodal feedbacks. AR-based rehabilitation systems are able to generate multiple feedbacks to assist the user when focusing on the training.

Enhancing memory ability is one of the major targets of cognitive rehabilitation (24). Kirner et al. (15) introduced the dGames-VI memory game to enhance associative memory based on an AR-assisted memory card game. This game is built on an artifact with holes. A user interacts with these holes to find two holes that have the same sound and image. This system facilitates short-term memory training using an entertaining game scenario. GenVirtual (16) is an AR music game that has been proposed to stimulate memory and concentration through interaction with virtual objects in association with musical notes. Virtual cubes with different colors are rendered on AR markers, and each cube represents one musical note. The user is required to remember the melody played by the system and interact with the correct cubes. This system can be used at home easily.

Educational AR systems have been reported to help users regain the capability of making decisions. Richard et al. (17) reported an AR application called AR to vegetal field (ARVe) that allows cognitively impaired children to handle plant entities. It involves a matching task, where plant entities are rendered on fiducial markers and visual, olfactory, or auditory cues are provided to aid the children in decision making. Experimental results showed that disabled children were enthusiastic when using ARVe (17). As this project requires several devices, it is relatively complex to set up. Therefore, it is not suitable for home use.

In addition, it has been documented that individuals with dementia tend to be excluded from labor markets (25). To improve this situation, researchers have used AR to enhance the job skills of people with cognitive impairments. ARCoach (18) is designed for vocational tasks through prompting users with cognitive impairments. Using this system, users can learn how to prepare a meal following prompts such as combinations of sound and images. This system frees the trainer from constantly being with the user as useful information is provided by AR. Therefore, in comparison with conventional interventions that are supervised by the trainers, AR-based approaches are low cost and efficient.

Some applications consider more than one feature for better rehabilitation effect. Artifact-AR (19) aims to enhance cognitive functions, including identification, memorization, and comparison. Physical artifact videos are overlapped with a 3D model in Artifact-AR. For training purposes, two exercises are implemented in this system. The first one allows the user to compare and associate pictures and sounds by selecting virtual images or sound clips. In the second exercise, the user is able to replicate patterns that are drawn on a reference image. Similarly, Frutos-Pascual et al. (20) proposed a mixed reality–based tangram game to contribute to the improvement of cognitive therapies. Traditional tangram pieces that are marked with AR markers are used for movement tracking.

The user places tangram pieces according to a reference provided by the system. This system has been tested on real users, and the results showed that AR elements enhance the entertainment effect of the training and help users to focus on the training (20).

Previous studies indicated that AR can provide cognitive stimuli to users to help reduce the risk of cognitive decline (22). Therefore, AR elements can be utilized to prevent cognitive impairments so as to decrease the risk of dementia. One of these applications is Eldergames (21), which uses a mixed reality–based solution to preserve cognitive functions in elderly people. In this system, AR markers are installed on pens to realize interaction with a table and remote communication with other players. This system involves a Memo game that improves the player's short-period memory, and five Minigames to train cognitive functions, including memory, reasoning, and selective attention. Due to the high costs of the touchable table applied in this system, it is not suitable for home use. Another application, the AR cube system (22), is designed for players at the initial stages of mild dementia to contrast cognitive impairment. Two games are implemented in this system, namely, a word game and a speed/shape-matching game. The word game seeks to recover logical reasoning by requiring the user to form words. The speed/shape-matching game trains response inhibition and information processing by matching shapes of different colors. However, when the user's hand obstructs the tracking of markers, the 3D model rendered on the screen disappears.

Generic System Structure for AR-Assisted Dementia Care Applications

Based on the overview of current AR systems, a generic architecture of AR-assisted dementia care applications can be extracted. This section discusses details of this structure, which is illustrated in Figure 5.3. Figure 5.3 also presents the devices and algorithms or toolkits for each module.

The monitoring module encompasses devices and software for tracking and interaction. Cameras are the most widely used tracking devices in AR-based applications due to their low cost. They are applied in vision-based tracking methods (e.g., marker-based tracking that determines the positions of the camera and poses of the camera with respect to an AR marker). For example, DARD (8) detects a given marker using a web camera. Some interaction methods that aim at collecting user data are also included in this module. Interactions in most AR-based dementia care systems are realized by moving or covering AR markers. Some AR applications offer more intuitive interfaces, such as data gloves. Image processing and signal processing are used to analyze the collected data.

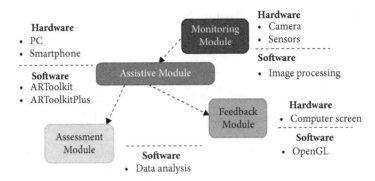

Figure 5.3 Structure for AR-assisted dementia care applications.

The assistive module is the core module. For rehabilitation systems, this module contains the exercises/games that have been designed to improve cognitive functions; for assistive applications, this module involves functions that process input data and provide corresponding assistance. The conventional device that performs the processing in this module is the personal computer (PC). PCs offer large storage space and high stability but have low portability. The adoption rate of smartphones for use in dementia care appears to be increasing as they expand the scope of activity (26). The assistive navigation system (11) provides outdoor spatial guidance using a smartphone. The assistive module is developed by using well-known AR software platforms, for example, ARToolKit (27) and ARToolKitPlus (28).

In the feedback module, visual, auditory, and other types of feedbacks are provided to facilitate users. The feedbacks of the majority of AR applications are provided in visual form, such as 3D models and text. This information is usually rendered on the screen by using OpenGL (GenVirtual (16)). Several systems provide voice prompts to reduce fatigue or provide auxiliary guidance (dGames-VI (15)). Tactile feeling can be provided using vibratory motor sensors (the wearable navigation system (13)) or physical objects. The incorporation of tactile feedback stimulates the users so as to avoid boredom and augments the immersive feeling.

To enhance the user's motivation, the assessment module in rehabilitation systems evaluates a user's performance with respect to his or her physical conditions and recovering progress. Data used for evaluation are extracted through sensors and analyzed to compute performance indicators. As rehabilitation systems aim to enhance a user's cognitive functions using serious exercises, one of the most popular indicators is the success rate. The ARCoach system (18) evaluates a user's improvement using the success rate as this indicator can be quantified easily. However, thus far, only limited applications in AR-based dementia care assess and evaluate a user's performance.

Although the structure in Figure 5.3 is commonly used among dementia applications, some of these applications may contain only two or three modules in this structure. For example, TARDIS (14) has no assessment module.

AR-Assisted Exercising System for the Enhancement of the Capability of Planning ADLs

This section illustrates how to build a dementia care system using AR. Assistive systems for activities of daily living (ADLs) (14) have been developed to assist users who have memory loss with everyday tasks using AR. However, no rehabilitation system has been established to enhance the user's capability of planning ADLs. Conventional assistive systems for ADLs continue to provide guidance when a user performs ADLs, which may add to the user's reliance on the system and further deteriorate his or her cognitive functions by underusing his or her existing abilities. As rehabilitation systems are proposed to increase the capability of planning ADLs, the number of prompts should be deliberated.

This section presents an AR-assisted system to illustrate the application of AR in dementia care. The objective of this system is to enhance a user's planning capability in ADLs. The proposed system, as shown in Figure 5.4, consists of two training phases: the virtual-object training phase and the real-object training phase. The virtual-object training phase encourages a user using visual stimulations and guides him or her to complete the tasks step by step. The real-object training phase provides visual and audio prompts only when the user

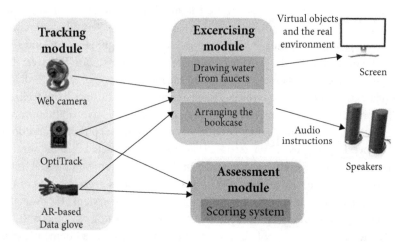

Figure 5.4 System architecture.

forgets the next step so as to allow the user to transfer skills learned from the virtual environment to reality.

The proposed system is composed of three modules: a tracking module, an exercising module (i.e., the assistive module introduced in the Generic System Structure for AR-Assisted Dementia Care Applications Section), and an assessment module. The feedback module introduced in the Generic System Structure for AR-Assisted Dementia Care Applications Section is part of the exercising module of this system. In the tracking module, the user is tracked by the OptiTrack system.[1] A web camera is used to obtain visual information, and physiological data are collected using an AR-based data glove. The AR-based data glove combines three types of sensors, namely, flex sensors, force sensors, and accelerometers, to simultaneously measure the bending degrees of the fingers, grip forces, and accelerations of the arm. Data acquired from the tracking module are applied in the exercising module for interaction. The exercising module involves two exercises that simulate two ADLs, namely, drawing water and arranging a bookcase. The exercise context, including virtual and real environment, is rendered on a computer screen. Audio instructions are generated and played using the speakers. The assessment module contains a scoring system that evaluates the user's performance. This system is developed using C++ and the ARToolKitPlus. 3D objects created from SolidWorks and video frames captured by the web camera are rendered using OpenCV and OpenGL. Details of this system are introduced in the following sections.

Drawing Water from Faucets

This exercise is designed based on a previous work that developed an AR-based rehabilitation system to train the upper extremity of stroke patients (29). In the virtual-object training phase, the task is separated into several steps, thereby ensuring a methodical way of carrying out the task. In the real-object training phase, the system would only let the user know the target of the task. The system would provide audio hints when necessary.

In the virtual-object training phase, the user sits behind a desk and wears the AR-based data glove on one arm. Reflective balls are attached on the data glove for positioning. Three OptiTrack cameras are positioned in front of the user to define the tracking volume. The computer screen is placed on the desk and the web camera is located above the screen, facing the user. This phase is composed of two tasks (Figure 5.5), and each task is split into two steps: (a) place a cup under the faucet and (b) draw water from the tap by grasping the faucet and rotating it. After completing the first task, the user only needs to wave his or her hand to signal to proceed onto the next task. When the exercise begins, the 3D

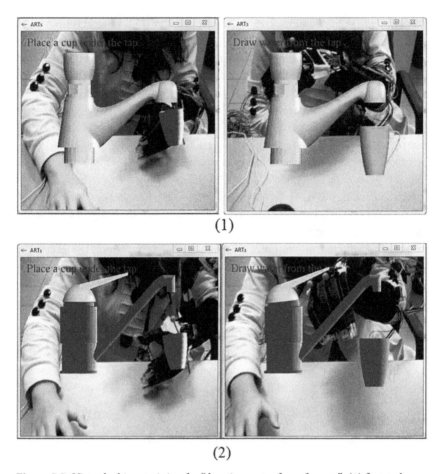

Figure 5.5 Virtual-object training for "drawing water from faucets": (1) first task; (2) second task.

coordinates of the user's hand are converted to the 2D coordinates in the screen coordinate system. Collisions between virtual faucets and the user's hand are determined based on their coordinates. Finger-bending angles are applied in this system to detect whether the user has grasped the faucet. Visual feedback, such as the water flow and the movement of the cup, is rendered on the screen.

A wooden board installed with two faucets is used in the real-object training phase (Figure 5.6). Reflective balls are glued near these two faucets to identify their locations. Figure 5.7 illustrates the flowchart of this training phase. A timer that will be triggered after 10 seconds is used in this phase. Audio instructions will be played only when the timer is triggered, as illustrated in the left part of Figure 5.7. Force sensors detect whether the user has picked up the cup. When the

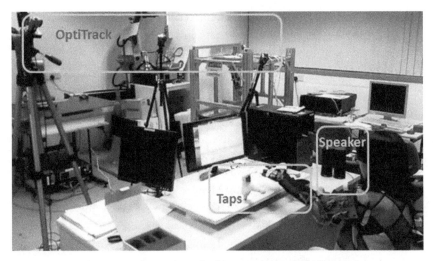

Figure 5.6 Real-object training phase for "drawing water from faucets."

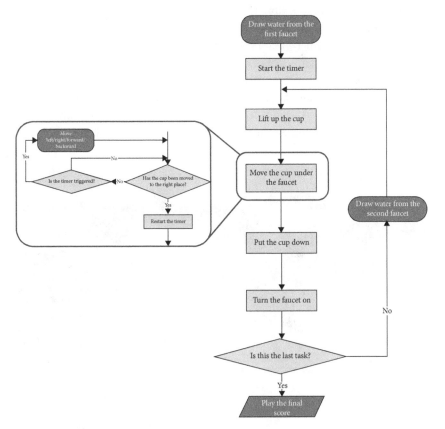

Figure 5.7 The flowchart of the real-object training phase.

user lifts the cup, the cup's position is monitored using OptiTrack. Data detected from the force sensors and OptiTrack are combined to determine whether the user has put the cup down and turned on the faucet.

Arranging the Bookcase

This exercise is able to improve the user's body coordination, planning capability, and language understanding. The implementation and mechanism of the virtual-object training phase are similar to that introduced in the Drawing water from faucets Section (Figure 5.8). This phase involves two tasks. The first one is manipulating a virtual book, in which the user would need to turn the virtual book 180 degrees counterclockwise. In the second task, the user "grasps" a book that lies on the desktop and places it on the bookcase. The system would assist the user to perform this task step by step.

A real bookcase with real books is used in the real-object training phase (Figure 5.9). This phase is able to improve the user's body coordination as it requires the user to walk around and place books with both hands. Three tasks are involved here, namely, put a dictionary on the top shelf, reposition an inverted folder, and arrange three books according to their serial numbers. The system would only announce the target of the task when the task begins. The positions of the hand and books, which are detected using OptiTrack, and the data, which are measured using force sensors, are used to determine whether the user has grasped the book. Audio hints would be played only when the timer is triggered.

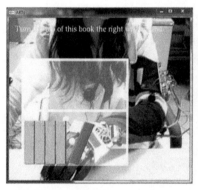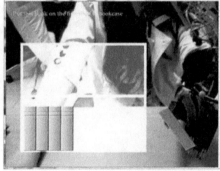

Figure 5.8 Virtual-object training phase for the exercise "arranging the bookcase."

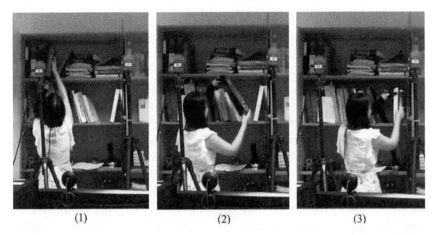

Figure 5.9 Real-object training phase for the exercise "arranging the bookcase": (1) put a dictionary on the top shelf; (2) reposition an inverted folder; (3) arrange three books according to their serial numbers.

Scoring System

The two exercises simulating the ADLs use the same scoring system. This scoring system involves two indicators, namely, task completion time (TCT) and the success rate. The TCT refers to the time spent on completing one task, and the score for TCT in each training phase is calculated using Equation (1). The success rate is determined by the number of mistakes made by the user. For example, the system will determine that it is a mistake if the user tries to turn on the faucet without placing the cup under it. Equation (2) calculates the score for the success rate in each training phase. In these two equations, thresholds represent the minimum scores indicating healthy movements, the full score represents the maximum score for the specific task, n represents the number of tasks in each training phase, s represents the number of steps, and m is the number of mistakes in each task. Thresholds are determined based on data measured from 10 healthy participants (four females and six males) whose ages range from 32 to 20.

$$\text{Score of TCT} = \sum_{i=1}^{n} \text{Full Score} \times \left(\text{Threshold} / \text{Data recorded}\right) \qquad (1)$$

$$\text{Score of success rate} = \left((s - m) / s\right) \times \text{Full Score} \qquad (2)$$

User Study

A user study was performed to evaluate the advantages of the proposed system on enhancing a user's capability of planning ADLs. Ten elderly adults with different degrees of memory loss were enrolled in this test. Their occupations range from teachers to cleaners, and their nationalities include Chinese, Malaysian, and Singaporean. Participants were four males and six females with ages ranging between 52 and 70. This experiment consisted of a pretest session, a training session, and a posttest session, as shown in Table 5.2. The pretest session involves two items. The first item is recording the time and procedure of completing the real-object training phase of drawing water from faucets. The second one is a pretest survey, which provides insights on the memory and capability of the elderly adults on planning ADLs. In the training sessions, subjects were trained by the virtual-object training phases of drawing water from faucets and the exercise "arranging the bookcase." Each phase was repeated twice. In the posttest session, the participants performed the real-object training phase of drawing water from the faucets again and filled in a questionnaire about the usability of the proposed system. Questionnaires for the pre- and posttests are presented in the appendix.

Based on the results of the pretest survey, participants were classified into four groups, which are illustrated in Figure 5.10. The numbers of participants in each group are four, two, two, and two, respectively. To normalize the results of the posttest questionnaire, the total number of participants in each group is set to be one. According to Figure 5.10, almost all participants agreed that this system is able to teach them the procedures of ADLs. Answers from question 5 reveal that this type of exercise can enhance the capability of remembering the procedures

Table 5.2 User Study Schedule

Session	Content	Repeat times
Pretest	The real-object training phase of drawing water from faucets	
	Pretest questionnaire	
Training session	The virtual-object training phase of arranging the bookcase	2
	The real-object training phase of arranging the bookcase	2
	The real-object training phase of drawing water from faucets	2
Posttest	The real-object training phase of drawing water from faucets	
	Posttest questionnaire	

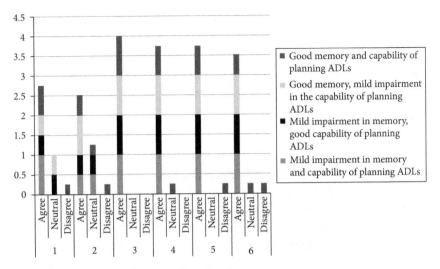

Figure 5.10 Normalized statistical results of posttest.

of ADLs. However, results from question 1 show that participants who have normal capability of planning ADLs are not easily attracted by these exercises. Moreover, results from question 6 justify that users with impaired memory or planning capability in ADLs prefer to use this system. In addition, several participants indicated that audio prompts can provide clearer instruction than visual hints rendered on the screen. They suggested adding audio instructions in the virtual-object training phase.

In the posttest, times spent on completing the real-object training phase of drawing water decreased from 12.78% to 31.07% from the pretest. Besides, some participants inquired about the next step during the pretest, which did not occur in the posttest. Meanwhile, in the training session, the scores of the first and the second trials of each phase were recorded. The improvements of these scores and relative standard deviations are presented in Table 5.3. All these results reveal that the proposed system can enhance the participants' capability of planning ADLs.

In conclusion, the proposed system is able to teach the users procedures of ADLs and enhance their capabilities of planning ADLs. The target users of this system should be the elderly who have impaired capability of planning ADLs.

Discussion

Applying AR to dementia care has many advantages due to core features of AR technology (e.g., highly controllable environment, intuitive interface, and

Table 5.3 Improvement of Scores of the First and the Second Trial of Each Exercise

Training phase	Improvement (%)
The virtual-object training phase of arranging the bookcase	8.09 ± 6.51
The real-object training phase of arranging the bookcase	5.04 ± 2.61
The real-object training phase of drawing water from faucets	3.86 ± 5.76

real-time feedback). First, the environment created using AR is highly control-lable. To improve the quality of life in dementia, the training environment should not be overchallenging or underusing the patient's existing abilities. Considering the continuous changes of the patient's condition, the environment should be adjustable and reconfigurable. However, modifying the real environment according to the patient's requirement is costly, sometimes even impossible. Due to the characteristic of AR technology, an enriched customized system can be constructed with a relatively low cost and less modeling time (30).

The second advantage is lessening the workload of caregivers and reinforcing the patient's independence. As there is a worldwide shortage of healthcare workers, taking care of dementia patients either is costly or affects the caregiver's normal life. AR-based dementia care systems are able to provide assistance in ADLs and monitor the user's status continuously. Therefore, incorporating AR into dementia care can improve the patient's personal autonomy and reduce the caregiver's work intensity.

Nevertheless, there are challenges in the application of AR in dementia care:

- Achieving balance between immersive feeling and portability

  Most hardware displays that could provide deeper immersion, such as immersive rooms and 3D TV, are not readily portable. The head-mounted displays (HMDs) are portable, but they are cumbersome and less socially acceptable. Mobile phones are the most widespread portable devices in daily life, but the users experience limited immersive feelings. Enhancing immersion by using multimodal feedbacks, such as audio information (10), may be one of the possible solutions.
- Tracking in an unprepared environment

  Although tracking in an unprepared environment is more suitable for assisting patients in outdoor activities, it is still a challenge as various factors need to be considered (31). Thus far, accurate tracking in an unprepared environment is achieved at a high computation cost and poor robustness.

- Providing training tools to caregivers

  Existing applications focus on assisting patients and rarely provide training for caregivers. Most caregivers are the patient's relatives who have no experience in taking care of dementia patients. AR-based training tools could be used to teach caregivers to develop day-to-day routines, communicate with their loved ones, and handle challenges in dementia care (32).

Conclusion

The number of individuals with dementia is growing rapidly due to an aging population. Thus, there is an ever-increasing interest in using computer technology to assist persons with dementia. AR has been utilized in dementia care, but only a few relevant studies have been reported. This chapter presents a survey on the current state-of-the-art studies on AR-based assistive and rehabilitation applications for persons with dementia. A system structure that is widely used in AR-based assistive and rehabilitation systems for dementia has been extracted from this survey. To illustrate the details of using AR in dementia care, an AR-assisted exercising system that aims to enhance the planning capability is presented. This innovative system uses a two-training-phase strategy that allows the user to transfer the capability learned from the virtual environment to reality. The research on using AR in dementia care is relatively new; more studies on assistive and rehabilitation applications are required. Moreover, with developments in smartphones, portable applications for dementia care will become more feasible.

Appendix: Questionnaire for the User Study

Pretest

1. Do you have any trouble remembering family members or daily tasks?
2. Can you complete every step of daily tasks correctly without any assistance?

Posttest

1. Do you agree that these exercises are interesting?
2. Do you agree that this system provides clear instruction?
3. Do you agree that you learned the procedure of ADLs from the first exercise?
4. Do you agree that the second exercise cements the skill you learned from the first exercise?

5. Do you agree that this exercise improves your capability of planning daily tasks?
6. Would you like to train your capability of planning ADLs using this system?

Note

1. http://www.optitrack.com/products/flex-3/

References

1. Lengenfelder J, Schultheis MT, Al-Shihabi T, Mourant R, DeLuca J. Divided attention and driving: a pilot study using virtual reality technology. Journal of Head Trauma Rehabilitation. 2002;17(1):26–37.
2. Ong SK, Yuan M, Nee AYC. Augmented reality applications in manufacturing: a survey. International Journal of Production Research. 2008;46(10):2707–42.
3. Garcia A, Andre N, Boucher DB, Roberts-South A, Jog M, Katchabaw M. Immersive augmented reality for Parkinson disease rehabilitation. In Ma M, Jain LC, Anderson P, editors. Virtual, Augmented Reality and Serious Games for Healthcare. Berlin: Springer; 2014, pp. 445–69.
4. Azuma RT. A survey of augmented reality. Presence-Teleoperators and Virtual Environments. 1997;6(4):355–85.
5. Garcia L, Kartolo A, Méthot-Curtis E. A Discussion of the Use of Virtual Reality in Dementia. Rijeka: INTECH; 2012.
6. Ong SK, Shen Y, Zhang J, Nee AYC. Augmented reality in assistive technology and rehabilitation engineering. In: Furht B, editor. Handbook of Augmented Reality. New York: Springer; 2011, pp. 603–30.
7. Dementia Guide. These Are the Dementia Symptoms That Identify Onset [documented on the Internet]. November 2009 [cited 2016 Apr 16]. Available from https://www.dementiaguide.com/community/dementia-articles/These_Are_the_Dementia_Symptoms_that_Identify_onset.
8. Sahar NM, MatNasir EMNE, Zainudin AH. Development Augmented Reality for Dementia Disease. Paper presented at the International Integrated Engineering Summit (IIES 2014); Johor, Malaysia; 2014 Dec 1–4.
9. Al-Khafaji NJ, Al-Shaher MA, Al-Khafaji MJ, Asmail MAA. Use BuildAR to help the Alzheimers disease patients. In: Proceedings of the International Conference on E-Technologies and Business on the Web (EBW '13); 2013 May 7–9; Bangkok, Thailand, pp. 280–84.
10. Quintana E, Favela J. Augmented reality annotations to assist persons with Alzheimers and their caregivers. Personal and Ubiquitous Computing. 2013;17(6):1105–16.
11. Hervás R, Bravo J, Fontecha J. An assistive navigation system based on augmented reality and context awareness for people with mild cognitive impairments. IEEE Journal of Biomedical and Health Informatics. 2014;18(1):368–74.
12. Zhang J, Ong S, Nee AYC. Design and development of a navigation assistance system for visually impaired individuals. In: Proceedings of the 3rd International Convention on Rehabilitation Engineering & Assistive Technology (i-CREATe); 2009 Apr 22–26; Singapore.

13. Zhang J, Zhao MY, Ong SK, Nee AYC. A wearable navigation system for visually impaired users. In: Proceedings of the 6th International Convention on Rehabilitation Engineering & Assistive Technology (i-CREATe); 2012 Jul 24–26; Singapore.

14. Wood S, McCrindle R. Augmented reality discovery and information system for people with memory loss. In: Proceedings of the 9th International Conference on Disability, Virtual Reality and Associated Technologies; 2012 Sep 10–12; Laval, France.

15. Kirner C, Cerqueira CS, Kirner TG. Using augmented reality artifacts in education and cognitive rehabilitation. In: Eichenberg C, editor. Virtual Reality in Psychological, Medical and Pedagogical Applications. Rijeka: InTech; 2012, pp. 247–70.

16. Correa AGD, de Assis GA, Nascimento Md, Ficheman I, Lopes RdD, editors. Genvirtual: an augmented reality musical game for cognitive and motor rehabilitation. In: Proceedings of Virtual Rehabilitation 2007 Conference; 2007 Sep 27–29; Venice, Italy, pp. 1–6.

17. Richard E, Billaudeau V, Richard P, Gaudin G. Augmented reality for rehabilitation of cognitive disabled children: a preliminary study. In: Proceedings of Virtual Rehabilitation 2007 Conference; 2007 Sep 27–29; Venice, Italy, pp. 102–108.

18. Chang Y-J, Kang Y-S, Huang P-C. An augmented reality (AR)-based vocational task prompting system for people with cognitive impairments. Research in Developmental Disabilities. 2013;34(10):3049–56.

19. Kirner C, Kirner TG. Development of an interactive artifact for cognitive rehabilitation based on augmented reality. In 2011 International Conference on Proceedings of Virtual Rehabilitation (ICVR '11); 2011 Jun 27–29; Zurich, Switzerland, pp. 1–7.

20. Frutos-Pascual M, García-Zapirain B, Méndez-Zorrilla A. Improvement in cognitive therapies aimed at the elderly using a mixed-reality tool based on Tangram game. In: Kim T-H, Cho H-S, Gervasi O, Yau SS, editors. Computer Applications for Graphics, Grid Computing, and Industrial Environment. New York: Springer; 2012, pp. 68–75.

21. Gamberini L, Martino F, Seraglia B, Spagnolli A, Fabregat M, Ibanez F, et al. Eldergames project: an innovative mixed reality table-top solution to preserve cognitive functions in elderly people. In: 2nd Conference on Proceedings of Human System Interactions, 2009 (HSI '09); 2009 May 21–23; Catania, Italy, pp. 164–69.

22. Boletsis C, Mccallum S. Augmented reality cube game for cognitive training: an interaction study. Studies in Health Technology and Informatics. 2014;200:81–87.

23. Subramanian S, Knaut LA, Beaudoin C, McFadyen BJ, Feldman AG, Levin MF. Virtual reality environments for rehabilitation of the upper limb after stroke. In: International Workshop on Virtual Rehabilitation; 2006 Aug 29–30; New York, pp. 18–23.

24. Bahar-Fuchs A, Clare L, Woods B. Cognitive training and cognitive rehabilitation for persons with mild to moderate dementia of the Alzheimer's or vascular type: a review. Alzheimers Research & Therapy. 2013;5(4):35.

25. Bond GR, Drake RE, Becker DR. An update on randomized controlled trials of evidence-based supported employment. Psychiatric Rehabilitation Journal. 2008;31(4):280.

26. Hartin PJ, Nugent CD, McClean SI, Cleland I, Norton MC, Sanders, C, et al. A smartphone application to evaluate technology adoption and usage in persons with dementia. In: 2014 36th Annual International Conference of the IEEE Engineering in Medicine and Biology Society (EMBC '14); 2014 Aug 26–30; Chicago, pp. 5389–92.

27. Kato H, Billinghurst M. Marker tracking and HMD calibration for a video-based augmented reality conferencing system. In: Proceedings of 2nd IEEE and ACM International Workshop on Augmented Reality (IWAR '99); 1999 Oct 20–21; San Francisco, pp. 85–94.
28. Wagner D, Schmalstieg D. Artoolkitplus for pose tracking on mobile devices. In: Proceedings of the Computer Vision Winter Workshop; 2007 Feb 6–8; St. Lambrecht, Austria, 139–46.
29. Zhao MY, Ong SK, Nee AYC. Augmented reality-assisted rehabilitation of activities of daily living. In: Proceedings of the 5th International Conference on Internet Technologies & Society 2014; 2014 Dec 10–12; New Taipei City, Taiwan, pp. 89–93.
30. Shen Y, Ong SK, Nee AYC. Hand rehabilitation based on augmented reality. In: Proceedings of the 3rd International Convention on Rehabilitation Engineering & Assistive Technology; 2009 Apr 22–26; Singapore.
31. Cagalaban G, Kim S. Projective illumination technique in unprepared environments for augmented reality applications. In: Kim T-H, Stoica A, Chang R-S, editors. Security-Enriched Urban Computing and Smart Grid. New York: Springer; 2010, pp. 17–23.
32. Russell D, Benedictis T, Saisan J. Dementia and Alzheimer's Care [document on the Internet]. 2015 [cited 2015 Oct 15]. Available from: http://www.helpguide.org/articles/alzheimers-dementia/dementia-and-alzheimers-care.htm

PART II
PSYCHOSOCIAL IMPLICATIONS

6

Caring for Older Adults with Dementia

The Potential of Assisted Technology in Reducing Caregiving Burden

Tenzin Wangmo

Introduction

Technological innovations and their deployment in healthcare have the potential to alleviate several concerns that our society faces, including caring for older persons with dementia and those with other health needs. This is critical in light of population aging and the growing number of older persons who live to much older ages with physical and neurological illnesses. For individuals with dementia and their families, scholars underline that technological innovations that are *user oriented* and *user codesigned* may be more appropriate in fostering users' wishes to remain as independent as possible, age in place, and reduce caregiving burden (Bharucha et al. 2009; Carswell et al. 2009; Ienca et al. 2017; Ienca et al. 2018). The goal of this chapter is to explore interconnections between informal caregivers of persons with dementia, innovations made in the area of assistive technologies for dementia, and the formal healthcare system/the state. Therefore, the chapter begins with a brief introduction on informal caregivers, followed by a discussion about caregiving burden associated with caring for persons with dementia. As caregivers for persons with dementia consist of various actors ranging from professional healthcare providers to paid support at home, as well as unpaid family members and friends, the focus of this chapter will be on informal caregivers, specifically those who are family members as they provide the bulk of the informal care (Jutkowitz et al. 2017). Thereafter, the chapter provides an up-to-date summary of the potential of assistive technologies in addressing the important concern of caregiving burden. Assistive technology is the umbrella term describing devices or systems that allow persons with cognitive, physical, and communicative disabilities to increase, maintain, or improve their capabilities (Ienca et al. 2017; Marshall 2000). Intelligent assistive technology (IAT) is also a type of assistive technology but with its own computation capability and the ability to communicate through a network. In this chapter, assistive technology is used to denote IAT as well. Differentiations are only made when necessary. Finally, the chapter makes a call for fair and ubiquitous deployment of assistive technologies to persons with dementia and their informal caregivers. This is critical to ensure that the former benefit from existing validated technological innovations and the latter are not overburdened, and thereby continue to contribute toward the sustainability of the healthcare system. This chapter will not discuss ethical issues associated with the use of technology, such as privacy, confidentiality, informed consent, or personhood, nor regulatory issues associated with assistive technologies. For these concerns, the readers are referred to other chapters of this volume.

Informal Caregivers of Persons with Dementia

Worldwide it is estimated that there are approximately 50 million persons living with dementia, of which 9 million people are living in Europe (Alzheimer's Disease International 2017). The global cost of dementia was $818 billion in 2015 (Alzheimer's Disease International 2017). In 2009, the total worldwide cost of dementia based on a dementia population of 34.4 million was $455 billion, of which $142 billion was attributed to informal care (Wimo, Winblad, and Jonsson 2010). The economic value of informal caregiving is vast. It is difficult to state the cost savings associated with the support informal caregivers provide for each and every country in this chapter. Thus, Switzerland and the United States are taken as examples to underpin the healthcare costs saved as a result of support informal caregivers provide in two Western countries with very different population sizes and healthcare systems.

In Switzerland, there are approximately 134,000 persons with dementia (Alzheimer Europe 2014). In 2013, approximately 170,000 informal caregivers in Switzerland contributed 64 million hours of unpaid work, which would have cost CHF 3.4 billion if formal caregivers had fulfilled those needs (Spitex Schweiz 2014). The total yearly cost of dementia in Switzerland in 2007 was CHF 6.3 billion, and the cost of dementia per year is lower for those living at home (CHF 55,000) than those living in an institution (CHF 68,000) (Kraft et al. 2010).

In the United States, it is estimated that there are 5.5 million persons with dementia (Alzheimer's Association 2017) and more than 15 million informal caregivers who provided 18.2 billion hours of unpaid care for a family member with Alzheimer's disease or other dementias in 2016 (Alzheimer's Association 2017), amounting to a price tag of $230 billion. A recent economical evaluation of lifetime cost of dementia concluded that families bear most of the financial costs (approximately 70%) and that the cost of caring for a person with dementia is greater than caring for someone without dementia (Jutkowitz et al. 2017).

The exact lifetime cost of caring for a person with dementia was estimated to be $321,780 and the total annual cost was estimated to be $89,000 per individual in 2015 (Jutkowitz et al. 2017). For the year 2010, the informal caregiving cost calculated ranged between $41,689 and $56,290 (Hurd et al. 2013).

In light of dementia's gradual progression, it is understandable that the role and responsibilities as an informal caregiver do not occur suddenly but gradually. This role becomes evident with increasing realization that the care recipient who has dementia displays unusual behaviors and limitations resulting in greater need for support with common activities from the caregiver (Czekanski 2017). Several qualitative studies have captured the difficult but rewarding experience of being an informal caregiver for a person with dementia (Czekanski 2017; Holthe et al. 2018; Kindell et al. 2014). These caregivers discuss challenges faced when moving from a role of being a partner or a child to that of being responsible for protecting and monitoring their spouse or parent (Kindell et al. 2014). Davis and colleagues (2011) illustrate the stress and sadness associated with the loss of relationship with the care recipient when dementia progresses and the conflicts that arose when having to make decisions for their loved one with dementia.

For persons with dementia, their family caregivers are the core of their support network. A recent study from the United States concluded that almost all older adults with dementia (>95%) living in the community were receiving care from a family member (Riffin et al. 2017). In many cases these family caregivers are spouses but also adult children and other relatives. In the United States, adult children make up a quarter of the caregiver population (Alzheimer's Association 2017). Another study found that 50% of the caregivers of patients with dementia were adult children (Riffin et al. 2017). When adult children are the care providers, it is likely that they are sandwiched between caring for an older parent with dementia and having to meet the needs of their young children. Moreover, female family members disproportionately carry the caregiving role, often resulting in higher feelings of burden (Chiatti et al. 2015; Riffin et al. 2017).

Care tasks that family caregivers provide consist of support with activities of daily living (ADLs), instrumental ADLs, undertaking activities associated with healthcare logistics (e.g., doctor's appointments), and healthcare management (e.g., medications) (Chiatti et al. 2015; Riffin et al. 2017). An Italian study found that informal caregivers of older persons with dementia spent on average 50 hours a week caring for that person with little support from public services (Chiatti et al. 2015). A nationally representative study from the United States revealed that caregivers of persons with dementia provide an average of 30 hours of support per week (Riffin et al. 2017). Depending on the severity of the dementia and the physical health of the person in need of care, caregiving for persons with dementia would mean providing support in all the tasks mentioned previously and possibly multiple times a day. When intensive care is required from these in-formal caregivers, it is likely that they will face more challenges in engaging with other activities such as gainful employment and social activities with friends and other members of the family.

Caregiving Burden and Dementia

Caregiving burden denotes the level of stress, depression, and pressure that caregivers perceive when fulfilling caregiving roles, responsibilities, and re-lated tasks. It points to the lack of balance between the demand of (or need for) care and the ability (and maybe even willingness) to address these demands, ultimately resulting in the perception of being burdened. Studies provide evidence on caregiving burden and its effects on the health of the caregiver (Cassie and Sanders 2008; Gitlin et al. 2003), including mortality (Schulz and Beach 1999). Not surprisingly, a comparative study of caregivers of persons with mild cognitive impairments and a control group concluded that the former was twice as likely to suffer from caregiving burden as the latter (Paradise et al. 2015). Furthermore, caregivers of persons with dementia spent more hours per day in caregiving activities and had more depressive symptoms than caregivers of persons with cognitive impairments but not de-mentia (Fisher et al. 2011).

Caregiving burden is associated with many factors, including the time of de-mentia onset—specifically early- or late-onset dementia (van Vliet et al. 2010); characteristics of the person with dementia, such as behavioral factors and psy-chological symptoms (Chiao, Wu, and Hsiao 2015; Chiatti et al. 2015; Koca, Taskapilioglu, and Bakar 2017; Sutcliffe et al. 2017; Werner et al. 2012b); gender of the caregiver (Akpinar, Kucukguclu, and Yener 2011; Sutcliffe et al. 2017); stigma associated with being a caregiver (Werner et al. 2012a); and intensity of caregiving required (Kowalska et al. 2017; Riffin et al. 2017). Specifically, a parent or spouse with dementia depicting difficult behavioral symptoms and greater need for ADL care would in many cases mean that the caregiver must be con-stantly on call to give all necessary support and thus is likely to perceive higher levels of caregiving burden. That female carers show greater caregiving burden could be attributed to them being sandwiched between different roles. In the case of adult children, it may mean responsibilities of a mother toward a young child and that of a daughter toward a parent with dementia (Hirschfeld and Wikler 2003–2004; Lai 2012; Pillemer and Suitor 2014), in addition to having other roles and responsibilities of an employee. Being sandwiched between different roles may mean that adult children feel more burden of care when compared to spouse caregivers (Chappell, Dujela, and Smith 2014); however, results are mixed as to whether adult children perceive caregiving burden more greatly than spouses (Pinquart and Sorensen 2011).

Furthermore, negative effects of caregiving have been noted on caregivers' psychological and physical health as well as their social lives (Pinquart and Sorensen 2007; Riffin et al. 2017). Both the psychological and physical health of caregivers were found to be worse than that of noncaregivers (Pinquart and Sörensen 2003). Psychiatric morbidity such as depression and anxiety is related to caregiving burden (Blieszner and Roberto 2010; Garand et al. 2005). Also, increased financial problems on the family are associated with greater caregiving burden (Lai 2012). A study of eight European countries also found similar results, highlighting caregiving burden due to financial constraints (Alvira et al. 2015).

However, recent studies concluded that caregiving can have a positive impact on the caregivers and that the negative picture of caregiving roles with an emphasis on caregiving burden is not justified (Fisher et al. 2011; Roth, Fredman, and Haley 2015; Stansfeld et al. 2017). An integrative review presented four domains that explain positive aspects of caregiving for family members with dementia (Yu, Cheng, and Wang 2017). These included (a) feeling a sense of accomplishment and gratification through competently supporting the person with dementia, (b) valuing the mutuality in the dyadic relationship, (c) perceiving family cohesion and functionality in caring for the person with dementia, and (d) finding it an opportunity to care for a loved one with dementia and thus seeing personal growth and purpose in life. Similarly, another review found that caregiving is associated with positive constructs such as self-efficacy, spirituality, residence, rewards, gain, and meaning of life (Stansfeld et al. 2017). Furthermore, a study revealed a negative association between positive aspects of care and caregiving burden even when controlled for age and marital status (Abdollahpour, Nedjat, and Salimi 2018). It thus reinforced that positive feelings such as caregiver gains, satisfaction, family relationship quality, and meaningfulness reduce feelings of being burdened by caregiving roles and responsibilities.

Interestingly, burden of care could be mitigated by perceptions and attitudes of the person with dementia prior to the onset of dementia (Chiriboga et al. 2014; Etters, Goodall, and Harrison 2008). That is, a previous positive perception of the family member or prior good family functioning leads to greater willingness to provide care, and thereby alleviate feelings of caregiving burden. Daley and colleagues (2017) found that dementia patients and their caregivers who viewed themselves as a team and expressed themselves using "we/us" depicted greater positive aspects of caregiving than those who referred to themselves as "I/me." In a similar vein, a scoping review of men as caregivers for persons with dementia underlined that relational factors are critical to caregiving experiences (Robinson et al. 2014).

Informal Caregivers, Caregiving Burden, and Assistive Technology

As stated earlier, for family carers of persons with dementia the burden of being the caregiver is higher than those of carers of persons without dementia, and caregiving often entails a negative impact on their overall health and well-being (Fisher et al. 2011; Paradise et al. 2015; Pinquart and Sörensen 2003; Riffin et al. 2017). Thus, the promises of assistive technology in reducing stress and worries of persons with dementia and their caregivers is a highly awaited phenomenon. Lindqvist and colleagues (2013) stated that the potentials of assistive technology will become evident if end-users are able to effectively adjust to assistive technology and use it appropriately. A few studies have sought to capture the landscape of assistive technology available to aid persons with dementia. The first review of available IATs for persons with dementia found 58 total technologies (Bharucha et al. 2009). These included cognitive aids to support memory, aphasia, and agnosia; physiological sensors to detect vitals and falls; environmental sensors to detect movement; and advanced integrated sensor systems such as security systems. Nevertheless, these technologies lacked clinical validation, which meant that they are yet to be widely deployed.

An update was carried out to produce a state-of-the-art technology list on available IATs for potential use in dementia care (Ienca et al. 2017). This comprehensive systematic review identified 539 IATs that have either been developed for patients with dementia or could be potentially used by this group. These technological innovations encompassed "distributed systems, robots, mobility and rehabilitation aids, handheld multimedia devices, wearables, human-machine interface, and software applications" (p. 1304). They were geared toward assisting a person with dementia in ADL needs, cognitive and emotional assistance, monitoring, interaction, engagement, and so forth. This review also concluded that 60% of the technologies were not user centered—that is, they were not designed in collaboration with the intended user of the technology. Similar to the previous review, clinical validation of IATs was available for almost half of them, but the quality of these validations was questionable since only three studies used randomized controlled trials.

In light of vastly growing technological innovations developed for dementia care, it is not surprising that there has been concurrent exploration to utilize such innovations to support family members of persons with dementia. The goals of deploying assistive technology to caregivers are not only to reduce caregiving burden and stress but also to improve the overall quality of life of both the caregiver and the care recipient. Czaja and Rubert (2002) revealed that telecommunications technology facilitated informational resources for caregivers of persons with dementia. Using a randomized study design and telephone support, another study found positive results (i.e., significant improvement on feelings of anxiety and depression), particularly for those caregivers who reported low mastery with their caregiving roles (Mahoney, Tarlow, and Jones 2003a). Home-based monitoring systems for persons with dementia has proven to be helpful in facilitating family caregiving (Kinney et al. 2004). A further study utilizing "Buddy," a handheld assistive technology to provide information and act as a source of reminders for different tasks (e.g., medication time), was useful for both older persons with dementia and their caregivers (Becker and Webbe 2008).

The innovative use of assistive technology for supporting caregivers has continued to target different facets of caregiving burden. For instance, a care-giver and patient with dementia dyad evaluated an in-home video monitoring system to be effective in communication and behavior management (Williams et al. 2013). A videophone psychological intervention for caregivers of persons with dementia improved their caregiving skills, reduced feelings of caregiving burden, and resulted in positive perceptions of their caregiving roles (Czaja et al. 2013). Similarly, another study demonstrated the clinical benefits (i.e., reduced burden, anxiety, and depression symptoms) of the Tele-Savvy technology for caregivers of dementia patients, which uses teleconferences and video modules (Griffiths et al. 2016).

Assistive technology such as a GPS tracking system is helpful in monitoring persons with dementia and to find them when they display wandering tendencies (Werner et al. 2012b). A pilot study using GPS with a small sample ($n = 33$) of dementia patients and their caregivers reported ease in using the GPS system, older patients felt higher levels of independence, and caregivers were less wor-ried (Pot, Willemse, and Horjus 2012). Tracking devices are also beneficial for users since it allows them to be independent and for caregivers to receive some respite (Landau et al. 2010; Pot, Willemse, and Horjus 2012).

Although there may be many effective technologies that are available for both persons with dementia and their caregivers, it is important that potential users know that these products exist and are able to use them effectively. Holthe and colleagues (2018) studied 13 family caregivers of patients with dementia and re-ported the benefits of different technologies (i.e., localization device, GPS, timer for stove and coffee machine) in easing their daily routines. However, the study participants highlighted that (a) it is critical for the technologies to be simple enough for patients to learn and relearn how to use them, (b) information about such technologies was not known to them previously, and (c) there was a time lag between information on the availability of such technology and when they actu-ally received the technology for use at home. Vouching for simple technology in facilitating caregivers' ability to support their family members, participants of a small-sample demonstration project valued simple aids and alarm systems over complex user interface systems (Nauha et al. 2018). A randomized controlled trial with a large sample of dyad participants (dementia patients and their caregivers) is currently underway that aims to evaluate the effectiveness of relatively simple information and communication technologies (e.g., home-leaving sensors, smoke and water leak sensors, bed sensors, and automatic lights) in alleviating caregiver burden (Malmgren Fange et al. 2017).

Existing evidence reveals the effectiveness of simple technologies in supporting caregivers in addressing their burden of caregiving. These technologies usually also include Internet-based and smartphone-based applications, which are effective in delivering interventions for caregivers to reduce burden associated with their roles (Coffman, Resnick, and Lathan 2017). Since the Internet and smartphones are vastly used, assistive technology designed to aid both caregivers and care recipients based on these modes of delivery may be very promising. That is, assistive technology using this source might be not only an effective mode of technology delivery because many users may already possess these devices but also one that could be learned and adjusted to quite easily. Studies to date have highlighted the benefits of incorporating the views of end-users to make them more effective (Mahoney, Mahoney, and Liss 2009; Mahoney et al. 2015). Interventions and design concepts of assistive technology should seek to further integrate the perspectives of carers in addition to that of persons with dementia, particularly female caregivers. Their inputs will ensure that developed and deployed technologies are better designed to reduce as much of the burden of caregiving as possible.

Interconnectedness Between Family and the Healthcare System

Caregiving is a responsibility not only of the family but also of the state. Depending on the support systems available within a country, caregiving burden may be felt differently. Alvira and colleagues (2015) found that caregiving burden varied by country, with the difference being most pronounced between Northern and Southern European countries. Specifically, informal carers in Spain had the worst scores for psychological well-being because caregiving was seen as a role of the family and limited formal services were available from the state. Conversely, in Sweden better quality of life of informal caregivers was found due to the presence of greater formal healthcare resources for families. In a similar way, Kotsadam (2012) showed how formal eldercare available universally in Norway meant that family caregivers are less burdened and do not suffer negative economic consequences of being caregivers.

Several policies exist at the level of the state that underpin its role in promoting the health and well-being of its population in need. These include old age benefits like Social Security in the United States and old age insurance in European countries. At the level of public health, it includes Medicare and Medicaid in the United States and mandatory social health insurance in many European countries. The existence of these security systems has allowed older persons and those who are ill to remain independent, and to not be thrown into poverty. At the same time, they enable younger generations to pursue their own lives and careers without being burdened to care for their aging parents. However, it is known that these security systems are experiencing great strain in many countries (e.g., United States, Germany, Italy), mostly as a consequence of population aging. That is, there are more older persons receiving old age benefits and for longer periods of time. In the same manner, the healthcare system today faces the challenge of caring for not only a greater number of older persons but also older persons who are sicker and for longer periods.

The interplay between macro-level policies and micro-level familial relationships is evident from studies examining intergenerational support between adult children and their older parents. These studies conclude that state support enables older parents to remain independent and for their children to decide when and what type of support they can provide to their parents (Haberkern and Szydlik 2010; Lowenstein and Daatland 2006). Evidence available to date thus underlines that state support does not reduce the obligation that children feel to care for their parents but makes the entire support system more symbiotic. Cross-national studies in Europe have carefully examined the role of the state and intergenerational relationships (Attias-Donfut, Ogg, and Wolff 2005; Daatland, Veenstra, and Herlofson 2012; Gierveld, Dykstra, and Shenk 2012; Herlofson et al. 2011). Their findings highlight variations evident in the level of support the state provides to its citizens and its influence on filial obligation as well as attitudes toward care provision between generations. Thus, families in Northern European countries provide and expect a different level of caregiving support when compared to those in Southern European countries. Irrespective of these differences, there are flows of support between generations of a family. Although these studies have not specifically examined parents with dementia, the core findings are relevant for a caregiving relationship that takes place between members of the family when a loved one suffers from dementia.

Without extensive support from family caregivers, the burden of care for persons with dementia will squarely fall on the healthcare system, making the latter unsustainable. It is in the interest of the healthcare system and thereby the state to ensure that family care providers are not overburdened since such feelings may drive them away from these important roles and responsibilities (Roth, Fredman, and Haley 2015). The sustainability of the healthcare system is deeply dependent on the web of informal care activities that are provided to persons with dementia (and other older persons in need). Furthermore, a healthcare system's sustainability is key for all countries, particularly those based on a collective willingness to pay for the overall system (de Meijer et al. 2013), so that the population does not withdraw from this model built on the solidarity principle. There is hence a dire need to balance willingness and ability to care for a family member with dementia and feelings of being (over) burdened.

Speaking in favor of the sustainability of the caregiving system is the positive role that formal support (from the healthcare system or government) plays for persons with dementia and their caregivers (Park et al. 2018). Such formal support could include respite for caregivers through social programs, providing the means and resources for caregivers to gain knowledge about additional support services, and making assistive technology available to support persons with dementia and their family caregivers. Several scholars highlight the potential of such technologies for dementia care (Bharucha et al. 2009; Ienca et al. 2017) and alleviation of caregiving burden (Czaja et al. 2013; Griffiths et al. 2016; Mahoney et al. 2003b). It is critical to ensure that there is fair and comprehensive access to clinically validated assistive technologies. This might be a very worthy policy initiative to implement on the part of the state. Moreover, in light of (a) population aging; (b) increasing development in assistive technologies that aim to improve quality of life and overall functioning, as well as postpone long-term care situations (Bharucha et al. 2009; Pollack 2007); and (c) the fact that institutionalization is more expensive than caring at home (de Meijer et al. 2013; Kraft et al. 2010), the state should be genuinely interested in ensuring that resources are in place so that patients with dementia and their families have ubiquitous access to such technologies.

The pervasiveness of assistive technology is important to eradicate the technological divide. That there could be a technological divide and that new and effective technology to support persons with dementia may be available only to those who can afford it have been raised in the literature (Bharucha et al. 2009; Ienca et al. 2017). Issues of justice and equity within the context of technology are significant and have been evaluated in depth in a recent work (Ienca et al. 2016). Furthermore, a descriptive review of ethical issues in the development of IATs found that justice, and thereby fair access to assistive technology, was the least-thought-about and discussed ethical concern (Ienca et al. 2018). It is crucial that the state takes responsibility for ensuring justice by making access to such technologies fair and ubiquitous so that the positive impacts of technological innovations can be enjoyed by all levels of society without discrimination. When new technologies are only available for those who have more resources, the benefits of such innovations are limited only to this group, furthering the cumulative disadvantage that those who are not able to afford such developments may already be suffering.

Conclusion

Economic costs saved by the overall healthcare system from the support that informal caregivers provide to persons with dementia are vast. The role of informal caregivers is integral not only for the well-being of the person to whom care is provided but also for the overall sustainability of the healthcare system. Engagement of family members in caring for their loved ones with dementia is an issue of personal responsibility and a task that brings forth both positive and negative impacts on caregivers' health and well-being (Chiao, Wu, and Hsiao 2015; Gitlin et al. 2003; Roth, Fredman, and Haley 2015; Yu, Cheng, and Wang 2017). Although it is generally accepted that adult children have and will continue to support their aging parents (Pillemer and Suitor 2014), it cannot be taken for granted that children and even other family members will always do so in the future and that they will be able to provide the level of care the care recipient requires. There is thus a need to ensure that informal caregivers receive the necessary support from the state (and the healthcare system) that enables them to fulfill their caregiving roles toward their family member with dementia without feeling that this relationship is a burden, and for them to meet other roles they may have. Providing fair and ubiquitous access to clinically proven assistive technologies to families of persons with dementia might be a valuable solution on the part of the state. Such state-level support could be operationalized in different ways, such as (a) recognizing that clinically validated assistive technologies are an integral part of enabling the health of persons with dementia and thus insuring them as part of health insurance plans; (b) providing tax incentives for expenditures made toward assistive technology when caring for a person with dementia; and (c) investing state resources in the innovation, validation, and deployment of clinically validated assistive technologies. This is critical in light of a lack of clinical evidence on the efficacy of assistive technologies. Thus, rigorous research is needed to validate available assistive technologies so that useful technologies can be deployed more rapidly. There is no doubt that legal and ethical concerns associated with such widespread deployment of assistive technologies must be addressed appropriately and without delay, at both the national and international levels.

References

Abdollahpour, I., Nedjat, S., and Salimi, Y. (2018), "Positive aspects of caregiving and caregiver burden: a study of caregivers of patients with dementia", *J Geriatr Psychiatry Neurol*, 31 (1), 34–38.

Akpinar, B., Kucukguclu, O., and Yener, G. (2011), "Effects of gender on burden among caregivers of Alzheimer's patients", *J Nurs Scholarsh*, 43 (3), 248–54.

Alvira, M. C., et al. (2015), "The association between positive-negative reactions of informal caregivers of people with dementia and health outcomes in eight European countries: a cross-sectional study," *J Adv Nurs,* 71 (6), 1417–34.

Alzheimer's Association. (2017). "2017 Alzheimer's disease facts and figures," https://www.alz.org/facts/overview.asp.

Alzheimer Europe. (2014). "Switzerland. 2013: the prevalence of dementia in Europe," http://www.alzheimer-europe.org/Policy-in-Practice2/Country-comparisons/2013-The-prevalence-of-dementia-in-Europe/Switzerland.

Alzheimer's Disease International, (2017) "Dementia statistics," https://www.alz.co.uk/research/statistics.

Attias-Donfut, C., Ogg, J., and Wolff, F. C. (2005), "European patterns of intergenerational financial and time transfers", *Eur J Ageing,* 2, 161–73.

Becker, S. A., and Webbe, F. M. (2008), "The potential of hand-held assistive technology to improve safety for elder adults aging in place", in K. Henriksen, et al. (eds.), *Advances in Patient Safety: New Directions and Alternative Approaches (Vol. 4: Technology and Medication Safety)* (Rockville, MD: Agency for Healthcare Research and Quality).

Bharucha, A. J., et al. (2009), "Intelligent assistive technology applications to dementia care: current capabilities, limitations, and future challenges", *Am J Geriatr Psychiatry,* 17 (2), 88–104.

Blieszner, R., and Roberto, K. A. (2010), "Care partner responses to the onset of mild cognitive impairment", *Gerontologist,* 50 (1), 11–22.

Carswell, W., et al. (2009), "A review of the role of assistive technology for people with dementia in the hours of darkness", *Technol Health Care,* 17 (4), 281–304.

Cassie, K. M., and Sanders, S. (2008), "Familial caregivers of older adults", *J Gerontol Soc Work,* 50 (Suppl 1), 293–320.

Chappell, N. L., Dujela, C., and Smith, A. (2014), "Spouse and adult child differences in caregiving burden", *Can J Aging,* 33 (4), 462–72.

Chiao, C. Y., Wu, H. S., and Hsiao, C. Y. (2015), "Caregiver burden for informal caregivers of patients with dementia: A systematic review", *Int Nurs Rev,* 62 (3), 340–50.

Chiatti, C., et al. (2015), "The UP-TECH project, an intervention to support caregivers of Alzheimer's disease patients in Italy: preliminary findings on recruitment and caregiving burden in the baseline population", *Aging Ment Health,* 19 (6), 517–25.

Chiriboga, D. A., et al. (2014), "Recalled attributes of parents with Alzheimer's disease: relevance for caregiving", *Health Psychol Behav Med,* 2 (1), 1038–52.

Coffman, I., Resnick, H. E., and Lathan, C. E. (2017), "Behavioral health characteristics of a technology-enabled sample of Alzheimer's caregivers with high caregiver burden", *Mhealth,* 3, 36.

Czaja, S. J., and Rubert, M. P. (2002), "Telecommunications technology as an aid to family caregivers of persons with dementia", *Psychosom Med,* 64 (3), 469–76.

Czaja, S. J., et al. (2013), "A videophone psychosocial intervention for dementia caregivers", *Am J Geriatr Psychiatry,* 21 (11), 1071–81.

Czekanski, K. (2017), "The experience of transitioning to a caregiving role for a family member with Alzheimer's disease or related dementia", *Am J Nurs,* 117 (9), 24–32.

Daatland, S. O., Veenstra, M., and Herlofson, K. (2012), "Age and intergenerational attitudes in the family and welfare state", *Adv Life Course Res,* 17, 133–44.

Daley, R. T., et al. (2017), "'In this together' or 'Going it alone': Spousal dyad approaches to Alzheimer's", *J Aging Stud,* 40, 57–63.

Davis, L. L., et al. (2011), "The nature and scope of stressful spousal caregiving relationships", *J Fam Nurs,* 17 (2), 224–40.

de Meijer, C., et al. (2013), "The effect of population aging on health expenditure growth: a critical review", *Eur J Ageing,* 10 (4), 353–61.

Etters, L., Goodall, D., and Harrison, B. E. (2008), "Caregiver burden among dementia patient caregivers: a review of the literature", *J Am Acad Nurse Pract,* 20 (8), 423–28.

Fisher, G., et al. (2011), "Caring for individuals with dementia and CIND: findings from the aging, demographics, and memory study", *J Am Geriatr Soc,* 59 (3), 488–94.

Garand, L., et al. (2005), "Caregiving burden and psychiatric morbidity in spouses of persons with mild cognitive impairment", *Int J Geriatr Psychiatry,* 20 (6), 512–22.

Gierveld, J. J., Dykstra, P. A., and Shenk, N. (2012), "Living arrangements, intergenerational support types and the older loneliness in Eastern and Western Europe", *Demographic Res,* 27, 167–200.

Gitlin, L. N., et al. (2003), "Effect of multicomponent interventions on caregiver burden and depression: the REACH multisite initiative at 6-month follow-up", *Psychology Aging,* 18 (3), 361–74.

Griffiths, P. C., et al. (2016), "Development and implementation of tele-savvy for dementia caregivers: a Department of Veterans Affairs clinical demonstration project", *Gerontologist,* 56 (1), 145–54.

Haberkern, K., and Szydlik, M. (2010), "State care provision, societal opinion and children's care of older parents in 11 European countries", *Ageing Society,* 30, 299–323.

Herlofson, K., et al. (2011), "Intergenerational family responsibility and solidarity in Europe", *Multilinks deliverable 4.3* 104.

Hirschfeld, M. J., and Wikler, D. (2003–2004), "An ethics perspective on family caregiving worldwide: justice and society's obligation", *Generations,* 27 (4), 56–60.

Holthe, T., et al. (2018), "Benefits and burdens: family caregivers' experiences of assistive technology (AT) in everyday life with persons with young-onset dementia (YOD)", *Disabil Rehabil Assist Technol,* 13 (8), 754–62.

Hurd, M. D., et al. (2013), "Monetary costs of dementia in the United States", *N Engl J Med,* 368 (14), 1326–34.

Ienca, M., et al. (2017), "Intelligent assistive technology for Alzheimer's disease and other dementias: a systematic review", *J Alzheimers Dis,* 56 (4), 1301–40.

Ienca, M., et al. (2018), "Ethical design of intelligent assistive technologies for dementia: a descriptive review", *Sci Eng Ethics,* 24 (4), 1035–55.

Ienca, M., et al. (2016), "Social and assistive robotics in dementia care: ethical recommendations for research and practice", *Int J Social Robotics,* 8 (4), 565–73.

Jutkowitz, E., et al. (2017), "Societal and family lifetime cost of dementia: implications for policy", *J Am Geriatr Soc,* 65 (10), 2169–75.

Kindell, J., et al. (2014), "Living with semantic dementia: a case study of one family's experience", *Qual Health Res,* 24 (3), 401–11.

Kinney, J. M., et al. (2004), "Striving to provide safety assistance for families of elders: the SAFE House project", *Dementia,* 3 (3), 351–70.

Koca, E., Taskapilioglu, O., and Bakar, M. (2017), "Caregiver burden in different stages of Alzheimer's disease", *Noro Psikiyatr Ars,* 54 (1), 82–86.

Kotsadam, A. (2012), "The employment costs of caregiving in Norway", *Int J Health Care Finance Econ,* 12 (4), 269–83.

Kowalska, J., et al. (2017), "An assessment of the burden on Polish caregivers of patients with dementia: a preliminary study", *Am J Alzheimers Dis Other Demen,* 32 (8), 509–15.

Kraft, E, et al. (2010), "Cost of dementia in Switzerland", *Swiss Medical Weekly,* 140, w13093.

Lai, D. W. L. (2012), "Effect of financial costs on caregiving burden of family caregivers of older adults", *SAGE Open*, 2 (4), 2158244012470467.

Landau, R., et al. (2010), "Families' and professional caregivers' views of using advanced technology to track people with dementia", *Qual Health Res*, 20 (3), 409–19.

Lindqvist, E., Nygard, L., and Borell, L. (2013), "Significant junctures on the way towards becoming a user of assistive technology in Alzheimer's disease", *Scand J Occup Ther*, 20 (5), 386–96.

Lowenstein, A., and Daatland, S. O. (2006), "Filial norms and family support in a comparative cross-national context: evidence from the OASIS study", *Ageing Society*, 26, 203–23.

Mahoney, D. F., Tarlow, B. J., and Jones, R. N. (2003a), "Effects of an automated telephone support system on caregiver burden and anxiety: findings from the REACH for TLC intervention study", *Gerontologist*, 43 (4), 556–67.

Mahoney, D. F., et al. (2015), "Prototype Development of a Responsive Emotive Sensing System (DRESS) to aid older persons with dementia to dress independently", *Gerontechnology*, 13 (3), 345–58.

Mahoney, D. F., et al. (2003b), "The Caregiver Vigilance Scale: application and validation in the Resources for Enhancing Alzheimer's Caregiver Health (REACH) project", *Am J Alzheimers Dis Other Demen*, 18 (1), 39–48.

Mahoney, D., Mahoney, E., and Liss, E. (2009), "AT EASE: Automated Technology for Elder Assessment, Safety, and Environmental monitoring". *Gerontechnology*, 8 (1), 11–25.

Malmgren Fange, A., et al. (2017), "The TECH@HOME study, a technological intervention to reduce caregiver burden for informal caregivers of people with dementia: study protocol for a randomized controlled trial", *Trials*, 18 (1), 63.

Marshall, M. (2000), *ASTRID: A Guide to Using Technology Within Dementia Care* (London: Hawker Publications).

Nauha, L., et al. (2018), "Assistive technologies at home for people with a memory disorder", *Dementia (London)*, 17 (7), 909–23.

Paradise, M., et al. (2015), "Caregiver burden in mild cognitive impairment", *Aging Ment Health*, 19 (1), 72–78.

Park, M., et al. (2018), "The roles of unmet needs and formal support in the caregiving satisfaction and caregiving burden of family caregivers for persons with dementia", *Int Psychogeriatr*, 30 (4), 557–67.

Pillemer, K., and Suitor, J. J. (2014), "Who provides care? A prospective study of caregiving among adult siblings", *Gerontologist*, 54, 589–98.

Pinquart, M., and Sorensen, S. (2007), "Correlates of physical health of informal caregivers: a meta-analysis", *J Gerontol B Psychol Sci Soc Sci*, 62 (2), P126–37.

Pinquart, M., and Sorensen, S. (2011), "Spouses, adult children, and children-in-law as caregivers of older adults: a meta-analytic comparison", *Psychol Aging*, 26 (1), 1–14.

Pinquart, M., and Sörensen, S. (2003), "Differences between caregivers and noncaregivers in psychological health and physical health: a meta-analysis", *Psychology Aging*, 18 (2), 250.

Pollack, M. E. (2007), "Intelligent assistive technology: the present and the future", in Cristina Conati, Kathleen McCoy, and Georgios Paliouras (eds.), *User Modeling 2007: 11th International Conference, UM 2007, Corfu, Greece, July 25–29, 2007. Proceedings* (Berlin, Heidelberg: Springer Berlin Heidelberg), 5–6.

Pot, A. M., Willemse, B. M., and Horjus, S. (2012), "A pilot study on the use of tracking technology: feasibility, acceptability, and benefits for people in early stages of dementia and their informal caregivers", *Aging Ment Health,* 16 (1), 127–34.

Riffin, C., et al. (2017), "Family and other unpaid caregivers and older adults with and without dementia and disability", *J Am Geriatr Soc,* 65 (8), 1821–28.

Robinson, C. A., et al. (2014), "The male face of caregiving: a scoping review of men caring for a person with dementia", *Am J Mens Health,* 8 (5), 409–26.

Roth, D. L., Fredman, L., and Haley, W. E. (2015), "Informal caregiving and its impact on health: a reappraisal from population-based studies", *Gerontologist,* 55 (2), 309–19.

Schulz, R., and Beach, S. R. (1999), "Caregiving as a risk factor for mortality: the Caregiver Health Effects Study", *JAMA,* 282 (23), 2215–19.

Spitex Schweiz (2017), "Zeitlicher Umfang und monetäre Bewertung der Pflege und Betreuung durch Angehörige", https://www.spitex.ch/files/62R5XI6/medienmitteilung_spitex_tag_2014.pdf, accessed December 26, 2017.

Stansfeld, J., et al. (2017), "Positive psychology outcome measures for family caregivers of people living with dementia: a systematic review", *Int Psychogeriatr,* 29 (8), 1281–96.

Sutcliffe, C., et al. (2017), "Caring for a person with dementia on the margins of long-term care: a perspective on burden from 8 European countries", *J Am Med Dir Assoc,* 18 (11), 967–73.e1.

van Vliet, D., et al. (2010), "Impact of early onset dementia on caregivers: a review", *Int J Geriatr Psychiatry,* 25 (11), 1091–1100.

Werner, P., et al. (2012a), "Family stigma and caregiver burden in Alzheimer's disease", *Gerontologist,* 52 (1), 89–97.

Werner, S., et al. (2012b), "Caregiving burden and out-of-home mobility of cognitively impaired care-recipients based on GPS tracking", *Int Psychogeriatr,* 24 (11), 1836–45.

Williams, K., et al. (2013), "In-home monitoring support for dementia caregivers: a feasibility study", *Clin Nurs Res,* 22 (2), 139–50.

Wimo, A., Winblad, B., and Jonsson, L. (2010), "The worldwide societal costs of dementia: Estimates for 2009", *Alzheimers Dement,* 6 (2), 98–103.

Yu, D. S. F., Cheng, S. T., and Wang, J. (2017), "Unravelling positive aspects of caregiving in dementia: an integrative review of research literature", *Int J Nurs Stud,* 79, 1–26.

7

The Predestined Nature of Assistive Technologies for Dementia

Taro Sugihara, Tsutomu Fujinami, and Osamu Moriyama

Introduction

Global aging is becoming a serious problem in this century, as human societies are facing aging-related issues such as dementia. According to a report by the World Health Organization, there are approximately 47.5 million people with dementia (PWD) in the world, and 7.7 million new cases each year [1]. For the first time in history, the elderly population is increasing at an alarming rate and can eventually surpass the younger generation. This causes many problems worldwide, with no known specific solutions.

Caregivers in care homes are often required to cope with the multifunctional nature of their work. Caregiving is a hybrid task that encompasses medical treatments, the support of daily activities, and psychological and social support through appropriate interactions. Caregiving tasks are often not easy and quick to complete and are usually challenged by unexpected actions of the residents. For example, if a resident stands up and begins to walk while a caregiver is assisting another resident to eat, the caregiver immediately has to stop the eating assistance and rush to the erratic resident to prevent falls or wandering. Unfortunately, human resources to look after residents are limited.

Assistive technologies for dementia will be a fruitful way to enhance resources in care homes, especially in the era of global super-aging. While assistive technologies are deployed across national boundaries, the end-users of these technologies, that is, the people who are cared for and their caregivers, are bound by the policies in their respective countries or regions. Consequently, even if a researcher or an engineer develops an extremely innovative and efficient technology, it may be challenging to deploy it into standard care. Researchers and/ or engineers have to pay attention to the local policies and organizational rules of the region where they plan to deploy the technology and narrow the gaps between the implementation and the setting of technology development.

This chapter examines how these issues affect healthcare policies and technology deployment by using a case study approach focused on Japanese care homes. A report subsidized by the Japanese Ministry of Health, Labour, and Welfare estimated that the number of PWD in Japan will increase by approximately 6.5 million to 7 million in 2025, 8 million to 9.5 million in 2040, and 8.5 million to 11.5 million in 2060 [2]—making Japan the most rapidly aging society in the world.[1] In light of these demographic trends, we describe several technologies for assisting elderly adults with dementia and assess their potential to improve care. Furthermore, we present the benefits and challenges of implementing such technologies into practice from the micro, meso, and macro perspectives.

The chapter is organized as follows:

1. An overview of the relationship between dementia, person-centered care, and assistive technologies
2. A discussion of the potential benefits of assistive technologies in resolving these challenges (this will be done using a case study approach based on the authors' investigation at a care home and a following summary of surveys conducted by the Japanese government to understand the need for assistive technologies among caregivers)
3. An analysis of the barriers to the adoption of assistive technologies based on governmental surveys and an assessment of the difficulties of deploying these technologies in the caregiving field

Dementia, Person-Centered Care, and Assistive Technologies

Dementia is characterized by a decline in memory, language, problem solving, and other cognitive skills that affect a person's ability to perform everyday activities [3]. The cognitive ability of PWD is predominantly impaired in two ways: memory and higher-brain functioning. If a person's memory is impaired, he or she has difficulty remembering recent events (as recent as the last few hours). Such a person may also have difficulty recognizing the consequences of his or her situation. In other words, a PWD may recognize what he or she is seeing, but cannot understand what the situation means.Person-centered care [4, 5] is a type of care, which includes dementia care, wherein the person who is cared for is central; the caregiver keenly observes and communicates with the patient to determine the type of tasks and the reasons such tasks should be performed. The caregiver can then help the patient accomplish his or her goals.

The core idea of person-centered care is to respect the "personhood" of patients, which includes an understanding of the individual needs and a consideration of their motivation and personal history. Person-centered care is regarded by many caregivers as the most suitable approach to dementia care because it allows one to assist PWD in relation to other stakeholders, especially in relation to caregivers [4].

However, person-centered care might generate conflicts due to possible mismatches between caregivers' needs and the behavior of PWD. In Japan caregivers often desire to provide quality care for the elderly in care homes and are dedicated to promoting the quality of life of residents. A report [6] examining caregivers' attitudes and values in relation to care provision revealed that the majority of caregivers attribute high importance to the value of being respectful to the older residents they care for (94% of the 214 respondents). They also regarded caregiving as a worthwhile job (84%) and considered themselves morally responsible for care recipients (81%). Additional recurrent themes included the wish to communicate with the elderly through daily-task interactions and to care for them in a relaxed manner. Unfortunately, their wishes often fail to be fulfilled because PWD can change their behavior suddenly and unexpectedly, regardless of the context of the caregivers' tasks. As we have seen before, caregivers are required to promptly react to the residents' dangerous actions (e.g., beginning to show signs of aimless wandering) even if they are assisting others (e.g., eating).

Technologies for assisting PWD and their caregivers can be classified into five groups: screening [7–9], memory aid, monitoring health or safety [10–13], information sharing and telecare [14–18], and communication support and therapy [19–24]. These technological types are thoroughly described in this study [25]; in contrast, other technologies such as powered assistive robots were excluded from the discussion on this study because the study focused on the characteristics of dementia itself instead of frailty by aging such as muscular weakness.

Although such assistive technologies are fruitful in helping caregivers, little attention has been given to assessing these technologies from the perspective of person-centered care. When a system is implemented, it is highly probable that its impact on person-centered care will be significant since it enables caregivers to have leeway to make a decision by monitoring PWD's actions in advance, to tell risky situations to other staff members beyond time and distances, or to concentrate their care under the calm atmosphere after therapeutic sessions. Although assistive technologies have huge potential to improve dementia care, they also might generate new conflict. Caregivers are professionals who look after vulnerable people. To improve caregiving services, it is important to implement assistive technologies efficiently and to consider necessary ethical concerns.

Benefits of Deploying Assistive Technology

Assessing Needs at the Micro and Meso Level

Interviews

Individual face-to-face semistructured interviews were conducted. Each interview was approximately 30 minutes long. Prior to the study, we obtained informed consent from the chief manager of the nursing home and the chief nurses. We received additional ethical approval from an institution the first author had belonged to. We interviewed 8 nationally qualified nurses and 14 caregivers without national qualification. Nurses in Japanese care homes are entitled to provide medical treatments (e.g., administering medicines) in addition to delivering physical and mental assistance. Interview questions addressed physical/mental hardships of caregiving tasks and their reasons.

The first author conducted the interviews on site. The coding was performed using MAXQDA 2010—a software for qualitative data analysis. The analysis was led by the first author, who has a PhD, specializes in human-computer interaction, and was a university lecturer of social research methods. All the interviews were recorded and transcribed verbatim. The first author carried out the interviews and took brief notes during the interview. None of the invited participants refused to participate in the interviews. The questions were almost the same as those of the preliminary investigation.

A constant comparison [26] method was used to analyze the transcripts. The transcripts were repeatedly read to identify commonalities and differences between the data, and similar data were classified into the same category. When a category was recognized as similar to another one, these two categories were combined into one single category. This analysis process was repeated until no new categories could be formed, that is, until a theoretical saturation was reached. All analyses were internally reviewed for validation with special focus on the consistency between data and conclusions. This part of the analysis was conducted by the third author, who is a cognitive scientist.

Ethical Considerations

The study was approved by the Japan Advanced Institute of Science and Technology. We strictly followed informed consent guidelines prior to data collection. We made every effort to convey the purpose of the study to the informants and managers of the care institution. After an explanation of the study's structure and objectives, all the informants agreed to be interviewed and have their responses recorded through a voice recorder. In addition to that, the manager obtained documented consent from all the participating residents' families.

Interview Results

Twenty respondents had worked in care facilities or hospitals as a nurse for 3 or more years. The number meant that this care house has kept skilled caregivers. According to a series of reports of caregiving in Japan [27–35], over 70% of the newcomers had at least 3 years' work experience. Therefore, if the employees continued working for 3 or more years in the same care house, it meant that the care houses provided better working conditions to their employees. Twenty-two subcategories were associated with mental hardships and nine subcategories were associated with physical hardships (some included both). Table 7.1 shows the results of the interview. In total, 8 categories and 26 subcategories were determined after theoretical saturation.

Comments related to mental hardships focused on how to cope with the individuality of the elderly. Remembering personal history, understanding personal needs, grasping the conditions of an elderly individual with a psychiatric problem, and establishing a desirable relationship with the individual after understanding his or her condition were the typical problems addressed by interviewees. PWD and persons with depression need individualized care, but not "cookie cutter" care. While there is no doubt that such care was provided to the residents, the interviewees' observed that it requires tremendous effort to collect residents' information and promptly react to their unexpected actions. Nursing and caregiving tasks were often reported as causes of mental fatigue.

The interviewees also referred to staff shortages and the nature of caregiving. Caregiving tasks inherently become reaction-based work during multitasking. Caregivers can never focus all their resources on one single care recipient, as they have to be aware of every resident in need. Therefore, caregivers struggle to achieve peace of mind during their daily tasks, as they always have to be alert.

Moreover, interviewees mentioned their reflective attitude toward their daily activities. The need for multitasking might cause mental conflicts originating from the difficulty in providing equal care to all residents. For instance, a caregiver was concerned that she might have occasionally chosen colloquial words after being suddenly approached by a resident asking for help with medications. Another caregiver regretted that she did not have enough time to talk with the residents, although she desired to chat with them in a friendly and informal way.

Physical hardships were also presented as a major challenge for caregivers, though in a smaller proportion compared to mental hardships. Caregivers' comments focused on actual activities such as assisting residents during bathing and responding to nurse calls. For safety reasons, the facility was equipped with several sensors and button-based nurse call stations located in residents' rooms and in corridors. Residents were permitted to push the button and call staff anytime if they needed help. The button directly connects patients to mobile phones worn by all working staff to which caregivers are required to respond

Table 7.1 Results of Care House Interviews

Categories	Subcategories	Mental Hardships	Physical Hardships
Assistance	Communication with residents	4	0
	Assistance with mobility, dressing, and face washing	1	0
	Assistance with taking a bath	5	4
	Meal assistance	1	1
	Toiletry assistance	0	0
Care house issues	Problems that stem from the care house's physical characteristics	1	0
	Special needs in the care house	1	0
	Differences in other care houses	1	0
Staff shortage	Overall difficulties	1	3
	Less leeway (caused by staff shortage)	7	2
Discretion to make decision	Definite cases	0	0
	Ambiguous cases	4	2
Caregiving attitudes	Colleagues' attitudes	1	0
	Criticism of himself/herself	7	2
Gaps between reality and ideals		2	0
Information-sharing issues	Care records	4	0
	Information transfer to the other workers	0	0
	Cell phone use	0	0
	Nurse call button use	2	4
	Knowing the other staff members' surroundings	6	4
Time-consuming tasks	Psychiatric issues	15	0
	Risk of falling down	4	0
	Dementia-related issues	12	0
	Others	7	0
Conflicts between reality and care house policies	Norms and management policies	2	1
	Responsibility as a manager	0	0

immediately. Moreover, other sensors connected to different nurse calls were installed in front of the restroom door for the most vulnerable residents. When the nurses receive a call, they are required to respond to them promptly. If the resident can communicate verbally, the nurse picks up the phone and asks about his or her needs. If the call is from a PWD, one of the nurses must stop his or her task immediately and rush to the sensor location. Examples of these demanding tasks are provided in Table 7.2.

It is important for elderly adults in Japan to take a bath on a regular basis to maintain sanitary conditions because the local humid environment is suitable for virus reproduction. Consequently, the facility ensures that residents will have a bath at least thrice a week. Before going into the bathtub, the person washes his or her body not only for personal hygiene but also to keep the water in the bathtub clean. This procedure is important for reducing the risks of infection from other persons who used the bathtub previously. The resident also has to dry himself or herself with a towel after leaving the bathtub. The caregivers have to assist residents during this procedure in a Japanese-style bathroom. Some of the

Table 7.2 Ratio of Caregiving Hardships

Need for Mitigating Hardships by Assistive Technologies	Care Houses		Family
	Managers (N = 114)	Caregivers (N = 106)	Caregivers (N = 696)
Assistance with sitting and standing	28.1	24.5	47.7
Assistance with transferring	64.9	66.0	48.3
Assistance with moving	19.3	20.8	37.8 (in home)
			19.4 (outside)
Assistance with eating	28.9	28.3	49.1
Assistance with toiletry activities	42.1	48.1	62.5
Assistance with bathing	53.5	59.4	58.3
Monitoring for safety	37.7	40.6	28.2
Dementia care and its improvement	47.4	52.8	28.9
Information sharing	29.8	29.2	N/A
Other caregiving issues	14.0	12.3	N/A
Improvement of rehabilitation effects	25.4	22.6	16.1
Improvement/maintenance for activities of daily living	43.0	42.5	N/A
Improvement/maintenance for motivation to live	42.1	52.8	N/A
Others	0.9	2.8	0.6

residents need special assistance when they use a bathing machine and a wheel stretcher. In any case, the caregivers go back and forth between the Japanese-style bathrooms and the rooms of residents. These tasks are physically demanding for them.

These tasks also caused mental hardships, as many elderly PWD refuse taking baths. This has caused mental exhaustion to the caregivers, as they often elicit strong emotional reactions from the patients while forcing them to bathe. Therefore, caregivers desired to know the mood of residents before assisting them during bathing tasks.

Knowing the situations of where colleagues are and what they do was significant for reducing redundant activities. As mentioned before, a caregiver often faced serious conflicts caused by multitasking and by uncontrollable actions from the residents. Although the caregivers desired a colleague's help in such situations, it was difficult to know whether their colleagues were available or capable to help. Caregivers commonly tried to call colleagues with a cell phone or walked to the staff room to find them. However, if they could not be located, then having limited resources for decision making became a cause of stress.

Table 7.2 displays survey results regarding caregiving hardships [36, 37]. The answers of professional caregivers and care managers strongly correlated ($r = 0.98$). The most difficult task was assisting while transferring; two-thirds of caregivers stated that this task was tough, although the respondents in our study did not report this issue. Caregiving issues associated with the residents' body movements were not reported as the most severe in our study; however, the needs for information sharing and knowing PWD were similar to our results [36]. The results of in-home care revealed that the task of moving a person's body created feelings of burden for family caregivers [37].

Needs at the Macro Level

From a macro standpoint, there is a need for assistive technologies in society. The Cabinet Office of Japan conducted a survey assessing the need for assistive robots in September 2013 [37]. According to this brief report, 59.3% of 1,842 respondents accepted robot use when they had to care for vulnerable people. Moreover, 65.1% of the caregivers responded that they would welcome the use of a robot if they themselves would be required to be cared for.

Worldwide aging trends (shown in Figure 7.1) potentially push for these needs to increase. Japan is the country with the highest proportion of aging population. The population ratio of adults aged 65 years and older is expected to increase to 36.7% in 2055. The Annual Report on the Aging Society 2015 [39] stated that the elderly population of Japan will reach an estimated 34.6 million (39.9% of the

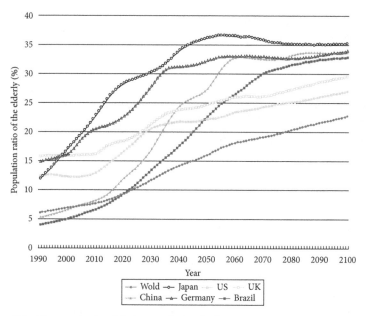

Figure 7.1 Changes in the elderly population [38].

total population), which is equivalent to 78.4% of the working population as in-dicated in Figure 7.2.

A shortage of caregivers accelerates this alarming situation. Figure 7.3 shows that 20% of care workers leave their jobs every year, and almost three-quarters of them do so within 3 years of commencing work at a care institution [27–35]. Therefore, it is difficult for care home managers to secure skillful, long-term caregivers. This means that care environments are being gradually affected by the enlarging gap between an increasingly higher number of elderly people and a shortage of caregivers. The Ministry of Health, Labour, and Welfare estimates that approximately 377,000 caregivers will be deficient in 2025 [40].

The government has lobbied for the use of assistive technologies, especially assistive robots, to support institutional care in nursing homes. The Ministry of Health, Labour, and Welfare and the Ministry of Economy, Trade, and Industry have collaboratively supported the development of assistive robots. With the purpose of mitigating caregiving burden and enhancing the market of assistive robots, the ministries have set five priority targets: powered assistive robots that transfer patients from beds and wheelchairs, assistive robots for personal mobility, toiletry assistance robots, bathing assistance robots, and monitoring robots for PWD's safety [41].

Interviews in a report [42] targeting rental and intermediary agents re-vealed that three types of assistive technology are particularly needed in care

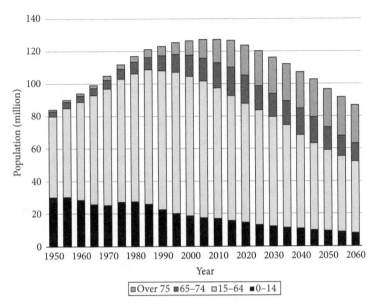

Figure 7.2 Population changes in Japan.

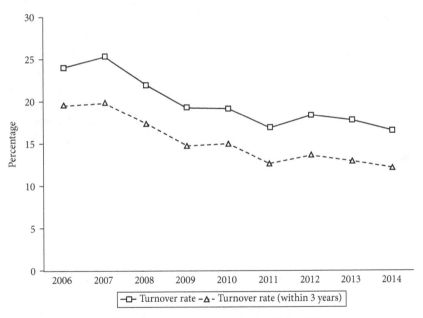

Figure 7.3 Changes of caregiver turnover ratio from 2006 to 2014.

homes: monitoring technologies, transferring assistants, and toiletry assistants. Participants from six care homes who had experience with assistive technologies noted that transferring-assistance robots were an important piece of technology that mitigated caregivers' waist pain. Despite the recognized significance of these three technologies, respondents observed that some structural barriers present an obstacle to their implementation.

These priority targets and the interview results are covered with the needs at the micro and meso levels, concerning residents' body movement and dementia care. However, the other significance, the need for information sharing to improve caregiving, is a noteworthy result when referring to the results in the previous section. While the government has not pushed for the problem to be solved, professional caregivers and managers in care houses, as reported in our investigation and a governmental report, pointed out its significance as a hardship.

Barriers to Assistive Technologies

Even though there is a need for technology assistance, assistive technologies for dementia have not been widely adopted. For instance, assistive robots, one of the most typical assistive technologies for caregiving support, have shown low adoption rates nationwide. According to a report from the Ministry of Economy, Trade, and Industry [43], the ratio of assistive robot sales to total robot sales was estimated to be 1.06% (approximately US $1.53 billion) in 2015, although the ratio is predicted to raise to 4.52% (US $39.3 billion) in 2035. Another report estimated that the sales range of assistive robots was from US $53 million to US $150 million in 2012 [42]. A report from the Ministry of Health, Labour, and Welfare [44] also revealed that both caregivers (81.1%) and managers (62.3%) hoped to accelerate the introduction of assistive robots into standard care if possible, even though introduction of some assistive technologies was piloted in only 16.7% of 114 care homes.

Challenges at the Micro and Meso Levels

For adequate person-centered care, care houses need to employ a sufficient number of caregivers, especially skilled ones. However, it is difficult to hire caregivers in Japan due to budget limitations. According to a report on labor conditions in the country [35], 59.3% of 6,230 respondents reported a lack of caregivers at their institutions. When questioned about the availability of skilled caregivers, 53.9% of 8,260 respondents answered that it was difficult to employ skilled caregivers, and 49.8% noted that managers could not pay employees a salary that is sufficient to retain them in the workforce because of inadequate government subsidies. Moreover, 29.1% indicated that it is impossible to improve their working conditions and environments due to financial limitations.

Caregivers are required to fulfil high-level intelligent tasks on a daily basis. Caregiving tasks heavily depend on contextual factors such as the needs of PWD, the type of care work, the equipment used, and the caregiver–care receiver relationship. Person-centered care is extremely demanding. Effective implementation of person-centered care requires caregivers to focus on everything that occurs in the facility. To fulfill their responsibilities, caregivers must carefully observe their patients, and based on their training and experience, they must try to discern the patients' needs and react appropriately. Caregivers have to respond to and alleviate various behavioral and psychological symptoms of dementia Behavioral and PsychologicalSymptoms of Dementia (BPSDs) to implement person-centered care.

In such cases, caregivers cannot have much leeway for incorporating new methods or tools into their daily workflow. The survey [44] revealed that over half of caregivers and managers believed that the installment, maintenance, and guidance of technology operations should not be increased in the introduction phase. If engineers underestimate these issues, assistive technologies will likely face rejection, a critical barrier for development and deployment.

In addition to that, financial costs are a major barrier to the adoption of assistive technologies. As noted before, care homes in Japan often struggle to pay employees a reasonable salary. Therefore, incorporating new technologies into care homes is heavily affected by budget limitations. Nonetheless, residents in care homes face many physical and psychiatric challenges that require technological assistance. The managers have to consider the trade-off between the positive effects these technologies have on patients' daily symptoms and the associated financial costs.

Individual PWD and their caregivers typically cannot purchase assistive technologies because of their high costs. Elderly adults typically receive 145,000 yen per month from the Welfare Pension or 54,000 yen per month from the National Pension [45]. The average cost of care expenditures for elderly who need to be cared for is 79,200 yen per month [46]. Furthermore, over 80% of the elderly rely on their pension money to live comfortably [30]. Care facilities face the same issue. In 2013, approximately 83.9% of the income in intensive care homes for the elderly and 75.7% of the income in group homes were supported by welfare benefits [47, 48]. This means that it is difficult for the elderly to purchase assistive technologies with their personal finances without welfare support schemes.

In addition to financial problems, caregivers also encounter ethical dilemmas in various situations. Typically, these situations involve having to prioritize among competing demands for assistance. For instance, if a caregiver who is helping a patient at the lavatory hears a sensor-detected alarm installed in a room occupied by a person with severe dementia, an ethical dilemma arises: deciding whether to respond to the alarm or not. These types of dilemmas frequently occur throughout the day and are extremely stressful. Kahn et al. describe this type of work stress as "role stress" [49]. Role stress, especially in its components of role ambiguity and role conflict, is a well-known predictor of burnout [50]. In healthcare settings, several studies show that role ambiguity and role conflict are causally related to emotional exhaustion [51–53].

The management of assistive technologies also generates new ethical dilemmas. Survey respondents (including caregivers and care home managers) pointed out that they faced the problem of reducing the costs of maintenance and system deployment. State-of-the-art assistive technologies are not routinely utilized for caregiving tasks. In addition, assistive technologies often require human supervision and hence require skilled health professionals who can engage in operationalization and maintenance, which are usually time-consuming. Caregivers have to spend time acquiring the knowledge and skills about the system's functions and operations, which takes away the time they spend interacting with residents. Consequently, conflicts between care and technological operation give rise to a new cause of role stress as the time invested in the technology's functionality might conflict with the time required at the bedside.

If caregivers have adequate knowledge and skill, they could learn to cope with the role stress that results from the various dilemmas they face. In contrast, less trained personnel and novices might hardly cope with it. While managers recognize the problem of budget limitations, there is little they can do to employ a sufficient number of skilled caregivers and alleviate the situation. Furthermore, individual group homes that are for dementia care, which are faced with a high separation rate as shown in Figure 7.3, are continually obliged to train new employees.

The Challenges at the Macro Level

In summary, the explosive aging of the Japanese population gave rise to needs for care homes, especially for the elderly and middle-aged workers who live away from their relatives. As described in section "Assessing Needs at the Micro and Meso Level", the government predicts a dramatic lack of caregivers by 2025. The increased need for care housing has resulted in a greater demand of caregivers. However, financial constraints in public finances make it difficult to employ more caregivers. Figure 7.4 shows that between 2004 and 2013 [54], the budget for elderly benefits has on average increased from 6,000 to 7,500 billion yen per year.

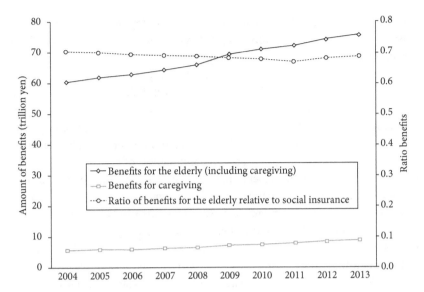

Figure 7.4 Care expenses from 2004 to 2012.

The ratio of benefits for the elderly relative to social insurance has also remained around 70%. The social benefits including medical care and pensions have been continuously raised, and this indicates that there is no room for the government to spend more money on increasing the number of caregivers. Assistive technologies are no exception; subsidies for the introduction of technologies to care houses are restricted due to the need to cut total expenses from social insurance.

Since the number of care institutions is increasing while the budget to employ new caregivers is not, the demand for caregivers is increasing dramatically. In addition, it is difficult for care institutions to provide high-quality caregiving services because many workers reportedly quit within the first 3 years of employment (see Figure 7.3), and inexperienced newcomers constitute a significant percentage of the workforce.

To solve these problems, there is a need to make caregiving more efficient and provide caregivers with systematic ways to acquire and improve their skills. Assistive technologies are a viable way to realize quality caregiving. Organizations can provide more efficient caregiving, counterbalancing the shortage of caregivers and funds if the technologies are embedded into the workflow efficiently.

As indicated in section "Needs at the Macro Level", the Japanese government fosters robot development and deployment under its determined five targets. As these technologies could mitigate hardships in care fields, it is important that the government takes an active role in promoting their deployment. However, it is debatable whether the government's *five targets* alone are sufficient to address this problem. We argue that it is also important to meet the patients' needs for mental and physical assistance to improve the quality of life.

Kitwood has identified five fundamental needs of PWD necessary to enhance their personhood from a person-centered care perspective: (a) attachment, (b) comfort, (c) identity, (d) occupation, and (e) inclusion [4]. These specific needs stem from the approach to dementia care inherent in person-centered care, which is focused on appreciating the uniqueness of each person. This approach is in contrast with conventional approaches where individuality is often disregarded in favor of optimizing performance. One significant requirement for assistive technologies in dementia care is to meet the needs for comfort, identity, and inclusion of PWD and enable caregivers to react adequately to these needs [55].

Information sharing within the care home plays a significant role in dementia care. Assistive technologies that facilitate information sharing enable caregivers to provide care without the restrictions of time and location. If an assistive device transmits information about the signs of aimless wandering to the first available caregiver on duty, the caregiver has the opportunity to promptly take adequate action. Survey results show that approximately 30% of respondents attribute significance to this issue [36]. Our interview showed similar results, as seen in Table 7.1.

However, assistive technologies for dementia have not been adopted as much as other medical technologies. The Association for Technical Aids, an organization that provides certification of assistive technologies, disclosed information about the online sales of assistive technologies. The association has collected and introduced over 9,500 items to people with disabilities, caregivers, and managers [56]. This retrieval system encompasses 11 broad categories that typically focus on safety monitoring, bathing assistance, toileting assistance, and physical support. However, there is no mention of technologies for information sharing. One of major reasons information-sharing technologies might have not appeared in the association's report is that these technologies, unlike the aforementioned technological types, are not covered by national subsidy. PWD and their caregivers need to spend their own savings if they wish to incorporate information-sharing systems into their homes or residential facilities. Therefore, financial factors might be responsible for the limited market growth of these technologies, despite remarkable progress at the research level [17, 18]. It is probable that the deployment and adoption of assistive technologies will be incomplete until these technologies are included in certified national schemes for financial subsidy.

Assistive technologies offer effective solutions to meet the needs of elderly adults with dementia and their caregivers, and their development has been promoted by the government. On the other hand, financial constrains pose a major barrier to the introduction of these technologies for the benefit of PWD and their caregivers. Although it is essential for these technologies to be subsidized by the government for their deployment, the government would have to meet an ambivalent requirement: generally suppressing the expenditures for caregiving and support to purchase assistive technologies. In addition, the government strongly fosters assistive technologies for physical assistance. In contrast, technologies for improving cognition and emotional well-being have not been given enough attention.

Conclusion

This chapter provided an analysis, from the Japanese perspective, of the emerging need for assistive technologies among elderly individuals with dementia and other age-related impairment, healthcare organizations, and society at large. In addition, it discussed the existing barriers to the deployment of assistive technologies in Japan. In spite of the urgent need for assistive technologies in the aging world, our results indicate that these barriers, if not successfully overcome through regulatory interventions, might undermine their introduction into standard care. As a result, we concluded that the governance and management of assistive technologies in Japan is more dependent on governmental subsidies than on the individual needs of patients and caregivers as governmental policies strongly affect the market sales and societal adoption of these technologies. This is the conspicuous and predestined nature of assistive technologies in dementia care.

Note

1. These figures are slightly different from those reported by the World Health Organization. For the purpose of consistency, we will refer to the figures provided by the ministries of Japan throughout this chapter.

References

1. World Health Organization, "Dementia," 2016 (2015). http://www.who.int/mediacentre/factsheets/fs362/en/, accessed February 5, 2016.

2.   Toshiharu Ninomiya, "Nihon ni okeru Ninchisho no Koueisha Jinkou no Shourai Suikei ni kansuru Kenkyu Soukatsu Houkokusho [in Japanese]," *Kousei Roudou Kagaku Kenkyuhi Hojokin* (2014).
3.   Alzheimer's Association, "2015 Alzheimer's disease facts and figures." https://www.alz.org/facts/downloads/facts_figures_2015.pdf, accessed February 5, 2016.
4.   Tom Kitwood. Dementia Reconsidered. Open University Press, 1997.
5.   Tom Kitwood, Kathleen Bredin. "Towards a theory of dementia care: Personhood and well-being," *Ageing and society* 12 (1992) 269–287.
6.   Chiharu Soga. "Yoriyoi group home ni surutameno jittai chosa houkokusho (in Japanese)," *Chingin to Shakaihosho* 1440 (2007) 10–29.
7.   James C. Mundt, Kae L. Ferber, Matthew Rizzo, John H. Greist, "Computer-automated dementia screening using a touch-tone telephone," *Archives of internal medicine* 161 (20) (2001) 2481–2487.
8.   David W. Wright, Felicia C. Goldstein, Patrick Kilgo, John. R. Brumfield, Tara Ravichandran, Melissa L. Danielson, Michelle Laplaca, "Use of a novel technology for presenting screening measures to detect mild cognitive impairment in elderly patients," *International journal of clinical practice* 64 (9) (2010) 1190–1197.
9.   Hyungsin Kim, Young Suk Cho, Ellen Yi-Luen Do, "Computational clock drawing analysis for cognitive impairment screening," *Proceedings of the Fifth International Conference on Tangible, Embedded, and Embodied Interaction*, ACM, 2011, pp. 297–300.
10. Yasushi Masuda, Takumi Yoshimura, Kazuki Nakajima, Masayuki Nambu, Tomihiro Hayakawa, Toshiyo Tamura. "Unconstrained monitoring of prevention of wandering the elderly," *Proceedings of the Second Joint EMBS/BMES Conference and the 24th Annual Conference and the Annual Fall Meeting of the Biomedical Engineering Society*, Vol. 3, IEEE, 2002, pp. 1906–1907.
11. Frank Miskelly, "A novel system of electronic tagging in patients with dementia and wandering," *Age and ageing* 33 (3) (2004) 304–306.
12. Chung-Chih Lin, Ming-Jang Chiu, Chun-Chieh Hsiao, Ren-Guey Lee, Yuh-Show Tsai, "Wireless health care service system for elderly with dementia," *IEEE transactions on information technology in biomedicine* 10 (4) (2006) 696–704.
13. Datong Chen, Ashok J. Bharucha, Howard D. Wactlar, "Intelligent video monitoring to improve safety of older persons," *Proceedings of 29th Annual International Conference of the IEEE EMBS* (2007) 3814–3817.
14. Sara J. Czaja, Mark P. Rubert, "Telecommunications technology as an aid to family caregivers of persons with dementia," *Psychosomatic medicine* 64 (3) (2002) 469–476.
15. Diane F. Mahoney, Barbara J. Tarlow, Richard N. Jones, "Effects of an automated telephone support system on caregiver burden and anxiety: Findings from the REACH for TLC intervention study," *The Gerontologist* 43 (4) (2003) 556–567.
16. Stuti Dang, Niber Remon, Julia Harris, Julie Malphurs, Lauran Sandals, Angeles L. Cabrera, Nicole Nedd, "Care coordination assisted by technology for multi-ethnic caregivers of persons with dementia: A pilot clinical demonstration project on caregiver burden and depression," *Journal of telemedicine and telecare* 14 (8) (2008) 443–447.
17. Naoshi Uchihira, Sunseong Choe, Kunihiro Hiraishi, Kentaro Torii, Tetsuro Chino, Yuji Hirabayashi, Taro Sugihara, "Collaboration management by smart

voice messaging for physical and adaptive intelligent services," *Proceedings of PICMET'13* (2013), 251–258.

18. Hiroyasu Miwa, Kentaro Watanabe, Takuichi Nishimura, "Computerized long-term care record effects on nursing-care service processes," *Proceedings of the 2nd International Conference on Serviceology (ICServ '14)* (2014) 111–114.

19. Gary Gowans, Jim Campbell, Norman Alm, Richard Dye, Arlene Astell, Maggie Ellis, "Designing a multimedia conversation aid for reminiscence therapy in dementia care environments," *Extended Abstracts of the 2004 Conference on Human Factors and Computing Systems (CHI '04)* (2004) 825–836.

20. Noriaki Kuwahara, Shinji Abe, Kiyoshi Yasuda, Kazuhiro Kuwabara, "Networked reminiscence therapy for individuals with dementia by using photo and video sharing," *Proceedings of the 8th International ACM SIGACCESS Conference on Computers and Accessibility (Assets '06)* (2006) 125–132.

21. Norman Alm, Richard Dye, Gary Gowans, Jim Campbell, Arlene Astell, Maggie Ellis, "A communication support system for older people with dementia," *Computer* 40(5) (May 2007) 35–41.

22. Noriaki Kuwahara, Kiyoshi Yasuda, Nobuji Tetsutani, Kazunari Morimoto. "Remote assistance for people with dementia at home using reminiscence systems and a schedule prompter," *International journal of computers in healthcare* 1 (2) (2010) 126–143.

23. Kazuyoshi Wada, Takanori Shibata, Toshimitsu Musha, Shin Kimura, "Robot therapy for elders affected by dementia," *IEEE Engineering in Medicine and Biology Magazine* 27 (4) (2008) 53–60.

24. Wan-Ling Chang, Selma Sabanovic, Lesa Huber, "Use of seal-like robot Paro in sensory group therapy for older adults with dementia," *Proceedings of the 8th ACM/IEEE International Conference on Human-Robot Interaction* (2013) 101–102.

25. Taro Sugihara, Tsutomu Fujinami, Rachel Phaal, Yasuo Ikawa, "A technology roadmap of assistive technologies for dementia care in Japan," *Dementia* 14 (1) (2015) 80–103 (published online before print June 27, 2013).

26. Barney G. Glaser, Anselm L. Strauss, The Discovery of Grounded Theory: Strategies for Qualitative Research," Aldine Transaction, 1999.

27. Kaigo Roudou Antei Centre (Care Work Foundation), "Kaigo Roudou Jittai Chousa (2006 Annual Reports on Care Work Environment in Japan) [in Japanese]," (2007). http://www.kaigo-center.or.jp/report/h18_chousa_03.html, accessed September 23, 2011.

28. Kaigo Roudou Antei Centre (Care Work Foundation), "Kaigo Roudou Jittai Chousa (2007 Annual Reports on Care Work Environment in Japan) [in Japanese]," (2008). http://www.kaigo-center.or.jp/report/h19_chousa_03.html, accessed September 23, 2011.

29. Kaigo Roudou Antei Centre (Care Work Foundation), "Kaigo Roudou Jittai Chousa (2008 Annual Reports on Care Work Environment in Japan) [in Japanese]," (2009). http://www.kaigo-center.or.jp/report/pdf/h20_chousa_point. pdf, accessed September 23, 2011.

30. Kaigo Roudou Antei Centre (Care Work Foundation), "Kaigo Roudou Jittai Chousa (2009 Annual Reports on Care Work Environment in Japan) [in Japanese]," (2010). http://www.kaigo-center.or.jp/report/pdf/h21_chousa_point. pdf, accessed September 23, 2011.

31.   Kaigo Roudou Antei Centre (Care Work Foundation), "Kaigo Roudou Jittai Chousa (2010 Annual Reports on Care Work Environment in Japan) [in Japanese]," (2011). http://www.kaigo-center.or.jp/report/pdf/h22_chousa_kekka. pdf, accessed September 23, 2011.

32.   Kaigo Roudou Antei Centre (Care Work Foundation), "Kaigo Roudou Jittai Chousa (2011 Annual Reports on Care Work Environment in Japan) [in Japanese]," (2012). http://www.kaigo-center.or.jp/report/h23_chousa_01.html, accessed November 4, 2012.

33.   Kaigo Roudou Antei Centre (Care Work Foundation), "Kaigo Roudou Jittai Chousa (2012Annual Reports on Care Work Environment in Japan) [in Japanese]," (2013). http://www.kaigo-center.or.jp/report/h24_chousa_01.html, accessed January 5, 2016

34.   Kaigo Roudou Antei Centre (Care Work Foundation), "Kaigo Roudou Jittai Chousa (2013 Annual Reports on Care Work Environment in Japan) [in Japanese]," (2014). http://www.kaigo-center.or.jp/report/h25_chousa_01.html, accessed January 5, 2016.

35.   Kaigo Roudou Antei Centre (Care Work Foundation), "Kaigo Roudou Jittai Chousa (2014 Annual Reports on Care Work Environment in Japan) [in Japanese]," (2015). http://www.kaigo-center.or.jp/report/h26_chousa_01.html, accessed January 5, 2016.

36.   Ministry of Health, Labour, and Welfare, "Heisei 23 nendo Fukushi Yougu Kaigo Robot JitsuyoukaShien JigyoHoukokusho [in Japanese]," (2014). http://www. techno-aids.or.jp/robo2012.05.28.pdf, accessed February 2, 2016.

37.   Cabinet Office, "Kaigo Robot ni kansuru Tokubetsu Seron Chosa [in Japanese]," (2013).   http://survey.gov-online.go.jp/tokubetu/h25/h25-kaigo.pdf,   accessed February 2, 2016.

38.   United Nations Population Division, "World Population Prospects: The 2015 Revision," (2015). http://esa.un.org/unpd/wpp/Download/Standard/Population/ , accessed February 6, 2016.

39.   Cabinet Office, "Annual Report on the Aging Society: 2015," (2015).

40.   Ministry of Health, Labour, and Welfare, "2025 nen ni muketa kaigo jinzai ni kakaru jukyusuikei (kakuteichi) ni tsuite [in Japanese]," (2015).

41.   Ministry of Health, Labour, and Welfare, "Fukushi Yougu Kaigo Robot Jitsuyouka Shien Jigyo [in Japanese]," (2013). http://www.mhlw.go.jp/file. jsp?id=147397&name=0000013456.pdf, accessed February 1, 2016

42.   Ministry of Economy, Trade, and Industry, "Robot Gijutsu no Kaigo Riyo ni okeru Jutenbunya" wo Kaitei shimashita [in Japanese]," (2013). http://www.meti.go.jp/ press/2013/02/20140203003/20140203003.html, accessed February 1, 2016.

43.   Ministry of Economy, Trade, and Industry, "Robot Gijutsu no Kaigo Riyou ni kansuru Needs oyobi Shuyoukoku Doukou Chosa Jigyo Houkokusho [in Japanese]," (2014). http://www.meti.go.jp/meti_lib/report/2014fy/E003969.pdf, accessed February 2, 2016.

44.   Ministry of Economy, Trade, and Industry, "2012-nen Robot Sangyo no Shijo Doukou [in Japanese]," (2013). http://www.meti.go.jp/press/2013/07/ 20130718002/20130718002-3.pdf, accessed February 2, 2016.

45.   Ministry of Health, Labour, and Welfare, "Heisei 26 nendo kousei nenkin hoken, kokumin nenkin jigyo no gaiyo [in Japanese]," (2015). http://www.mhlw.go.jp/

file/04-Houdouhappyou-12509000-Nenkinkyoku-Chousashitsu/H26gaikyou.
pdf, accessed February 10, 2016.

46. Japan Institute of Life Insurance, "Heisei 27 Nendo 'Seimei Hoken ni kansuru
     Zenkoku Jittai Chosa" (Sokuhoban) [in Japanese]," (2015). http://www.jili.or.jp/
     press/2015/pdf/h27_zenkoku.pdf, accessed February 10, 2016.

47. Mayune Okubo, "Heisei 25 Nendo Tokubetsu Yogo Roujin Home no Keiei Jokyo
     [in Japanese]," Welfare and Medical Service Agency (2015).

48. Mayune Okubo, "Heisei 25 Nendo Ninchisho Koreisha Group Home no Keiei
     Jokyo nitsuite [in Japanese]," Welfare and Medical Service Agency (2015).

49. Robert L. Kahn, Donald M. Wolfe, Robert P. Quinn, Jiedrick D. Snoek, Robert A.
     Rosenthal, Organizational Stress: Studies in Role Conflict and Ambiguity, John
     Wiley (1964).

50. John R. Rizzo, Robert J. House, Sidney I. Lirtzman, "Role conflict and ambiguity in
     complex organizations," *Administrative science quarterly* 15 (2) (1970) 150–163.

51. Clifton E. Barber, Mieko Iwai, "Role conflict and role ambiguity as predictors of
     burnout among staff caring for elderly dementia patients," *Journal of gerontological
     social work* 26 (1996) 101–116.

52. Jeanne A. Schaefer, Rudolf H. Moos, "Effects of work stressors and work climate
     on long-term care staff's job morale and functioning," *Research in nursing & health*
     19 (1) (1996) 63–73.

53. Esme Moniz-Cook, Dip Clin, Dawn Millington, Miriam Silver, "Residential care
     for older people: job satisfaction and psychological health in care staff," *Health &
     social care in the community* 5 (2) (1997) 124–133.

54. National Institute of Population and Security Research, "Dai 18 Hyo Koureisha
     Kankei Kyufuhi no Suii (1973–2013 Nendo) [in Japanese]," (2015). http://www.
     ipss.go.jp/ss-cost/j/fsss-h25/4/H25-18.xlsx, accessed February 8, 2016.

55. Taro Sugihara, Tsutomu Fujinami, "Emerging triage support environment of
     care with camera system for persons with dementia," in: Ergonomics and Health
     Aspects, M.M. Robertson (Ed.), HCII 2011, LNCS, vol. 6779, Berlin: Springer
     (2011) 149–58.

56. The Association for Technical Aids, Technical Aids Information System [in
     Japanese], (2016). http://www.techno-aids.or.jp/TaisCodeSearch.php, accessed
     February 2, 2016.

8

Shaping the Development and Use of Intelligent Assistive Technologies in Dementia

Some Thoughts

Elisabeth Hildt

In many nations worldwide, an increase in the prevalence of age-related disorders such as dementia can be observed. "Dementia" is a broad term to describe neurocognitive disorders including Alzheimer's disease, vascular dementia, and Lewy body dementia (Moga et al. 2017). Dementia is characterized by a decline in mental ability including impaired memory and communication and problems with orienting in time and space. This leads to impairments in daily activities and relationships and an increasing need to rely on others. In 2015, worldwide, around 46 million individuals were affected by dementia (GBD 2015 Disease and Injury Incidence and Prevalence Collaborators 2016).

Technology can be seen as a factor that may help us come to terms with dementia-related challenges. Among others, intelligent assistive technologies (IATs) have been used as one way to support persons with dementia and their caregivers and relatives.

This chapter aims to offer some general thoughts on the development and use of IATs in dementia, that is, in the care for people with dementia and in dementia-related research. Based on an analysis of ethical principles and concepts, guidelines, recommendations, and codes of conduct in the field broadly construed, the text argues for an approach that takes the user's perspective, in particular the users' abilities, wishes, and goals, more clearly into consideration in IAT development and use. Although the reflections may have implications for caregivers, family members, and others involved in the care of persons with dementia, they are not so much intended to guide individual, patient-directed decision making as to address future directions for technology development and use in a more general way.

Assistive Technology in Dementia

When it comes to the use of assistive technology in dementia, and in particular to the question of access to assistive technology, the way the disease category is understood matters. Alzheimer Europe, an umbrella organization of Alzheimer associations from over 30 countries, assumes a holistic perception of dementia, an important part of which is to recognize that individuals with dementia have impairments that often result in disability (Alzheimer Europe 2010a). Alzheimer Europe stresses that understanding dementia as a disability or potential disability is a first and important step in ensuring that individuals with dementia have access to adequate assistive technology (AT). An Alzheimer Europe (2010b) report on the ethical use of AT for/by people with dementia states: "*Dementia* should be recognised as a disability. Consequently, the entitlement of people with *dementia* to AT should be recognised." Legally, however, countries differ in whether or not they officially recognize dementia as a disability (Alzheimer Europe 2010c).

In the United States, the Assistive Technology Act of 2004 encompasses disabilities that affect the ability of individuals "to see, hear, communicate, reason, walk, or perform other basic life functions" (Assistive Technology Act 2004, Sec. 2 (a) Findings). It goes on to state:

> Disability is a natural part of the human experience and in no way diminishes the right of individuals to (A) live independently; (B) enjoy self-determination and make choices; (C) benefit from an education; (D) pursue meaningful careers; and (E) enjoy full inclusion and integration in the economic, political, social, cultural, and educational mainstream of society in the United States.

The Assistive Technology Act seeks to improve the provision of AT to individuals with disabilities and to increase access to AT. It distinguishes between and stresses the need to provide both AT devices and AT services.

According to the Assistive Technology Act, Sec. 3 (4), an AT device is "any item, piece of equipment, or product system, whether acquired commercially, modified, or customized, that is used to increase, maintain, or improve functional capabilities of individuals with disabilities." Sec. 3 (5) defines an AT service to be "any service that directly assists an individual with a disability in the selection, acquisition, or use of an assistive technology device." This includes the need to evaluate the AT needs of an individual with a disability; provide for the acquisition of AT devices; select, customize, maintain, repair, and replace AT devices; coordinate AT device–based therapies, interventions, and services; make available training or technical assistance for individuals with disabilities, family members, or representatives; provide training or technical assistance for professionals and caregivers; and expand the availability of access to technology.

While the Assistive Technology Act covers all kinds of AT for individuals with disabilities, IATs form a specific subgroup.[1] IATs are a special group of ATs capable of computation and communicating information through a network (Ienca et al. 2017a). Often, they are able to sense the environment and provide adaptive responses to the users' needs. Bharucha et al. (2009, glossary) define IATs as "technologies that sense and respond to user needs [and] are adaptable to changing situations and compensate either for physical or cognitive deficits."

Marcello Ienca and colleagues (2017a) group IATs into the following categories: distributed systems, robots, mobility and rehabilitation aids, handheld multimedia devices, wearables, human-machine interfaces, and software applications. IATs serve to support and empower individuals with dementia in activities of daily living, have monitoring functions, provide (a feeling of) safety and security, give physical or cognitive assistance or emotional support, enable users to stay longer at home, facilitate communication, promote interaction and social engagement, and facilitate care and rehabilitation (Bharucha et al. 2009; Olsson et al. 2012; Novitzky et al. 2015; Ienca et al. 2017a).

Furthermore, it has been stressed that IATs could help face the manifold challenges of dementia at various levels, especially in view of the widely held expectation that dementia and dementia-related costs will increase considerably in the future. According to Ienca et al. (2017a, 1302), IATs

> could (i) mitigate the burden on public finances through the delay or obviation of institutional care, (ii) reduce the psychological burden on formal and informal caregivers, (iii) compensate for the progressive scarcity of human caregivers while enhancing and optimizing quality of care, and (iv) empower older adults with dementia and thereby improving their quality of life.

While it cannot be denied that overall, when it comes to IAT use in dementia, the reduction of healthcare-related costs and burdens does matter, from an ethical point of view the individual users and the way IATs may benefit the users are the primary concern. That is why, as a first and important step in thinking about ways to shape future IAT use, the next section will discuss ethical principles and concepts relevant to AT development and use in dementia and analyze how these concepts and principles are addressed in guidelines, recommendations, and codes of conduct in the field.

Ethical Principles and Concepts

Which ethical principles and concepts are central in IAT use by persons with dementia? Generally speaking, beneficence, nonmaleficence, autonomy, and justice are fundamental ethical principles that matter here, as in all fields of medicine (Beauchamp and Childress 2013). In addition, researchers, professionals, caregivers, and support groups have reflected more specifically in their publications on the ethical aspects of AT use in dementia (e.g., Landau and Werner 2012; Novitzky et al. 2015; Ienca et al. 2017b). Even more specific guidance can be found in a number of guidelines, ethics codes, and recommendations that have been developed in several fields of assistive technology use (e.g., Virginia Department of Education 2008; Alzheimer Europe 2010a, 2010b; RESNA 2008; Santa Clara County 2013). Some of these guidelines, codes, and recommendations are directed primarily toward members of a certain profession, group, or professional association, while other texts are directed to a broader audience involved in caring for persons with dementia.

Overall, in the documents, there is consensus that, in assistive technology use, the user should be central. ATs should not be utilized to primarily meet the caregivers' or family members' needs or to save costs (Olsson et al. 2012).

Several authors and guidelines stress that the individual user and his or her interests, well-being, and preferences are the focus of all considerations and at the center of all decisions (Landau and Werner 2012; RESNA 2008; Alzheimer Europe 2010a). For example, Alzheimer Europe (2010a) states: "The interests and wellbeing of the person with *dementia* must always come first in decisions relating to the use of AT for or by people with dementia."

A related aspect put forward by authors is that assistive technology can always be only part of a solution—it only serves to complement existing care (Wey 2007; Alzheimer Europe 2010b; Ienca et al. 2017a). This implies the idea that assistive technology should not lead to a decrease in human-delivered care and services or a reduction in interpersonal contact, communication, and contact time. Overall, it is necessary to ensure that the assistive technology serves the user's quality of life and to avoid extra burden by the need to manage the technology.

But access to technology is crucial—an aspect that clearly is the focus of the Assistive Technology Act (2004). Making sure that individuals in need of technology have access to it is a matter of justice. Distributive justice is complicated by the fact that the more complex the assistive technology, the higher the risk that financial factors limit access for many individuals suffering from dementia and other disabilities (Alzheimer Europe 2010b). In view of these financial aspects, it will be necessary to avoid a digital divide and to find ways so that existing socioeconomic inequalities will not be increased. This may be achieved by offering highly efficient low-technology solutions, by developing technologies with a broad spectrum of users that can be marketed broadly, or by ensuring that individuals have easy access to and financial support within the healthcare system.

According to an article by Peter Novitzky and colleagues (2015), who give a review of the literature discussing ethical issues in research and development, clinical experimentation, and clinical application of ambient assisting living technologies for people with dementia, the ethical issues most often discussed in the literature are safety, security, and privacy.

In the current literature, users' safety and the need to avoid risk often play a crucial role (Landau and Werner 2012; Olsson et al. 2012; Ienca et al. 2017b). For example, the Rehabilitation Engineering and Assistive Technology Society of North America (RESNA) Standards of Practice (2008), written from the perspective of assistive technology providers, say in paragraph 12: "Individuals shall provide technology that minimizes consumers' exposure to unreasonable risk. Individuals shall provide adjustments, instructions or necessary modifications that minimize risk." In addition to avoiding risks, this approach involves carefully balancing the expected benefits and possible problems and risks of IAT use.

Also, respect for privacy and confidentiality are of central importance in the use of IATs by persons with dementia. Their relevance is particularly obvious when it comes to the use of tracking or monitoring devices and to the question of where, when, and under which conditions these devices could be installed and who may have access to the monitoring information they provide (Alzheimer Europe 2010b; Landau and Werner 2012). "Maintain the confidentiality of privileged information" is one of the principles mentioned by the RESNA Code of Ethics. Directly related to privacy are the topics of data protection, information security, and the need to avoid and prevent misuse of information.

With dementia patients who experience smaller or larger limitations in their competence to consent, most authors consider it very important to attempt to involve the persons with dementia in decision making as much as possible, including consulting with them and achieving informed consent for technology use whenever possible (Wey 2007; Alzheimer Europe 2010a, 2010b; Landau and Werner 2012; Olsson et al. 2012; Novitzky et al. 2015; Ienca et al. 2017a). There is substantial concern that monitoring devices or other forms of technology may restrict the privacy or freedom of persons with dementia without having obtained their informed consent.

Notwithstanding the fact that avoidance of risks undoubtedly is of central relevance in IAT use, in many contexts it is not easy to find an adequate balance between safety and risk avoidance on the one hand and individual autonomy on the other hand, especially when it comes to surveillance technology. Ruth Landau and Shirli Werner (2012) concede that safety and avoiding risks is important, but emphasize that autonomy is equally important, and explicate details concerning individual decision making and informed consent, advance care plans, and advance directives. Against this background, Landau and Werner's Recommendation 1 reads: "It is crucial to maintain balance between the needs of persons with dementia for protection and safety and their need for autonomy and privacy" (Landau and Werner 2012, 361).

While these publications often focus on informed consent and health-related decision making when it comes to autonomy, it is important to stress that the concept of autonomy is much broader. It encompasses following one's wishes, pursuing one's self-chosen plans and goals, and shaping one's life in a self-determined way (Hildt 2006). For example, Joseph Raz (1986, 407) describes autonomy as follows: "One is autonomous if one determines the course of one's life by oneself."

Seen from this perspective, to respect and promote the autonomy and integrity of individuals with dementia is not merely a matter of obtaining informed consent but includes supporting independence and an independent life as much as possible. Accordingly, in addition to supporting individual health-related decision making and seeking informed consent, an autonomy-based approach to IAT use should focus on the user's life plans, wishes, and abilities. This approach involves assessing a user's plans, wishes, and abilities and reflecting on how IATs can be used to support the user to achieve those goals. Central questions to be asked include: Which activities is the person able to accomplish independently, without additional help? What does the person want to accomplish? What can a person realistically achieve, if adequately supported by IATs? How can the time somebody is able to live independently be extended?

From this point of view, the user's wishes and abilities are considered central. Details of this autonomy-based approach to IAT use that focuses on the user's abilities and wishes will be outlined in the following section.

Toward an Abilities-Focused Approach in IAT Development and Use

In what follows I will argue for an approach that takes the abilities and wishes of the users more clearly into consideration. According to this approach, in IAT development and use it is important to focus on what persons with dementia are able to do independently and what they want to achieve with the help of IAT (see section User Abilities.

Directly related to this is the question of which technology should be used and developed to best support the users to achieve their goals and accomplish the tasks they consider relevant. This will be discussed in the section Technologies.

User Abilities

While there undoubtedly is broad agreement that assistive technologies should benefit users, often it may not be clear what this means in detail. For example, consider a GPS tracking device: in practice, the way it is handled will differ considerably whether it is seen as being primarily useful to prevent accidents or health risks, to prevent a person with dementia from leaving a building, or to track somebody who tends to wander around and get lost, or whether the device is considered to allow an individual to have his or her range of activities supported or to enable independent, self-determined activities. Depending on the respective situation, any of these may be considered legitimate motivations for having a tracking device in place. Overall, however, the motivation behind using or installing a tracking device (and whether or not informed consent has been sought) will considerably influence its use.

While avoiding risks is central in assistive technology use, it seems that for many IATs the focus often is too much on risk avoidance and safety and too little on the question of what the user may want to accomplish. Stephen Wey, writing for the charity At Dementia, puts this user-centered viewpoint as follows (Wey, 2007, 3): "try and think about how technology could be used to help a person achieve things they are finding harder to do. Or how it can raise their quality of life and the quality of their relationships."

In the United States, assistive technology use in education is a field that has a considerable history of focusing on empowering users to accomplish tasks independently, as federally mandated through the Individuals with Disabilities Education Act (IDEA). Several guidelines on assistive technology use in education deal with this question in an exemplary way, for example, the guidelines by the Virginia Department of Education (2008), Connecticut State Department of Education (2013), or Santa Clara Council (2013). A closer look at some of these guidelines may prove helpful for dealing with the question of how to better take user abilities into consideration in IAT development and use for people with dementia.

The text "Assistive Technology: A Framework for Consideration and Assessment" published by the Virginia Department of Education directly links assistive technology to the goal of allowing the student to participate and act independently (Virginia Department of Education, 2008, 4): "Technology is considered as assistive technology if the student with a disability would be less able or unable to independently participate in a task or independently access the resources in the environment relevant to his/her [Individualized Education Program] goals without the technology."

In the education-related guidelines mentioned previously, the focus is on assistive technologies to ensure that students with a disability receive a free and appropriate public education (FAPE). This includes supporting the user to achieve functional tasks required in schools such as writing and reading, helping the user meet common standards, facilitating active participation with same-age peers, and so forth. Overall, the guidelines serve to ensure that students with disabilities get the technological support they need to succeed in their educational context, to promote independence, to enhance feelings of self-worth, and to increase quality of life.

Assistive technology support is considered to be a very individual strategy oriented toward a specific individual. The Santa Clara County guidelines (2013, 5) describe a series of identification tasks whose goal is to help find out whether or not a student is in need of assistive technology devices or services. These include identifying the tasks the student performs or wants to perform but is unable to perform; identifying special strategies or accommodations the student avails himself or herself to complete tasks; describing available assistive technologies that could be used to support the student completing the tasks; describing new or additional technologies that could be tried; and transferring the decision to the student's Individualized Education Program. Starting from the question of which tasks the person wants to be able to complete, the Santa Clara County guidelines offers a structured approach to find a way to facilitate task completion. Remarkably, the guidelines offer elaborated and detailed resource guides and worksheets that help the team in decision making.

Furthermore, these guidelines consider ongoing reassessment of the students' assistive technology needs and of possible changes in the students' needs over time as very important (Virginia Department of Education 2008; Santa Clara County 2013).

The Virginia Department of Education Guidelines (2008, 9) recommend an interdisciplinary team to find out the needs of the user. In the educational context, the interdisciplinary team encompasses somebody who is familiar with the individual user, a teacher or similar person knowledgeable in the area of curriculum, a person experienced in the area of language, a person considering the motoric abilities, somebody representing the financial side and possibilities of implementation, and additional persons from other fields. The basic idea here is that the various relevant aspects of the user's life; his or her needs, wishes, and goals; and the familial environment and existing support options or possible difficulties are taken into consideration.

The need for individual assessment is also seen by various guidelines outside the field of education. For example, the RESNA Standards of Practice (2008) stress the role of assessment and consumer needs when they specify in paragraph 9: "Individuals shall verify consumer's needs by using direct assessment or evaluation procedures with the consumer." Directly relating to the use of assistive technology in dementia, Alzheimer Europe (2010b) underlines and discusses in detail the need for comprehensive and constant assessment. The organization recommends the establishment of a system to review the use of assistive technology and suggests, among other things, that the reviews should involve the views of the persons with dementia, caregivers, and professionals.

While there are undoubtedly a number of differences between assistive technology use in educational contexts and in dementia care, there are also considerable similarities. For persons with dementia, the focus is not to provide FAPE. Unlike in educational contexts, for persons with dementia there is not a list of tasks required, nor are there common standards to be fulfilled. However, what is relevant for persons with dementia is their ability to manage activities of everyday life as independently as possible; to actively participate in familial, cultural, and social life; and to counteract (possible future) loss of abilities and functions. What matters is to find out, together with the persons with dementia, what abilities they consider most important, what functions they want to uphold or achieve, and how IATs may help them achieve their goals.

As in the educational context, in assistive technology use in dementia the focus should be on the users' abilities and wishes- and on the tasks to be accomplished with the help of assistive technologies. To achieve this, a detailed assessment is necessary in each individual case of what kinds of abilities or activities reasonably can be expected to be supported or achieved with the help of assistive technologies.

Furthermore, detailed reassessments of user needs are required throughout the duration of IAT use. Reassessment of IAT needs over time allows caregivers, health professionals, and technology designers to find out about the person's views toward the technology, the usefulness of the devices in place, and possible changes over time that require technology adaptations.

An interdisciplinary team to assess user needs is also advisable for persons with dementia. It may be adequate to include medical practitioners, neurologists, caregivers, family members, physical therapists, speech therapists, assisted living representatives, and other persons.

Based on material developed in the educational context, for example, the Resource Guide and Worksheet included in the Santa Clara County guidelines (2013), it seems promising to consider developing similar resource guides and worksheets for IAT use for persons with dementia.

With a strategy like this in place, the focus of IAT use in dementia is less on avoiding risks or on finding easier or cheaper ways of handling individuals with dementia and more on the abilities and wishes of the individual users. It will also help to avoid mismatches between the user's needs and the technologies offered or the devices in place.

Technologies

Another central question is which type of technology to use and develop to best support the users' abilities and goals. Overall, authors agree that technology use is just one part of a broader approach and that customization is needed that carefully adapts the technology to every individual user.

A high-tech approach may not always be helpful as it may be very complex and complicated and may burden users more than it is useful. Sometimes lower-tech options that are easier to use and maintain and are less expensive may be preferable. This may prove especially true for persons with dementia, who due to their age may be more reluctant to use technology than members of younger generations. In several contexts, off-the-shelf items and basic assistive technology may prove sufficient, straightforward, and of avail. There may also be a need for more specialized devices and services.

Technologies that can be deployed by a broad spectrum of users and in various contexts seem particularly interesting and may offer various advantages. The concept underlying this type of technology is called "universal design." The Assistive Technology Act (2004, Sec. 3) defines "universal design" as follows:

> The term "universal design" means a concept or philosophy for designing and delivering products and services that are usable by people with the widest possible range of functional capabilities, which include products and services that are directly accessible (without requiring assistive technologies) and products and services that are interoperable with assistive technologies.

In the educational context, the Virginia Department of Education (2008, 5) stresses the need to consider accessibility during the planning phase and to make access features a built-in part of the overall design. This includes giving users multiple ways of acquiring information, multiple ways of expression, and multiple ways of engagement.

Seen from the perspective of universal design, flexibility is important. Technology that offers various input and output modes and multiple ways of using it is considered highly advantageous. Accordingly, intelligent assistive devices for use by persons with dementia should not aim at targeting a narrow population of adults with a more or less specific form or stage of dementia, but should be open to individuals of all ages, with all kinds of dementias, or with disabilities resulting from a broad spectrum of diseases. In view of this, it seems questionable whether devices designed so that they specifically target one form of dementia are needed at all.

Following this approach, instead of devising IATs that aim at targeting specific stages of Alzheimer's disease or specific symptoms of individuals with Alzheimer's disease, it is advisable to target a broader spectrum of people. This is in accordance with the findings of Marcello Ienca and colleagues (2017a), who reported in their review that most IAT devices were designed not exclusively for individuals with dementia but also for the general elderly population with neurocognitive disability. However, in contrast to the concept of universal design, Ienca et al. (2017a) consider this a disadvantage and suggest that devices designed for more specific target populations that selectively address specific stages of dementia would be more useful. They speculate that the lack of specificity of a considerable part of the IATs "could represent a significant obstacle toward the massive adoption of IATs for dementia and could add an additional reason to the limited uptake of IATs" (1336). The future will show which approach will be more successful. It seems plausible, however, not to aim to develop too many different devices and IATs for the various forms or stages of dementia but to devise IATs that can be flexibly used. This will also make things easier for users who will not have to adapt to different technologies at various times as the disease progresses.

In addition, there is a clear need for clinical validation of IATs. As Ienca et al. (2017a) found out in their systematic review of IAT for dementia, more than 50% of IATs for dementia are without clinical validation through clinical trials with human subjects. They concluded that studies assessing the clinical effectiveness and safety of IATs in various clinical and nonclinical contexts are urgently required.

A promising step in this direction was taken by Phil Joddrell and Peter Cudd (2015), who suggested and tested guidelines for evaluating digital technologies for people living with dementia. Central to their user-centered approach is to consider both the person living with dementia and the caregiver as users. These evaluation guidelines provide support for protocol preparation for studies evaluating digital technologies for people with dementia. The guidelines consist of 10 sections including "Background," "Consultation," "Funding," "Participants," "Duration," "Environment," "Outcome measures," "Ethics and consent," and "Method." Of particular interest here is the section "Consultation," which suggests establishing a consultation group to consider the needs of persons with dementia and to involve relatives, caregivers, and professionals in the design process. Overall, for researchers designing evaluation protocols, these guidelines may serve as a very helpful point for orientation.

Shaping the Process of IAT Development

As has been argued throughout this chapter, there is a clear need to better take into consideration user abilities and user perspectives in IAT development and use. This is in line with the concept of user-centered design, the importance of which several authors underline in the context of (intelligent) assistive technology development (Bharucha et al. 2009; Alzheimer Europe 2010b; Thorpe et al. 2016; Ienca et al. 2017a, 2017b). Bharucha et al. (2009, 8) characterize user-centered design as follows: "User Centered Design is a product development philosophy and multistage problem solving-process that aims to take into account user needs, preferences, and values upfront to optimize user acceptance of the end product."

While Thorpe et al. (2016) gave an example of a user-centered design approach, according to a review by Ienca and colleagues (2017a), only around 40% of current IATs in dementia were designed through a user-centered approach.

A related but broader approach has been developed at the European level by the European Commission, where the concept of "responsible research and innovation" has been coined to guide the technology innovation process. René von Schomberg (2013, 63) described the concept as follows:

> Responsible Research and Innovation is a transparent, interactive process by which societal actors and innovators become mutually responsive to each other with a view to the (ethical) acceptability, sustainability and societal desirability of the innovation process and its marketable products (in order to allow a proper embedding of scientific and technological advances in our society).

Central to this approach is the idea that the various stakeholders involved in the technology should participate in the development process. Concerning IATs in dementia, this should include persons with dementia, physicians, caregivers, and other healthcare providers actively involved in the technology development phase. Accordingly, they should have joint reflections on possible future uses of the technology in question, have users test the devices at early developmental stages and later on, and consider their feedback. Not least, this approach involves having a public debate about priorities of IAT use in dementia, values and ethical principles, financial costs, and social goals.

Furthermore, for professional associations, patient organizations, or other stakeholders involved in assistive technology and dementia, the act of devising guidelines and policies for the development and use of IATs in dementia may prove beneficial. It may help them shape the process based on fundamental ethical principles. The Assistive Technology Act (2004) gives a definition of consumer-responsive policies, which are consistent, among others, with the principles of respect for individual dignity, personal responsibility, self-determination, privacy, rights, and equal access of individuals with disabilities, as well as inclusion, integration, and full participation in society and support for the involvement of others, if such involvement is desired.

As exemplified with education-related guidelines, guidelines from adjacent fields of technology use may serve as a guide, when it comes both to reflecting on the central ethical issues to guide IAT development and use and to specifying detailed aspects of handling IATs. Some existing guidelines have been in place for several years. It may prove very beneficial to learn about their history, relevance, and usefulness in the respective fields and about experiences made with them. Not least, the process of designing guidelines and policies is a chance to have a debate about the guiding principles in IAT use and development.

Overall, a user-centered approach that better takes user abilities and perspectives into consideration may also help to strengthen practicability and attractiveness of IATs and may finally lead to an increase in user adoption. In spite of the broadly shared assumption that IATs can be beneficial to persons with dementia, user adoption seems rather low (Thorpe et al. 2016; Ienca et al. 2017a). Possible reasons for low user adoption may include resistance of older individuals to use technology, the impression that the devices currently available for persons with dementia are rather immature and do not really meet the needs of persons with dementia, the high costs of IATs, limited access to IATs, lack of awareness, and others.

While the hope has been expressed that the use of IAT in dementia will increase in the future (Ienca et al. 2017a), it is important not to aim at increasing technology use for the sake of increasing technology use. Neither should the primary motivation be to reduce healthcare-related costs. Instead, the focus should be directed to identifying ways IATs may support the abilities and needs of persons with dementia. The approach outlined in this chapter will help to find out how far and in which contexts IATs can serve to support persons with dementia and which types of IATs may be most useful, but it may also encourage stakeholders to think about what can be changed at the societal level.

Note

1. A related term, with a focus on an individual's direct living environment, is ambient assisted living technologies (AAL technologies) (cf. Novitzky et al. 2015).

References

Alzheimer Europe (2010a): The ethical issues linked to the use of assistive technology in dementia care—An ethical framework for making decisions linked to the use of AT: http://www.alzheimer-europe.org/Ethics/Ethical-issues-in-practice/2010-The-ethical-issues-linked-to-the-use-of-assistive-technology-in-dementia-care/An-ethical-framework-for-making-decisions-linked-to-the-use-of-AT

Alzheimer Europe (2010b): The ethical issues linked to the use of assistive technology in dementia care—Our guidelines and position on the ethical use of AT for/by people with dementia: http://www.alzheimer-europe.org/Ethics/Ethical-issues-in-practice/2010-The-ethical-issues-linked-to-the-use-of-assistive-technology-in-dementia-care/Our-guidelines-and-position-on-the-ethical-use-of-AT-for-by-people-with-dementia#fragment2

Alzheimer Europe (2010c): The ethical issues linked to the use of assistive technology in dementia care—AT, ethical issues and legislation: http://www.alzheimer-europe.org/Ethics/Ethical-issues-in-practice/2010-The-ethical-issues-linked-to-the-use-of-assistive-technology-in-dementia-care/AT-ethical-issues-and-legislation#fragment5

Assistive Technology Act (2004): H.R. 4278. https://www.govtrack.us/congress/bills/108/hr4278/text

Beauchamp, T.L., Childress, J.F. (2013): Principles of Biomedical Ethics, Seventh Edition, Oxford University Press.

Bharucha, A.J., Anand, V., Forlizzi, J., Dew, M.A., Reynolds III, C.F., Stevens, S., Wactlar, H. (2009): Intelligent assistive technology applications to dementia care: Current capabilities, limitations, and future challenges, American Journal of Geriatric Psychiatry 17(2): 88–104.

Connecticut State Department of Education (2013): Connecticut Assistive Technology Guidelines, http://www.sde.ct.gov/sde/lib/sde/pdf/publications/atguide/atguide.pdf

GBD 2015 Disease and Injury Incidence and Prevalence Collaborators (2016): Global, regional, and national incidence, prevalence, and years lived with disability for 310 diseases and injuries, 1990–2015: A systematic analysis for the Global Burden of Disease Study 2015, Lancet 388(10053): 1545–1602.

Hildt, E. (2006): Autonomie in der biomedizinischen Ethik. Genetische Diagnostik und selbstbestimmte Lebensgestaltung. Campus: Frankfurt/M.

Ienca, M., Jotterand, F., Elger, B., Caon, M., Pappagallo, A.S., Kressig, R.W., Wangmo, T. (2017a): Intelligent assistive technology for Alzheimer's disease and other dementias: A systematic review, Journal of Alzheimer's Disease 56: 1301–1340.

Ienca, M., Wangmo, T., Jotterand, F., Kressig, R.W., Elger, B. (2017b): Ethical design of intelligent assistive technologies for dementia: A descriptive review, Science and Engineering Ethics, published online: September 22, 2017; doi:10.1007/s11948-017-9976-1.

Joddrell, P., Cudd, P. (2015): Applying guidelines for evaluating digital technologies for people living with dementia: A case study, in: Sik-Lanyi, C. et al. (Eds.): Assistive Technology, IOS Press, 204–211.

Landau, R., Werner, S. (2012): Ethical aspects of using GPS for tracking people with dementia: Recommendations for practice, International Psychogeriatrics 24(3): 358–366.

Moga, D.C., Roberts, M., Jicha, G. (2017): Dementia for the primary care provider, Primary Care 44(3): 439–456.

Novitzky, P., Smeaton, A.F., Chen, C., Irving, K., Jacquemard, T., O'Brolchain, F., O'Mathuna, D., Gordijn, B. (2015): A review of contemporary work on the ethics of ambient assisted living technologies for people with dementia, Science and Engineering Ethics 21: 707–765.

Olsson, A., Engström, M., Skovdahl, K., Lampic, C. (2012): My, your and our needs for safety and security: Relatives' reflections on using information and communication technology in dementia care, Scandinavian Journal of Caring Sciences 26: 104–112.

Raz, J. (1986): The Morality of Freedom, Oxford University Press.

Rehabilitation Engineering and Assistive Technology Society of North America (RESNA) (2008): RESNA Standards of Practice for Assistive Technology Professionals, http://www.resna.org/sites/default/files/legacy/certification/Standards_of_Practice_final_10_10_08.pdf

Rehabilitation Engineering and Assistive Technology Society of North America (RESNA) (undated): RESNA Code of Ethics, http://www.resna.org/sites/default/files/legacy/certification/RESNA_Code_of_Ethics.pdf

Santa Clara County (2013): Santa Clara County Special Education Assistive Technology Guidelines and Resources, https://www.sccoe.org/depts/selpa/SELPA%20Doc%20Library/Assistive%20Technology%20Guidelines.pdf

Thorpe, J.R., Ronn-Andersen, K.V.H., Bien, P., Özkil, A.G., Forchhammer, B.H., Maier, A.M. (2016): Pervasive assistive technology for people with dementia: A UCD case, Healthcare Technology Letters 3(4): 297–302.

Virginia Department of Education (2008): Assistive Technology: A Framework for Consideration and Assessment, http://www.doe.virginia.gov/special_ed/iep_instruct_svcs/assistive_technology/framework_assistive_technology.pdf

von Schomberg, R. (2013). A vision of responsible research and innovation, in: Owen, R., Bessant, J., Heintz, M. (Eds.): Responsible Innovation: Managing the Responsible Emergence of Science and Innovation in Society, John Wiley, pp. 51–74.

Wey, S. (2007): The Ethical Use of Assistive Technology, AT Dementia, https://www.atdementia.org.uk/content_files/files/The_ethical_use_of_assistive_technology.pdf

PART III
ETHICAL AND REGULATORY IMPLICATIONS

9

Ethical Concerns About the Use of Assistive Technologies

How to Balance Beneficence and Respect for Autonomy in the Care of Dementia Patients

Bernice S. Elger

Introduction

Ethical concerns about the use of assistive technology for patients suffering from dementia (Alzheimer Europe 2010) have been discussed for more than two decades, with a particular focus on monitoring and tracking technologies (McShane et al. 1998; McShane, Hope, and Wilkinson 1994). McShane et al. (1994, 1274) claimed that "used in the right circumstances, such devices could enhance the liberty and safety of people with cognitive impairment from wandering off and getting lost." They criticized that the development of this type of assistive technology is "being held back because of ethical worries that the use of such devices would interfere with personal liberty and fears that adverse publicity might result." (McShane, Hope, and Wilkinson 1994, 1274)

Is ethics creating unethical barriers that deprive dementia patients of beneficial assistive technology? "What benefit will new technologies offer if they are inadequately or not used?" (Mahoney 2010, 66). Indeed, despite the fact that tracking technologies such as those relying on GPS have been widely implemented in other sectors and that monitoring technologies have been routinely used in hospitals, in particular in intensive care units, these assistive technologies are still the exception when it comes to the care of older people and dementia patients. For example, in a recent podium discussion between representatives of public health authorities, health care personnel in charge of homes for older persons, and gerontology experts in a rich European country with high technological standards (Prudente 2017), the invited experts stated that regional authorities are convinced that there is no role for more sophisticated assistive technologies in the care of older adult and dementia patients, except for wrist emergency buttons that a patient can press actively in the case of a fall or need for help for other reasons. Thus, the authorities expressed their more or less firm opposition to the routine use of other monitoring technologies such as sensors placed in private homes or care institutions for older adults that would signal whether a person is moving normally, opening the fridge door, eating, and so forth. Multiple reasons were mentioned for the lack of use of these assistive technologies. Beside privacy concerns, the most important seemed to be that assistive technologies are perceived as false incentives in society which encourage unethical trends of egoism and isolation instead of reinforcing social bonds and mutual helping, a feeling of responsibility for each other, and the search for a better-organized system of mutual care and support between different players in society, such as, for example, neighbors caring for each other or younger family members supporting older ones. Furthermore, the experts argued that most technologies increase the problems of monitoring rather than solving them. For example, the use of sensors posed the problem of a threshold for when a system should initiate an automatic alarm. A dementia patient at home who does not move could be sleeping or could have had a fall. After which lapse of time of lack of sensor-transmitted activities should formal or informal caregivers contact the patient? Contacting them after 2 hours might mean waking the patient too early, but it could also mean that the patient has been in pain for 2 hours after a fall. If the intervention after a fall is not immediately started, it could even mean that a patient who could have been rescued by an early intervention instead dies from a treatable medical complication. Video surveillance of the entire surroundings might be of help but would not solve the problem of defining alarm thresholds. The reluctance of public health authorities to invest in or recommend technologies seemed thus to rely on the conclusion that technologies are costly without sufficient evidence that they improve the quality of life of patients or their caregivers, while bringing with them an ethically wrong incentive to neglect human interactions in a society that can find more "human" alternatives to care for older patients with cognitive and physical limitations. One should favor those alternatives, according to the public health specialist, because they have additional emotional benefits by reinforcing mutual help and human interactions. The invited assistive technology specialist argued that such reluctance might be due to the fact that public health decision makers lack experience with the technologies and that there is an ethical imperative to inform all involved stakeholders about the different technologies to enable them to choose whether they use it or not.

It is widely recognized that knowledge about available assistive technologies is rather limited among formal and informal caregivers for dementia patients (Ienca et al. 2018; Malinowsky, Rosenberg, and Nygard 2014; Newton et al. 2016). To avoid unjustified generalization and rejection, it is important to examine the ethical issues raised by distinct types of existing technologies in more detail, in order to obtain a more nuanced judgment about whether public health authorities and health care personnel should inform about them, offer patients and their informal caregivers more choice, or even actively recommend some of them. The present chapter will focus on four examples of assistive technologies that, despite having been available for some time and being relatively simple to use, are not widely implemented: memory aid technology, "smart dresser" devices designed to help dementia patients with getting dressed, GPS tracking devices, and sensors to monitor patients in their private homes, such as an intelligent wireless sensor system (IWSS) for the rapid detection of health issues (Cohen, Kampel, and Verloo 2016). The first two technologies are chosen as examples for "aid" technology where the risk of harm is very low compared to significant benefits for patients, caregivers, and society. The second two are chosen because of their ethically relevant characteristic of control: their aim is to enable patient surveillance and monitoring. The ethical issues related to these technologies will be discussed and conclusions drawn concerning the appropriate balance between beneficence (and nonmaleficence) and respect for patient autonomy.

The present ethical discussion aims to show that it is important to clearly distinguish among distinct types of technologies and to avoid unethical barriers that may result from "ethical contamination" of one type of technology by the controversies related to others.

Balancing Beneficence and Respect for Autonomy

Dementia prevalence is increasing with age (Charness, Best, and Souders 2012). The group of patients who could benefit from various assistive technologies thus consists of two significantly overlapping populations: older adults and patients suffering from dementia. We will refer to both without particular distinction. When we address benefits for "aging adults," it will be implied that this means those older adults who experience at least some cognitive or some physical impairment due to age interfering with their abilities to carry out activities of daily living (ADLs).

In principle, assistive technologies do not raise fundamentally new ethical issues.

> Exercising control over elderly people with dementia seems to be necessary and may be the best way to ensure wellbeing. Faced with the social and economic burdens of an aging population, if monitoring systems advance further understandings of dementia, help caregivers manage their responsibilities, and keep the elderly safe, how concerned should the public be about issues that have

always plagued caregiving relations—control, privacy, autonomy, and power asymmetries? (Kenner 2008, 266)

What is needed for any type of assistive technology is a thorough evaluation of its benefits and risks in order to carry out an evidence-based balancing between beneficence and respect for autonomy for each type of use.

Before discussing appropriate ways to balance beneficence and respect for autonomy, it is important to examine more closely the definition of "benefit." As shown earlier, different concepts are used to refer to the benefit of three types of stakeholders: patients, their caregivers, and society. Autonomous persons (in legal terminology, competent persons) have the right to define what they consider beneficial. They might value quality of life higher than safety and accept risks to a variable extent to increase quality of life. For example, some older, somewhat cognitively impaired patients might prefer (at a moment when they are legally competent to make this decision) to take long walks outside and risk getting lost or being run over by a car. By contrast, their caregivers might give a higher value to safety than quality of life because they feel at fault if the person for which they feel responsible is harmed during an outside walk. In this and other examples, the well-being of caregivers might conflict with the well-being of patients. Benefit for society is most often measured in financial costs, for example, the burden of care to the health care system and individual households, and less often in moral costs, referring among other things to the preservation of important ethical values and the encouragement of morally prized types of behavior.

It should be noted that we understand the discussion on benefit to include the principles of both beneficence and nonmaleficence. The understanding is that harm to persons will diminish their well-being and thus reduce the balance of overall benefit.

Respect for autonomy consists of autonomy rights related to physical and mental integrity as well as privacy rights related to health data and information about behavior. These rights are strongly protected by the European Parliament and in international human rights law, which has been ratified by many countries (Council of Europe 1950; Council of Europe 1997a, 1997b; European Parliament 1995, 2016; United Nations (1948), and there are only a few exceptions that must all be specified by legal dispositions (see, e.g., Swiss penal code Art. 321).

Most current democracies have been significantly influenced by anti-paternalistic philosophy:

The only purpose for which power can be rightfully exercised over any member of a civilized community, against his will, is to prevent harm to others. His own good, either physical or moral, is not a sufficient warrant. He cannot rightfully be compelled to do or forbear because it will be better for him to do so, because it will make him happier, because, in the opinions of others, to do so would be wise, or even right. These are good reasons for remonstrating with him, or reasoning with him, or persuading him, or entreating him, but not for compelling him, or visiting him with any evil in case he do otherwise.

It is justified to use control and coercion to avoid harm to others, but autonomous people should not be coerced for their own good or any other good. The latter would represent unjustified paternalism, which has been strongly criticized in modern bioethics (Elger 1995, 1998a, 1998b, 2010; Elger and Chevrolet 2000).

Some authors distinguish between hard paternalism and soft paternalism (den Hartogh 2016; Elger 2010; Gostin and Gostin 2009; Hill 2017; Rajczi 2016). Hard paternalism refers to coercion of competent people and is in principle never justified, while soft paternalism (i.e., exercising control over patients suffering from impaired decision-making capacity) can be justified under certain conditions (e.g., to avoid harm to others) (Elger 2010).

When discussing ethical issues related to assistive technologies and balancing beneficence and respect for autonomy, we will therefore distinguish whether they are used to avoid harm to others or harm to the patients themselves (paternalistic avoidance of harm). It is also particularly important to note that decision-making capacity in patients suffering from dementia can fluctuate over short time periods and, in particular in mild to moderate dementia, will by definition differ at the same time point according to each single decision to be made. Thus, except in the early stages of dementia, giving predominance to autonomy by relying on informed consent will not solve the ethical issues of justifying or not various degrees of soft paternalism later in the disease. To justify soft paternalistic uses in the majority of cases, it is necessary to reflect on the balancing of beneficence and respect for autonomy. In addition, when evaluating benefit, one must take into account that overriding preferences of incompetent patients comes with costs on their well-being and quality of life, as most people will react adversely to any type of coercion.

Low-Risk Technology

Given the low risk and promising benefit profile of memory aid and memory training devices as well as "smart dresser" devices, it is surprising that they are not routinely recommended and more widely implemented.

Memory Aid and Memory Training Devices

It is well known that an age-related decline exists for certain subtypes of memory functions. This is one of the reasons dementia prevalence increases with age. In particular, episodic and working memory processes are prone to

age-related decline. Other subtypes show significantly less decline, such as semantic, procedural, and meta-memory (Charness, Best, and Souders 2012).
Even in the absence of a diagnosis of dementia, older patients may suffer from
age-related "normal" memory decline: prospective memory failures interfere
with daily functioning, and retrospective memory decline represents a loss
of their social embeddedness and self-definition and decreases quality of life
(Haslam et al. 2011; Iyer and Jetten 2011; Jetten et al. 2010). Loss of memory can
be mitigated using mnemonics training, which may or may not use any technological devices. In addition, a number of low- and high-tech external devices
exist to help patient compensate for memory failures. The effectiveness and reliability of many of these devices have been tested and are promising (Charness,
Best, and Souders 2012). However, the most recent systematic review shows
that sample sizes of studies are too often very small, resulting in limited generalizability of the findings. In addition, studies are rarely carried out in users'
home environments, and outcomes for users, in particular, improved daily
functioning, quality of life, or social connectedness, are not addressed (King
and Dwan 2017).

The lack of widely generalizable research findings on the outcome of such
devices is regrettable but would not as such present an ethical barrier. This is
the case because the probability of any risk from using these devices is low.
Thus, from an ethical point of view, respect for autonomy of patients and their
caregivers would mean that health professionals should routinely explain the existence of these technologies to enable patients and families to make an informed
choice, at least in the case of low-cost, low-technology devices (Charness, Best,
and Souders 2012), where economic harm is minor. Other relevant harmful
consequences are related to stigma. Any visible aids signal to others that a person
suffers from a disability (e.g., needing a wheelchair or a hearing or memory aid).
Concerning memory aids, this harm can clearly be minimized through the design of the devices.

"Smart Dresser" Devices

Dementia interferes with self-care abilities of patients and affects, among other
things, the multiple daily tasks of dressing and undressing. The difficulties related to dressing are a recognized source of conflict between patients and their
informal caregivers in different cultural backgrounds (Mahoney, Coon, and
Lozano 2016a) and are known to present a major stressor for both (Mahoney
et al. 2015): "Caregivers voiced the need for tangible dressing assistance to reduce their frustration from time spent in repetitive cueing and power struggles
over dressing" (Mahoney et al. 2015, 345).

Tasks such as dressing can be a significant source of humiliation and privacy interference to patients because they feel infantilized for not being able to carry out such a basic task or stigmatized if they are seen by others in inappropriate clothing (Mahoney, Coon, and Lozano 2016a). Assistive technology that helps patients dress themselves (Mahoney et al. 2016b) can significantly reduce stress. This type of assistive technology has a clear benefit in that it enhances the privacy of dementia patients related to dressing (Mahoney et al. 2015; Mahoney, Coon, and Lozano 2016a). Indeed, privacy is known to be a major critical concern to older adults (Yusif, Soar, and Hafeez-Baig 2016).

Similarly to memory aid assistive technologies, although evidence-based data on the outcomes of "smart dresser" devices are even more limited than in the case of the former, it is quite obvious that the risks of harm are very low, while the potential for benefit is noteworthy.

Balancing Beneficence and Respect for Autonomy in Low-Harm Assistive Technologies

Dementia patients, similar to other vulnerable groups of patients suffering from diseases where effective treatments are absent, are at risk of exploitation by those who profit from selling unproven treatments. They and their families might spend significant resources on treatments with marginal or without proven benefits. However, at present there seems to be an ethically unjustified way of prioritizing some treatments over others: although current medications for the treatment of dementia are known to only marginally alleviate some of the symptoms (e.g., by enhancing cholinergic signaling) without any curative effects, they are widely prescribed (Hung and Fu 2017) and represent significant costs to patients and/or society (e.g., in the case of treatments reimbursed by society). Similar to existing medications, the assistive technologies described previously are noncurative but relieve symptoms, acting as a form of prosthesis that replaces brain functions such as dressing abilities and defective memory (Novitzky et al. 2015). These assistive technologies can be a lot less costly and present higher benefits than existing medications but are less widely used in spite of this ethically more favorite profile of risks and benefits. One of the reasons to provide medical treatment routinely but neglect low-risk assistive technologies could be that deprivation of medication is perceived as a lack of appropriate care, while the use of assistive technologies is less associated with the idea of medical care and judged rather to represent some form of superfluous or futuristic technological "gewgaw." Thorough ethical analysis can help to point out the lack of justification to prioritize medication over nonpharmaceutical prosthetic aids. There is no ethical reason to invest resources predominantly in one form of treatment if the harm-benefit ratios are similar. There is a clear ethical imperative to invest similar amounts of resources in research to improve the evidence about benefits of both medication and low-risk assistive technologies. It is also clearly ethically inappropriate to disrespect or conceal patients' and their representatives' and informal caregivers' autonomy by not informing them about these existing technologies.

Finally, low-risk assistive technologies such as memory aids and "smart dresser" technologies illustrate not only that it is possible to minimize harm and increase well-being of patients but also that beneficence and respect for autonomy are not necessarily in conflict but rather maximize each other as respect for patient choices will increase the benefits gained from use of the devices.

Surveillance and Monitoring Technologies

In contrast to the low-risk technologies discussed previously, surveillance and monitoring technologies present additional types of harm. While the technology as such, that is, GPS and wireless sensors, is of low physical risk, it presents significant interference with privacy and may be physically and mentally intrusive to a variable degree, as well as dangerous in some instances because of false-positive and false-negative signals or interpretations of signals. Violation of privacy, as well as intrusiveness, varies depending on which data are measured, transmitted, and stored and where the device is placed. Examples of these devices are sensors placed within a room (i.e. at some bodily distance), wearable devices such as GPS bracelets, and implantable GPS or other similarly placed sensors (Foster and Jaeger 2008). The interference with privacy, although it does not directly result in physical harm, has to be taken seriously. If—as we argued earlier—the most important ethical priority is to not cause avoidable harm to persons living with dementia, such as harm inflicted by insufficiently tested treatments, and as patients place a high value on privacy (Yusif, Soar, and Hafeez-Baig 2016), there is a significant obligation to focus on these risks. That means in particular that we must evaluate very carefully technologies at high risk of invading privacy (Mulvenna et al. 2017).

GPS Tracking of Dementia Patients

GPS tracking devices have possible benefits: they can enhance the safety of people with cognitive impairment and avoid harm if the patient or resident wanders off and gets lost (McShane, Hope, and Wilkinson 1994). The devices could also increase liberty because the alternative, in order to maintain safety, would be to either keep patients locked in safe environments such as their home or specially designed institutions or to only let them go out if they are accompanied by a caregiver. Both alternatives interfere with patient autonomy to move around, and the latter could be perceived as interfering with patient privacy as they are constantly observed. GPS, on the other hand, is less privacy invading as it only monitors location.

GPS bracelets may cause psychological harm because they can be associated with stigma and loss of dignity. For example, it has been pointed out that, besides constituting an unacceptable intrusion on the privacy of the wearer, they affect dignity because adult patients are treated like children and criminals (Eltis 2005; Hughes et al. 2008; Sandman and Heintz 2014).

There seems to be some evidence indicating that "cognitively intact older people favor the idea of tracking people with dementia. . . . They value the safety of people with dementia above preserving their autonomy" (Landau et al. 2010a, 1301, see also Landau et al. 2010b) Studies have tried to evaluate whether privacy concerns are lower in older people and seem to indicate that "older adults are generally less concerned than younger cohorts about privacy related to information . . . and specifically health information" (Charness et al. 2016, 5, see also Beach et al. 2009), although this effect was more pronounced in men than in women. While "older males indicated greater comfort with privacy related issues compared to younger and middle-aged males and all females . . . [t]here were no age or cohort trends discovered in females" (Charness, Best, and Evans 2016, 237).

In line with the rejection of paternalism, using tracking devices without explicit consent to prevent harm to others can be justified by the harm principle, but not by referring to beneficence to patients themselves (the latter would amount to unjustified paternalism if legally competent patients were willing to accept this harm). Wandering dementia patients rarely present a threat to others, except if they are prone to unusual behavior such as setting fire to things or if they drive cars and do not have appropriate cognitive abilities. Thus, the main justification for using these devices in incompetent dementia patients is paternalistic. The most frequently used way to justify their use is to make sure autonomy is respected by obtaining some form of real-time, advance, or proxy consent. "The decision whether, when and how to use GPS for tracking people with dementia should be made at the time of diagnosis jointly by the person with dementia, his/her family and professional caregivers. This decision should be made in formal structured meetings facilitated by a professional team" (Landau and Werner 2012, 358).

If proxy consent is used, it is important to remember that the balancing of beneficence with respect of autonomy does not depend only on individual balancing preferences, but is—in the same individual—influenced by emotional closeness and feelings of responsibility.[1] Relatives and healthcare personnel prefer nonpaternalistic attitudes toward themselves if they are asked to imagine themselves in the role of patients. If both nonpatients and healthcare personnel are asked how they think their relatives or patients should be treated if they suffer from dementia, both groups tend to justify significantly more paternalistic attitudes toward the patients than themselves (Elger 1998a, 2010; Johnson, Bouman, and Pinner 2000; Marzanski 2000a, 2000b). These studies indicate that the perception of what is ethically appropriate is influenced by some form of human "reflex" depending on the degree of perceived responsibility for others. This human reflex is mainly a feeling of responsibility and concern to care for relatives of patients and, in some cases—but generally much rarer and depending on the country (more frequently in the United States)—fear of litigation. This "responsibility reflex" has been confirmed in studies implying caregivers. Indeed, a more recent study suggests that

> caregivers' views change according to the locus of responsibility of the caregivers for the safety of people with dementia. The caregivers give preference to patients' safety more than autonomy when they are responsible for the patients. When the patients are under the responsibility of other caregivers, they give preference to patients' autonomy more than their safety. (Landau et al. 2010a)

Intelligent Wireless Sensor Systems for the Rapid Detection of Health Issues

Various terms exist to refer to different kinds of IWSSs. The simplest forms of sensors detect movement in a patient's home, opening of refrigerator doors, or the quantity and quality of food contained in refrigerators. This permits "tele-caregivers" to detect from a distance whether the patient presents health problems, for example, has suffered from a fall (Cohen, Kampel, and Verloo 2016, 2017), or might be at risk for hospital admission (Boumendjel et al. 2000). While some use abbreviations such as IWSSs to describe such sensors (Cohen, Kampel, and Verloo 2016, 2017), others refer to "telecare" (Mitseva et al. 2012) or "video surveillance" devices (Mulvenna et al. 2017), which fulfill similar purposes. Existing studies and experience from different countries (see "Introduction") confirm that public health authorities and caregivers for aging patients are reluctant to implement such intelligent sensor systems in patients' homes and care institutions (Cohen, Kampel, and Verloo 2017; Prudente 2017). Preference is clearly given to wearable emergency call devices where a patient has to press a button to call for help. Attitudes expressed by caregivers in a recent study seem to indicate that reluctance diminishes when used in care of more advanced dementia patients (quote from interviewee 5 from this study):

> For me, the only type of case where the IWSS would be useful, would be with an Alzheimer patient who doesn't know that he has to push his button anymore; with a person who doesn't know how to ask for help. (Cohen, Kampel, and Verloo 2017)

A recent review indicates that there

> is no evidence that smart homes and home health monitoring technologies help address disability prediction and health-related quality of life, or fall prevention.... The level of technology readiness for smart homes and home health monitoring technologies is still low. The highest level of evidence found was in a study that supported home health technologies for use in monitoring activities of daily living, cognitive decline, mental health, and heart conditions in older adults with complex needs. (Liu et al. 2016, 44)

Even more than GPS tracking devices, such intelligent sensors interfere significantly with privacy as they record sensitive information about patient activities and health. Among the older adult participants in the Intelligent Systems for Assessment of Aging Changes (ISAAC) study carried out by the Oregon Center for Aging and Technology (ORCATECH) who were questioned about their attitudes toward home sensor systems, a

> majority (60%) reported concerns related to privacy or security; these concerns increased after one year of participation. Few differences between participants with MCI [mild cognitive impairment] and those with normal cognition were identified. Findings suggest that involvement in this unobtrusive in-home monitoring study may have raised awareness about the potential privacy risks of technology. (Boise et al. 2013, 428)

Given this increased risk of harm to privacy, the lack of robust generalizable and reliable data on benefits and harms weighs more heavily in the benefit-harm balance for sensors and tracking devices than for the low-risk assistive technologies discussed earlier. Similarly, as for GPS sensors, paternalistic arguments are not sufficient to justify the use of these systems against the wishes of patients. However, they might be justified to prevent harm to others, that is, if the aim is to detect resident-to-resident violence associated with dementia (Sifford and Bharucha 2010).

If robust data on benefits and harms are lacking, the willingness to use devices will depend on subjective evaluations. Studies have shown that acceptance of monitoring devices varies widely. Cohen found low to moderate acceptability of IWSSs: informal caregivers were more satisfied than were patients (Cohen, Kampel, and Verloo 2016). In another study, one-third of elderly participants agreed that they would "feel invaded by technology" and that "the equipment would be in the way in the home".

> They used terms that suggested the system would "see them" and "know about their personal activities" despite repeated assurance it could not. . . . The majority of the participants (67%) expressed concerns that their privacy would be lost, with "big brother" watching them (50%). Moreover, concerns that their relatives would find home monitoring intrusive predominated, with 100% agreeing with this statement. (Mahoney 2010, 72)

Another study demonstrated that satisfaction with telecare was generally good. The study setting offered telecare for elderly persons (EPs) with cognitive impairments and their informal caregivers (ICGs) in the form of "intelligent home support services" and involved regions from four European countries. In a controlled setting, a long-term pilot-controlled study was carried out in real-life conditions. Acceptance of the technology and the services and quality-of-life outcomes that resulted from utilizing the services appeared to be promising in this study. The authors note that

> during the whole process of piloting the services in real life, we observed that even when EPs and ICGs were skeptical in the beginning, after giving them time to get used to the technology, the older adults and their relatives accept the technology and can see the opportunities for positive impact. (Mitseva et al. 2012, 16)

They underline the importance of involving patients early in their disease progress: "Since the targeted population have cognitive impairments or mild dementia, we found that it is most beneficial if the services are introduced as early in the disease progression as possible and it takes about 4–6 weeks for EP to get used to the system" (Mitseva et al. 2012, 16).

Older interviewees in another qualitative study were willing to balance beneficence and autonomy rights in favor of safety. If it was made clear to them that they were not able to function independently at home anymore, they were willing to use assistive sensor technology to stay at home and not lose their independence. "For elders, it is at that nexus point that activity-monitoring technology became the preferred means to reduce family and building-staff safety concerns and prolong their aging-in-place. Residents were willing to trade-off privacy for protection—protection of their independence" (Mahony 2010, 72, see also Mahoney and Goc 2009).

Finally, it should be taken into account that privacy-related harms caused by these assistive technologies can be reduced by careful design (Ontario Information & Privacy Commissioners 2011) and policies limiting data storage. The abuse of data by those who should not have access can be limited if data are available for real-time monitoring, where data can be "automatically analyzed to set alerts when parameters move out of range, and also viewed by a primary care provider," but are not stored (Charness, Best, and Evans 2016; Charness et al. 2013).

Balancing Beneficence and Respect for Autonomy in Intelligent Assistive Technologies Used for Tracking and Monitoring

Assistive technologies used for tracking and monitoring promise benefits but are associated with higher possible risks than external memory aids and "smart dresser" devices. The balancing between risks and benefits, as well as between beneficence and autonomy, is more difficult to carry out because individual preferences for balancing may vary significantly. A major argument against all forms of telecare is that it leads to less human contact and more isolation (Sorell and Draper 2012), independently of privacy risks. Indeed, there could be a risk that telecare is used based on unfair discrimination, for example, only for those patients who lack family or friend caregivers or depending on patients' wealth (although it is not clear whether wealthier patients prefer to buy expensive technology or rather pay human caregivers). However, even in the worst-case scenario that telecare adds significant privacy risks because telecare data are hacked and used for unlawful purposes, it remains questionable whether—besides subjectively variable negative feelings related to shame and stigmatization and discrimination of patients based on their disease—strong tangible harms can be expected.[2] Thus, there seems to be no justification to recommend use of these technologies routinely, but there is equally no justification not to inform patients and caregivers about their existence as this information will increase their choices about how to organize care.

The argument that the use of such devices will discourage society from finding alternative care options that rely on human resources is valid but difficult to evaluate in a long-term perspective based on consequentialist evaluations. If the demographic changes and increases of life expectancy continue, there could be more patients living with cognitive impairments than persons available to care for them. Of course, not all people with cognitive impairments need care, and cognitive impairments as such should not be used as an excuse to treat all older people the same and to monitor them. Given this context, it is clearly ethically preferable to carry out much-needed outcome research on assistive technologies now to be able to make informed choices when such a point is reached where human care is not sufficiently available.

In the meantime, it is important to increase efforts to minimize harm of these technologies and to avoid decision making under direct or indirect pressure. The latter occurs when patients feel they need to accept the use of technologies against their original preferences because otherwise they become a burden to society or their relatives. It also occurs when patients are forced to leave their homes if they refuse technology. Indeed, rational individuals have the right to be left alone. They might prefer to stay at home without technologies and take increased risks that might shorten their lives, and they also have a right to die in peace (Delgado Fontaneda and Lopez Sainz 2009).

As long as decisions are clearly in line with competent patients' wishes and their advance directives and there is no harm to others, there is no justification for paternalism in our present legal and ethical frameworks.

Conclusions

The use of assistive technologies for patients with cognitive impairments including dementia raises a number of important ethical issues.

Balancing between risks and benefits and between beneficence and respect for autonomy can only be done if all stakeholders are sufficiently informed. This is at present not the case, neither among possible users nor among professional caregivers. As explained earlier, studies have shown that a number of factors influence judgments, such as being introduced to technologies early in the disease (more favorable attitudes) rather than late, the existence of prejudices, and whether a person is the patient or the caregiver or relative who feels responsibility for the patient. These possible biases influence decision making and balancing and must therefore be made more transparent.

Another bias could be an "all or nothing" assumption by public authorities or caregivers in favor of or against introduction of assistive technologies, instead of selected use of it where appropriate. Indeed, it is clearly unethical (a) *not to* carefully distinguish different types of assistive technologies and (b) *not to* examine each of them and the specific context of use separately. The balancing is highly specific for each device: dignity and privacy can be maintained and are even increased with some assistive technologies such as smart dresser devices. Indeed, there are assistive technologies where the balance of risks and harms is clearly favorable. It would be unethical not to recommend memory training and not to use external memory devices in dementia patients because increasing patient decline is predictable, there is no hope of durable improvement, and thus the investment of technology does not have sustainable benefits.

For the same reasons, it is unethical to reject all technologies for fear of discouraging mutual human care interactions and isolating patients. The discussed assistive technologies may provide additional benefits and benefit could be maximized when they are combined with direct human interventions.

Finally, the question remains as to which technology is a medical device and which is not. There is a risk to medicalize problems that represent individual or social lifestyle choices. Whether medical or not, to make ethical choices, better knowledge about benefits and harms of technology is a *must*. As it is possible to reduce harms, including privacy harms, by further testing and improving assistive technologies, an ethical imperative exists to encourage more empirical and ethical research in this field.

Notes

1. We presume here that most relatives and healthcare personnel want to truly care for the aging or demented patients. There could of course be conflicts of interests and erroneous perceptions—some relatives might wish to preserve an estate or simply like control of an older person or make an erroneous assumption about his or her abilities.
2. If it is feared that telecare data could be used by criminals to break into houses or drain estates, one should keep in mind that those criminals usually get enough information on who is at home from simple outside observations. Telecare data could be used to enhance security by linking them to security personnel of a neighborhood or special housing areas.

References

Alzheimer Europe (2010), "Ethical issues linked to the use of specific forms of AT": http://www.alzheimer-europe.org/Ethics/Ethical-issues-in-practice/2010-The-ethical-issues-linked-to-the-use-of-assistive-technology-in-dementia-care/Ethical-issues-linked-to-the-use-of-specific-forms-of-AT#fragment1 (accessed January 12, 2017).

Beach, S., et al. (2009), "Disability, age, and informational privacy attitudes in quality of life technology applications: results from a national web survey," *ACM Transactions on Accessible Computing*, 2 (1), 1–21.

Boise, L., et al. (2013), "Willingness of older adults to share data and privacy concerns after exposure to unobtrusive in-home monitoring," *Gerontechnology*, 11 (3), 428–35.

Boumendjel, N., et al. (2000), "Refrigerator content and hospital admission in old people," *Lancet*, 356 (9229), 563.

Charness, N., Best, R., and Souders, D. (2012), "Memory function and supportive technology," *Gerontechnology*, 11 (1), 1–20.

Charness, N., Best, R., and Evans, J. (2016), "Supportive home health care technology for older adults: attitudes and implementation," *Gerontechnology,* 15 (4), 233–42.

Charness, N., et al. (2013), "Metrics for assessing the reliability of a telemedicine remote monitoring system," *Telemed J E Health,* 19 (6), 487–92.

Cohen, C., Kampel, T., and Verloo, H. (2016), "Acceptability of an intelligent wireless sensor system for the rapid detection of health issues: findings among home-dwelling older adults and their informal caregivers," *Patient Prefer Adherence,* 10, 1687–95.

Cohen, C., Kampel, T., and Verloo, H. (2017), "Acceptability among community health-care nurses of intelligent wireless sensor-system technology for the rapid detection of health issues in home-dwelling older adults," *Open Nurs J,* 11, 54–63.

Council of Europe. (1950), "The European Convention on Human Rights": http://www. echr.coe.int/Documents/Convention_ENG.pdf (accessed June 10, 2016). German translation: http://www.echr.coe.int/NR/rdonlyres/F45A65CD-38BE-4FF7-8284- EE6C2BE36FB7/0/Convention_DEU.pdf (accessed June 20, 2012).

Council of Europe. "Convention for the Protection of Human Rights and Dignity of the Human Being with Regard to the Application of Biology and Medicine: Convention on Human Rights and Biomedicine": https://rm.coe.int/CoERMPublicCommonSear chServices/DisplayDCTMContent?documentId=090000168007cf98 (accessed June 10, 2016).

Council of Europe. "Recommendation No.R(97) 5 on the protection of medical data of the Committee of Ministers to member states (13 February 1997)": http://www.coe. int/t/dghl/standardsetting/dataprotection/legal_instruments_en.asp (accessed June 5, 2016).

Delgado Fontaneda, A. J., and Lopez Sainz, M. I. (2009), "[Ethical and legal problems in severe dementia. The right to die in peace]," *Rev Esp Geriatr Gerontol,* 44 Suppl 2, 43–47.

den Hartogh, G. (2016), "Do we need a threshold conception of competence?," *Med Health Care Philos,* 19 (1), 71–83.

Elger, B. S. (1995), "L'information du patient oncologique dans un service de médecine interne," *Cahiers médico-sociaux,* 39 (4), 391–400.

Elger, B. S. (1998a), "Le concept de paternalisme—aspects éthiques et philosophiques." Thèse de doctorat à la Faculté de Médecine, Genève.

Elger, B. S. (1998b), "Protectionnisme versus l'autonomie bien dosée: quel est le meilleur intérêt de l'adolescent? Controverse en éthique sur le thème de 'La médecine prédictive et les enfants,'" *Médecine et Hygiène,* 56, 485–90.

Elger, B. S. (2010), *Le paternalisme médical: mythe ou réalité? Aspects philosophiques et empiriques d'un phénomène persistant* (Geneva: Editions Médecine & Hygiène).

Elger, B. S., and Chevrolet, J. C. (2000), "Beneficence today, or autonomy (maybe) to-morrow?," *Hastings Cent Rep,* 30 (1, Jan–Feb), 18–19.

Eltis, K. (2005), "Predicating dignity on autonomy? The need for further inquiry into the ethics of tagging and tracking dementia patients with GPS technology," *Elder Law J,* 13, 387–411.

European Parliament. (1995), "Directive 95/46/EC of the European Parliament and of the Council of October 24, 1995": http://eur-lex.europa.eu/legal-content/EN/TXT/ ?uri=URISERV%3Al14012 (accessed June 4, 2016).

European Parliament. (2016), "Protection of Personal Data. Reform of Data Protection Rules in the EU": http://ec.europa.eu/justice/data-protection/index_en.htm and http://

eur-lex.europa.eu/legal-content/EN/TXT/?uri=uriserv:OJ.L_.2016.119.01.0089.01. ENG&toc=OJ:L:2016:119:TOC (accessed June 15, 2016).

Foster, K. R., and Jaeger, J. (2008), "Ethical implications of implantable radiofrequency identification (RFID) tags in humans," *Am J Bioeth,* 8 (8), 44–48.

Gostin, L. O., and Gostin, K. G. (2009), "A broader liberty: J.S. Mill, paternalism and the public's health," *Public Health,* 123 (3), 214–21.

Haslam, C., et al. (2011), "'I remember therefore I am, and I am therefore I re-member': exploring the contributions of episodic and semantic self-knowledge to strength of identity," *Br J Psychol,* 102 (2), 184–203.

Hill, A. (2017), "Why nudges coerce: experimental evidence on the architecture of regulation," *Sci Eng Ethics,* 24 (4), 1279–95.

Hughes, J. C., et al. (2008), "Ethical issues and tagging in dementia: a survey," *J Ethics Ment Health,* 3 (1), 1–6.

Hung, S. Y., and Fu, W. M. (2017), "Drug candidates in clinical trials for Alzheimer's disease," *J Biomed Sci,* 24 (1), 47.

Ienca, M., et al. (2018), "Health professionals' views on intelligent assistive technology for dementia and elderly care." *Gerontechnology,* 17(3), 139–50.

Iyer, A., and Jetten, J. (2011), "What's left behind: identity continuity moderates the effect of nostalgia on well-being and life choices," *J Pers Soc Psychol,* 101 (1), 94–108.

Jetten, J., et al. (2010), "Declining autobiographical memory and the loss of identity: effects on well-being," *J Clin Exp Neuropsychol,* 32 (4), 408–16.

Johnson, H., Bouman, W. P., and Pinner, G. (2000), "On telling the truth in Alzheimer's disease: a pilot study of current practice and attitudes," *Int Psychogeriatr,* 12 (2), 221–29.

Kenner, A. M. (2008), "Securing the elderly body: dementia, surveillance, and the politics of aging in place," *Surveillance & Society Journal,* 5 (3), 252–69.

King, A. C., and Dwan, C. (2017), "Electronic memory aids for people with dementia experiencing prospective memory loss: a review of empirical studies", *Dementia (London),* 1471301217735180 [Epub ahead of print].

Landau, R., and Werner, S. (2012), "Ethical aspects of using GPS for tracking people with dementia: recommendations for practice," *Int Psychogeriatr,* 24 (3), 358–66.

Landau, R., et al. (2010a), "What do cognitively intact older people think about the use of electronic tracking devices for people with dementia? A preliminary analysis," *Int Psychogeriatr,* 22 (8), 1301–9.

Landau, R., et al. (2010b), "Families' and professional caregivers' views of using advanced technology to track people with dementia," *Qual Health Res,* 20 (3), 409–19.

Liu, L., et al. (2016), "Smart homes and home health monitoring technologies for older adults: a systematic review," *Int J Med Inform,* 91, 44–59.

Mahoney, D. F. (2010), "An evidence-based adoption of technology model for remote monitoring of elders' daily activities," *Ageing Int,* 36 (1), 66–81.

Mahoney, D. F., and Goc, K. (2009), "Tensions in independent living facilities for elders: a model of connected disconnections," *J Hous Elderly,* 23 (3), 166–84.

Mahoney, D. F., Coon, D. W., and Lozano, C. (2016a), "Latino/Hispanic Alzheimer's caregivers experiencing dementia-related dressing issues: corroboration of the Preservation of Self model and reactions to a "smart dresser" computer-based dressing aid," *Digit Health,* 2, 1–12.

Mahoney, D. F., et al. (2016b), "Accuracy and stability testing of a 'smart dresser' for persons with dementia," *Gerontechnology,* 15 (Suppl), 88s.

Mahoney, D. F., et al. (2015), "Prototype Development of a Responsive Emotive Sensing System (DRESS) to aid older persons with dementia to dress independently," *Gerontechnology,* 13 (3), 345–58.

Malinowsky, C., Rosenberg, L., and Nygard, L. (2014), "An approach to facilitate health-care professionals' readiness to support technology use in everyday life for persons with dementia," *Scand J Occup Ther,* 21 (3), 199–209.

Marzanski, M. (2000a), "On telling the truth to patients with dementia," *West J Med,* 173 (5), 318–23.

Marzanski, M. (2000b), "Would you like to know what is wrong with you? On telling the truth to patients with dementia," *J Med Ethics,* 26 (2), 108–13.

McShane, R., Hope, T., and Wilkinson, J. (1994), "Tracking patients who wander: ethics and technology," *Lancet,* 343 (8908), 1274.

McShane, R., et al. (1998), "The feasibility of electronic tracking devices in dementia: a telephone survey and case series," *Int J Geriatr Psychiatry,* 13 (8), 556–63.

Mill, J. S. (1859), "On liberty. The Online Library of Liberty." Collected Works of John Stuart Mill, ed. J. M. Robson (Toronto: University of Toronto Press; London: Routledge and Kegan Paul, 1963–1991), 33 vols.: http://oll.libertyfund.org/index.php?option=com_staticxt&staticfile=show.php%3Ftitle=165&Itemid=28 and http://oll.libertyfund.org/titles/mill-the-collected-works-of-john-stuart-mill-volume-xviii-essays-on-politics-and-society-part-i?q=on+liberty#Mill_0223-18_14 (accessed September 5, 2017).

Mitseva, A., et al. (2012), "Gerontechnology: providing a helping hand when caring for cognitively impaired older adults-intermediate results from a controlled study on the satisfaction and acceptance of informal caregivers," *Curr Gerontol Geriatr Res,* 2012, 1–19.

Mulvenna, M., et al. (2017), "Views of caregivers on the ethics of assistive technology used for home surveillance of people living with dementia," *Neuroethics,* 10 (2), 255–66.

Newton, L., et al. (2016), "Exploring the views of GPs, people with dementia and their carers on assistive technology: a qualitative study," *BMJ Open,* 6 (5), e011132.

Novitzky, P., et al. (2015), "A review of contemporary work on the ethics of ambient assisted living technologies for people with dementia," *Sci Eng Ethics,* 21 (3), 707–65.

Ontario Information & Privacy Commissioners (2011), "Privacy by Design. Strong Privacy Protection—Now, and Well into the Future." A Report on the State of PbD to the 33rd International Conference of Data Protection and Privacy Commissioners: https://www.ipc.on.ca/wp-content/uploads/Resources/PbDReport.pdf (accessed January 12, 2017).

Prudente, A. "Nouvelles technologies et qualité de vie des seniors: font-elles bon ménage?" Colloque Leenaards âge & société, November 23, 2017: http://www.leenaards.ch/wp-content/uploads/2017/11/Communique_FLeenaards_agesociete2017.pdf (accessed August 12, 2017).

Rajczi, A. (2016), "Liberalism and public health ethics," *Bioethics,* 30 (2), 96–108.

Sandman, L., and Heintz, E. (2014), "Assessment vs. appraisal of ethical aspects of health technology assessment: can the distinction be upheld?," *GMS Health Technol Assess,* 10, Doc05.

Sifford, K. S., and Bharucha, A. (2010), "Benefits and challenges of electronic surveillance in nursing home research," *Res Gerontol Nurs,* 3 (1), 5–10.

Sorell, T., and Draper, H. (2012), "Telecare, surveillance, and the welfare state," *Am J Bioeth,* 12 (9), 36–44.

United Nations (1948), "Universal Declaration of Human Rights. UN Document Series Symbol: ST/HR/ UN Issuing Body: Secretariat Centre for Human Rights, United Nations": http://www.hri.ca/uninfo/treaties/1.shtml (accessed June 30, 2005).

Yusif, S., Soar, J., and Hafeez-Baig, A. (2016), "Older people, assistive technologies, and the barriers to adoption: a systematic review," *Int J Med Inform*, 94, 112–16.

10

Issues of Informed Consent from Persons with Dementia When Employing Assistive Technologies

Peter Novitzky, Cynthia Chen, Alan F. Smeaton, Renaat Verbruggen, and Bert Gordijn

Introduction

Informed consent is one of the cornerstones and requirements sine qua non of modern medical research and clinical practice. It developed relatively quickly to gain great importance, despite initial setbacks. The requirement of informed consent applies to all subjects of medical research and therapy, including persons with dementia (PwDs), whose impaired competence to provide valid informed consent poses particular challenges. While assistive technologies (ATs)[1] provide opportunities for better care with novel techniques for obtaining informed consent, many of the ethical challenges need further consideration and deeper ethical analysis to be addressed satisfactorily.

This chapter, first, describes the purpose of informed consent, with a short historical overview. Second, it defines and specifies the requirements of informed consent, highlighting the issues of obtaining valid informed consent from PwDs. Third, this chapter reviews traditional and innovative methods of obtaining informed consent from PwDs. Fourth, it summarizes outstanding ethical issues that may emerge during research or application of ATs with PwDs. Finally, it proposes recommendations on how to tackle key ethical issues of informed consent with PwDs.

Purpose of Informed Consent

It may be argued that the requirement for informed consent is a logical consequence of the requirement of respecting every person's autonomy to make and be responsible for decisions [7, Art. 5]. Both these requirements are founded on the concept of human dignity, stipulated by *The Universal Declaration of Human Rights* [8, Art. 1] and the *Universal Declaration on Bioethics and Human Rights* (UDBHR) [7, Art. 3], applicable to every human being.

This origin of the requirement for informed consent in *UDBHR* [7] defines its three main purposes: (a) protection against undue paternalism by physicians, (b) avoidance of undue or uninformed influence from others (e.g., authorities), and (c) provision of a voice to the person concerned, to facilitate their self-determination [9].

Historical Milestones of Informed Consent

Informed consent was first mentioned in response to public outcry over injuries inflicted upon human participants through nontherapeutic interventions in 1891 in Germany. Later, in 1900, a German ministerial directive requiring informed consent was issued as a result of the Neisser case, where a clinical trial was conducted on people who were not asked for consent [10].

The informed consent standard was first internationally recognized in the *Nuremberg Code* [11], a response to Nazi research conducted on concentration camp prisoners. The first paragraph stipulates that voluntary consent from participants in any type of medical experiment is absolutely essential. The rigorous phrasing of the code delegitimized research with humans incapable of providing consent.

Thus, the strict standard of the code obstructed research and development (R&D) of novel therapies for people affected by some of the most serious conditions. Consequently, it needed to be liberalized. This occurred in two stages. First, the *Declaration of Helsinki* [12] distinguished therapeutic from nontherapeutic research, allowing therapeutic research on incompetent persons (albeit under special circumstance), while still prohibiting nontherapeutic research. However, early-phase research, that is, where direct benefits to the participant are uncertain, remained excluded. Further liberalization occurred in the 1990s. With strict safeguards,[2] the possibility of research without direct benefit to incompetent participants was gradually accepted [13].

Later bioethical documents, such as the *International Ethical Guidelines for Biomedical Research Involving Human Subjects* [14], the *Convention on Human Rights and Biomedicine* [15], and the *UDBHR* [7] reflect this development.

General Problems of Consent from Persons with Dementia

Beauchamp and Childress categorize the traditional requirements of informed consent into three groups [16]:

1. Consent threshold elements—including *competence* and *voluntariness*
2. Information elements—*disclosure* of relevant information, provision of recommendations, *understanding*
3. Consent elements—*decision, authorization*

PwDs may have issues with all these elements. Their competence may be diminished, for example, by cognitive impairment. The voluntariness of PwDs may also be negatively affected in research studies because PwDs tend to want to please researchers and are afraid of offending them [17].

The information elements represent a group of issues in their own right. One key issue is that it is generally difficult to ascertain whether a patient or research participant has sufficiently understood the information disclosed [9].[3] It is the professional's duty to find a correlation between the information to be disclosed and the background knowledge of the participant. Comprehensible language must be used to help ensure understanding. Information disclosed to PwDs may not be fully understood if the language used is too technical [18]. Furthermore, participants should not be overloaded with information or underinformed [19]. When in doubt regarding the understanding of the information provided about the objectives, risks, and benefits of the intervention, a mediator (e.g., independent adviser, responsible for protecting the safety, welfare, and interests of the PwDs) can be employed to assist the person in understanding the information [20].

The understanding of information by PwDs cannot be fully ascertained in the same way as with competent patients/research participants. Thus, the issue of understanding by PwDs remains unresolved.

The situation is similar with the consent elements. Due to cognitive impairment, PwDs become increasingly unable to provide consent, either as an ultimate decision or as a formal authorization for research participation or treatment. As such, the three essential elements of valid informed consent may pose problems for PwDs, who may fulfill some but rarely all of the necessary requirements.

As a person's competence deteriorates, the chances of obtaining explicit and express consent reduce. Therefore, other forms of consent may become relevant, such as substituted consent (as with the terminally ill) or presumed consent (as in emergencies [21]).

The case of PwDs is, however, very specific. Although progressive cognitive impairment eventually renders PwDs incompetent, their capacity to provide informed consent may not be completely diminished during the early stages of this condition. Competence is usually understood as a legal term, where the loss of competence refers to the loss of the legal right to decide in important matters [13]. The bioethical interpretation of loss of competence is much more nuanced. It still refers to the inability of a person to make decisions but without "artificial binary certainty" [22, pp. 51–52]. This means that for PwDs, competence to provide informed consent is not necessarily an "all-or-nothing 'on-off' switch" [23, p. 72], but rather a fluctuating state. Thus, capacity is a continuum, dependent on external variables that have the power to alter, diminish, or enhance the PwD's capacity to consent [22].

The capacity of a person is usually described as a capability in two domains: cognitive and volitive. For informed consent, the assessment of volitive capability, which also assesses the capacity to make judgments (*capacité de discernment*), is decisive [24]. The instrument currently considered the most valid for assessing PwDs' capacity [25] is the MacArthur Competence Assessment Tool (MacCAT) [26–28]. The MacCAT is available for both research and clinical application,[4] and shows good validity and reliability. However, it is time-consuming (30 to 60 minutes) and requires prior training and familiarity. It and other assessment instruments are also unable to measure moral and/or emotional capacity to make a meaningful decision consistent with one's life history [25]. Therefore, Vorm and Rikkert [25] recommend using the MacCAT in combination with specific questions regarding the hopes, beliefs, and personal history of the patient/research participant.

In addition, the proportionality principle should be applied as a criterion of the capacity to consent in research with PwDs. The riskier and more burdensome the trial, the higher the level of capacity for consent needed from research participants and the higher the standards required for consent [25].

As the disease progresses, PwDs may be considered incompetent and yet retain some decision-making capacity. This state introduces a "gray zone" into informed consent.[5]

It is notable that not long ago, physicians believed that a diagnosis of dementia automatically rendered PwDs incompetent in expressing their advance directives (approximately 72% in a US survey [29]). It is important to determine specific dementia subtypes [29].[6] Different dementia subtypes affect different areas of the brain and, therefore, different functions. Knowing which functions are affected helps professionals identify which PwDs may be considered competent [23].

Specific Problems of Consent from Persons with Dementia and ATs

Specific Consent Problems in Clinical Research with Competent Persons with Dementia

To enhance research participants' understanding of the nature, elements, and goals of a research study, it is advisable that the researchers repeat the information several times and, if appropriate, in smaller, more digestible portions [20]. The disclosure of information is a particularly interactive process. The condition for repeated provision of information has also been proposed during the drafting process of the *UDBHR* articles [7] concerning informed consent. The rationale behind this reiterative step is the general recognition that informed consent, by focusing on the fulfillment of its essential elements, is a procedural concept [9]. Aspects of this interpretation of informed consent are also noticeable in one of the first drafts of Art. 6 of *UDBHR* [7], where the committee interpreted informed consent as an "ongoing participation" [21, p. 9]. Ongoing participation in research necessitates a more active role on the part of the participants, where the disclosure of information is no longer a one-step unidirectional requirement but rather a continuous and mutual effort to communicate and understand the information throughout the duration of the research participation [21].

Additional ethical challenges regarding clinical research with ATs are presented by issues with data ownership, data handling, and the reuse of previously collected data. Ethical issues from the context of biobanks and genetic data research may be relevant to research with ATs. It is commonly accepted that the owners of genetic data gathered from participants are the institutions that host databanks. These institutions are accountable for the proper management of this data. However, the research results are the property of individual researchers, unless otherwise specified in the consent forms [18]. Similarly, questions regarding data ownership and management also arise during the R&D of ATs, when vast amounts of private, confidential, medical data are collected. The R&D process may involve many researchers and different research institutions, often in multiple countries with different legislative frameworks. This can be further complicated in geographic regions that have "tiers" of legislative frameworks, such as Europe, where European and national legislative frameworks interact, or in the United States, where both federal and state laws must be respected. These conditions increase the complexity of data ownership and data handling, both key issues for researchers and participants, which are scrutinized when considering consent.

New technologies also offer a great opportunity for reusing samples and data in new research studies. The requirement to recontact previous participants for informed consent is an issue that is still not completely resolved [18]. A similar issue may be encountered with the data gathered from PwDs with ATs, after they have been anonymized. For genetic data in databanks, a specific authorization model has been developed by Caulfield et al. [30], which enables participants to preserve a certain amount of control over their data for future analysis [18]. Similar or alternative frameworks may emerge in the future regarding recorded data of PwDs by ATs.

Specific Consent Problems in Clinical Practice with Competent Persons with Dementia

The challenges related to ongoing participation and understanding of information by PwDs also apply in clinical practice, because PwDs are free to refuse treatment. Stanton-Jean et al. highlight that a refusal of one particular treatment does not automatically mean a refusal of all treatments. Therefore, reasonable alternatives should always be communicated and explained in detail [18].

Specific Consent Problems in Clinical Research with Incompetent Persons with Dementia

Clinical research with incompetent persons such as PwDs requires special justification. Such justification is usually based on the premise that it would be unjust and unacceptable to abandon certain groups that are unable to provide informed consent. Exclusion from research studies also means the exclusion from the potential benefits of research studies [24].

Alzheimer Europe[7] and the European Dementia Consensus Network (EDCON) support the involvement of PwDs in research [25, 31]. Naturally, such research must fulfill certain conditions.

Art. 7b of the *UDBHR* [7] requires—as a general rule—that research studies should have a direct health benefit for the participants, although it permits exceptions to that rule. Research without a direct health benefit is only permitted when the risk is minimal. Also, incompetent participants should only be included in studies where there are no alternatives of comparable effectiveness with competent participants.[8] In exceptional cases, the *UDBHR* [7] allows research studies with incompetent participants without direct benefit for the participants. Such studies should, however, contribute to the health benefit of persons with the same condition, while exposing participants to minimal risks and burdens. As neither the *UDBHR* [7] nor the *Explanatory Memorandum on UDBHR* [21] define minimal risk, the definition of minimal risk used in the *Additional Protocol* to the *Convention on Human Rights and Biomedicine* [32] may be applicable. It defines minimal risk as a "very slight and temporary negative impact on the health of the person concerned" [32, Art. 17.1]. This includes procedures such as taking saliva, small tissue samples, blood, one X-ray exposure, or undergoing magnetic resonance imaging without contrast medium [13].

Groves [33] highlights that research conducted with PwDs, in search of pathophysiological foundations of the disease, often offers no therapeutic benefit for the research participant.[9] The author warns that there might be a "conspiracy of silence" [33, p. 20] about the phenomenon where the research results favor, to some extent, the interests of the researchers rather than those of the participants. Moreover, if participants and proxies were consistently to be informed about the lack of therapeutic benefits (e.g., in Phase I studies), there might be a decline in enrollment rates. This contributes to the controversial nature of clinical research on cognitively impaired adults [33].

Specific Consent Problems in Clinical Practice with Incompetent Persons with Dementia

In Art. 7 of the *UDBHR* [7], the term "medical practice," with regard to informed consent and incompetent persons, is mentioned only in relation to research authorization. An incompetent person incapable of consent may provide assent and should be involved as much as possible in the decision-making process. For legally incompetent persons (e.g., children), the institution of *assent* is widely applied. While giving consent refers to an "agreement *to* a proposal," assent indicates only "agreement *with* a proposal" [34, p. 313]. The former is a normatively transformative act (in a sense of action), and the latter is a state of mind or attitude (in a form of feelings or thoughts [34]). Assent is different from consent because it reflects the limitations of understanding in a person. The process of obtaining assent should consider the mental capacities, levels of maturity, and overall development of the person concerned. Assent is also accepted by the *Declaration of Helsinki* [35] as a valid way of including a person into the consenting process [18]. The fact that full competency has not been acquired yet (children) or has been lost (dementia) seems to be morally irrelevant for the process of assenting. In both cases the *UDBHR* [7] requires the greatest possible involvement of the incompetent person.

With PwDs of limited decision-making capacity, Vorm and Rikkert [25] favor the dual-consent procedure. Dual consent involves acquiring consent from the authorized representative, followed by the assent (or consent, if the participant is capable to provide it) from the PwD.

Regarding refusal or withdrawal of treatment, the requirements for intellectual capacity, including judgment, are generally less strict than those required for providing consent to clinical treatment. However, small signs of opposition (e.g., gestures, weeping, fear of hospitals, etc.) should not immediately be considered as refusals. As a guiding rule, it should be borne in mind that the more adverse the effect of withdrawing treatment, the stricter the requirements should be toward the capacity of judgment of the individual concerned. Any failure to respect autonomy, no matter how limited the autonomy, should be minimized. Consideration of the patient's whole situation (history, circumstances, previous care) should determine the best way of preserving the person's integrity, health, and dignity [24].

Informed Consent Procedures for Persons with Dementia

This section presents various methods of acquiring informed consent from PwDs. Rolling informed consent and advance directives represent more traditional methods, while delayed consent and dynamic consent are new methods that are currently under development.

Rolling Informed Consent

Rolling informed consent is a method of obtaining informed consent adjusted to the conditions of PwDs [36]. The method involves three aspects:

1. Repeatedly providing information (i.e., not only when requested) and asking for consent during various stages of treatment or research
2. Listening to the content and nuances of the speech of the PwD and continuously assessing whether participation is voluntary and not subject to coercion, persuasion, manipulation, or simple distress, which, if so, should be sufficient reason for the researcher to end the session, without needing the expressed request of the participant [37]
3. Repeatedly communicating the possibility of opting out or withdrawing from treatment or research at any given stage

Rolling informed consent has the potential to reflect the specific conditions of PwDs by ensuring that consent is regularly checked and confirmed, while also regularly monitoring the cognitive functions of the PwD. However, this method may be considered burdensome and time-consuming by professionals.

Advance Directives

A key issue with advance directives of PwDs is that of ruptures between previous desires expressed in advance directives and current wishes expressed during times of limited competency. Healthcare professionals can choose between two extremes. One is the application of the pure "best interest" standard[10] in every case with PwDs. However, doing this could bring negative consequences. One such consequence may be on PwDs who rely on caregivers to help them implement their decisions, whereby the caregivers may only help implement the decisions that they consider in the PwD's best interests. As such, PwDs would be a class of people that would be unable to occasionally make a reckless decision. Moreover, the PwD's assessment of his or her best interest would always be considered less valuable than an assessment made by other "competent" people. This may result in the coercion of PwDs, which is unlikely to restore (or, in the case of PwDs, maintain) one's sense of self except for the sense of a *powerless* self [39].

The other extreme solution is to always follow the advance directive of the patient.[11] This would be based on the respect for the human dignity of the person and his or her autonomy to make decisions. This translates into invariably following the previously expressed decisions to the full extent. The problem now is that the present interests of PwDs might conflict with earlier wishes expressed in advance directives [38].[12]

Both solutions offer satisfactory results in only a limited number of cases. In lucid states, PwDs may be competent enough to express genuine wishes that might overcome their advance directive, and vice versa. Moreover, consistent guidance of any of these two standards would overburden caregivers. A possible resolution of such cases has been provided by Huxtable [43] in the form of principled compromise.

Delayed Consent

Art. 6 and 7 of the *UDBHR* [7], other international documents, and recommendations from expert groups suggest that direct consent from the patient/research participant should always be preferred over any form of substituted judgment. PwDs who experience bouts of transient incapacity and temporary lucidity are in a "gray zone," where they are at times able to provide informed consent. For situations like this, which can occur during ongoing research, researchers have two possible options. The first is of temporarily interrupting the research and waiting until the person recovers lucidity. However, this might impede the continuity of the research, causing gradually increasing delays. The second option is to use a form of "retrospective consent" (used in the case of life-saving treatments of mature minors [34]), which involves seeking consent after the research activity has been performed (without prior consent), when the person recovers from the incapacitated state (e.g., [44]). This method is used in cases where the research could not be performed with competent participants, either because of time constraints or the permanent condition of the participant [45].[13]

It may be argued that in the case of PwDs and in nonemergency circumstances, researchers may delay the process of obtaining (rolling) informed consent from PwDs until they regain lucidity. This argument may be based on the likelihood that some PwDs have temporary nonlucid states (e.g., mild dementia). Delayed consent may in such cases respect the autonomy of the PwD to a greater extent than the substituted consent of a proxy. There is, however, a dearth of academic literature providing any further insight into the possibilities of retrospective or delayed consent specifically in relation to PwDs.

The issue with delayed consent for PwDs is that there is no way of knowing in advance whether the nonlucid state is temporary. Moreover, delayed consent may significantly and unpredictably extend the timeframe needed for obtaining consent from PwDs. Therefore, it would be prudent to define an upper limit for the timeframe.

Dynamic Consent

Dynamic consent is currently developed and investigated in biobank projects. Kaye et al. [47], however, propose using this approach or concept more widely within clinical research or other fields. It is defined as "a new approach for engaging individuals about the use of their personal information . . . [by] an interactive personalised interface that allows participants to engage as much or as little as they choose and to alter their consent choices in real time" [47, p. 2]. The consent of an individual is enclosed in an encrypted information container. Employing asymmetric cryptography, the consent, together with other personal information, can be publicly shared with a trusted research center through a trusted authority. Thus, it is also ensured that the research center has access only to the information that it has approval for ([47] and the documentation of the EnCoRe Project).[14] The research center thus gains access to the most recent consent and other necessary sensitive medical information of the participant relevant for the study while preserving the privacy of the participant. The flexibility and relative ease of receiving information is also beneficial for the participant. The participant may easily alter or withdraw consent, follow-up on the use of his or her data and the results of the study, or be available for subsequent contact for data reuse [47]. Eventually, other personal preferences or advance directives may also be included in this information container. The container would then serve as a logbook of information over the lifespan of a person.

When used in relation to research with PwDs, dynamic consent may introduce more data into the process of obtaining consent. Having more data may be beneficial by providing a record of the PwD's former wishes either as a form of advance directive or to inform decisions made with substituted consent. Having more data may also generate more issues and unresolvable complexities in the decision-making process. Therefore, even such a long-term record of the preferences and evolution of a PwD's advance directive provided by the dynamic consent framework is unlikely to provide solutions for the specific issues with PwDs already described.

Dynamic consent may be interpreted as a merger of rolling informed consent and advance directives with the utilization of modern technologies. The benefit of using technology is that it may alleviate some of the burdens of healthcare professionals. However, the use of technology always involves the danger of unidirectional information disclosure and consent, without the presence of a trained professional. This may generate additional issues in relation to the cognitive impairment of PwDs.

Outstanding Informed Consent Issues

This section highlights some further ethical issues related to informed consent from PwDs that need more attention and analysis in future medical research and clinical practice with ATs.

Informed Consent of Third Parties

ATs with recording abilities have boosted research with participant-created data, allowing the shift from researcher-created datasets to more automated participant-created datasets. ATs deployed in the dwellings of research participants may also capture data on visitors or other persons who have not consented to participate in a research study. The presence of third parties (e.g., family, cohabitants, friends, etc.) is an issue because these people are not given the opportunity to provide informed consent before their presence is captured within the dwelling of the research participant, where the research is being conducted. In cases like these, third parties may not be fully aware of the ongoing recording. Kelly et al. [48] concede that this might pose serious ethical and legal issues. However, a distinction is often applied regarding the focus of the research, which is on the participant and not on any third parties incidentally recorded. Kelly et al. [48] note that, nevertheless, the ethical standard of respect for autonomy directs that the privacy of third parties must be protected. Even if the study is designed to investigate the influence on the research participant by third parties (e.g., behavior in group settings), the anonymity of these third parties should be preserved [48].

To tackle such unwanted recordings, Kelly et al. suggest that participants must be given the chance to review and delete unwanted recordings before the researcher views them [48]. However, PwDs may unavoidably become ignorant about the lack of consent from third parties or may forget to review the recordings. The lack of additional literature on this issue suggests that further investigation is needed into alternative approaches to solving the problem of informed consent from third parties in research using data capture.

Autonomous Technology

One of the crucial attributes of certain ATs, especially AAL technologies, is their ability to disappear into the background of the environment. Sensor technologies may collect data and respond to certain events or states in an automated manner. PwDs using ambient technologies may forget their presence, during which time ATs may perform undesirable tasks.

The automated and autonomous nature of these technologies poses ethical risks to the PwDs [49]. They might expose PwDs, due to their inability to fully comprehend the extent of the data collection and transmission by information and communication technology (ICT), to misuse, criminal activities, privacy breaches, or dehumanizing treatment [49]. In addition, PwDs could be stripped of their freedom to make decisions, making them the only group of people without this right [39]. Undesired activity by ATs may also be detrimental in dementia management, as it could cause anxiety in PwDs (e.g., issues of "false alarms" [50], ICT's "life of their own" [51], etc.).

Even if ATs were to require consent from the PwD, the danger persists that, within a shared dwelling, consent is provided illegitimately by somebody else (e.g., carer). Thus, an unobtrusive authentication of the PwD for consent will be needed.[15] Even by introducing these precautionary measures, the question of autonomous ICT and the requirement for consent remain unresolved. Therefore, further research is required for more focused and detailed insight into the extent to which the needs of PwDs can be served by autonomous decisions made by ICT. The research should target the use of autonomous devices in particular contexts, that is, when such activity is acceptable for the person compared with when it is not (e.g., when it results in disturbing the person). Also, more research is needed to establish valid proportionality between the need for (and the degree of) autonomous ICT and the requirement of informed consent from PwDs for certain actions. Such research should also seek to identify how often consent should be sought from PwDs during research and/or clinical practice.

Information Overload

PwDs are more vulnerable to information overload [52, 53], which may occur during the acquisition of informed consent. Information overload might be addressed to some extent by the division of information into smaller, more digestible blocks, distributed across a longer timeline. However, despite all these efforts, information overload cannot be completely avoided, due to the condition of PwDs. One consequence of information overload may be the problem of routinization [54]. Studies show that even healthy volunteers often provide or refuse informed consent as a result of an unreflective, habitual act performed on electronic devices [54–56].

Therefore, during the acquisition of informed consent, there needs to be an appropriate, and personalized, balance of information, tailored to every individual PwD. Such a requirement also means that the information should be interactively and dynamically adjusted to the actual state of the PwD, taking into consideration his or her competence and other faculties, in order to successfully and ethically obtain informed consent.

More research is needed into how routinization affects PwDs. Further research is also required to more precisely determine what represents underinformation and information overload for PwDs.

The Seemingly Infinite Memory of Lifelogs

ATs may also function as lifelogs.[16] Lifelogs, due to their "seemingly infinite memory" capabilities, are not only perfect for logging information about health status, physiological data, or other relevant health information but also useful for storing the consent and previously expressed wishes and preferences of individuals. While one might expect this to be especially beneficial for forgetful PwDs, this may not be necessarily so.

Generally, forgetting is an intrinsic form of controlling one's memory [57]. With the utilization of lifelogs, this control may be lost. As an intrinsic part of human nature, one might prefer to forget certain memories. However, lifelogs may prevent people from forgetting. This might result in distress, depression, and/or anxiety. Analogously, if the previous consent of the PwD is always remembered and recorded, it may not be easily changed in cases of diminishing competency. Therefore, it would be important to regularly renew the consent of PwDs. Regular requests for consent can reinforce the PwD's feeling of control over the ATs, and their own care, and reaffirm their feeling of security. However, seeking consent too often may be burdensome and upsetting for PwDs. Therefore, an individually tailored approach that strikes the right balance needs to be developed for the consent-seeking process, with emphasis on avoiding causing anxiety, avoiding routinization, or reducing acceptability. These conditions impose high requirements on researchers and developers of ATs.

More research is required on how an adequate amount of relevant information can be provided by ATs while respecting the PwD's personal needs and condition.

Compelling Security Upgrades and Remote Updates

Recent developments in ICT revealed other issues related to consent, the level of control of ICT devices, and the security of their users. A series of recently discovered security issues (i.e., bugs, security vulnerabilities)[17] forced operating system developers to encourage their users to upgrade to newer systems. These newer operating systems come with higher security protection, official support, upgraded user interfaces, new functionalities, and different behaviors compared with their previous versions. These changes require study and adjustments of workflows for users, which PwDs cannot perform. Being single rather than corporate users, PwDs lose the official support from IT companies by not upgrading their systems. Due to their inability to upgrade the systems on their devices, they also lose control over their private and medical data that are stored in these devices, thus exposing these to hackers. These issues should be included in consent forms when offering treatment with ATs.

Moreover, there is the issue of autonomous technology. To provide end-users with the strongest security protection possible, companies offer remotely controlled automatic updates to their operating systems.[18] A PwD, unaware of the differences introduced by the new system into his or her workflow, may face extreme difficulties after such pseudo-intentional consent. Although PwDs may have "consented" to such an upgrade (in hope of greater security), in the end they may find themselves so unfamiliar with the upgraded system that it becomes unusable. This may result in increased anxiety, poorer dementia management, a greater digital divide, and the loss of computer-using functionality in PwDs. The support behind ATs must therefore include the need for long-term and system-wide support of the ICT devices deployed to PwDs.

More research is needed into the provision of ICT for PwDs, including how to address the digital divide. This should involve an investigation of how to better provide security updates and long-term ICT support and maintain the PwD's familiarity with ICT systems, and development of easy-to-use technologies for cognitively impaired persons.

Placebo Effect of ATs

Informed consent is closely related to the issue of using placebos in research. Placebos are inert substances or treatments used in both treatment and clinical research [58]. The term "placebo effect" is the result of all verbal and nonverbal communication and rituals of therapy, where the efficacy is not derived from any pharmacological or physiological intervention [59]. Despite the fact that the *UDBHR* [7] does not explicitly specify the role of informed consent in the use of placebo during treatment or research, studies involving ATs may have outcomes that could be identified as placebo effects.

One example may be the well-publicized robotic harp seal, PARO (com-PAnion RObot), which interactively responds and expresses emotions to a patient, just as a real animal does during animal-assisted therapy [60]. These therapies have demonstrated reductions in emotional, behavioral, and psychological symptoms, lowering agitation levels and improving the mood of PwDs [60]. However, the validity of these treatments may be questioned because they are assumed to have placebo effects or novelty effects, demand characteristics, experimenter expectancy effects, or informant bias [60].

There is a dearth of literature investigating the placebo effect of ATs. Research is needed to determine whether ATs have placebo effects and, if so, what consequences this would introduce into the care of PwDs using ATs.

Recommendations

As a result of the analysis presented in this chapter, the following recommendations are proposed. Informed consent interpreted solely on the basis of legal requirements should be avoided, especially with PwDs. The diagnosis of dementia should not automatically imply lack of competence to provide informed consent. Incompetent PwDs, in the "gray zone" of informed consent, may retain sufficient capacity to provide consent or assent. Strict adherence to regulations can result in harmful and unethical consequences.

If research can be conducted with healthy, or at least competent, volunteers instead of vulnerable populations, such as PwDs, it should be. In accordance with the *UDBHR* [7], research with persons who lack the capacity to consent should only be allowed if there is a direct health benefit to those participants, and if no comparable study can be undertaken with participants able to consent.

Traditional (rolling informed consent, advance directives) and alternative methods (delayed informed consent, dynamic informed consent) should be used to obtain informed consent from PwDs. Combining informed consent methods (and modern technologies) may prove helpful in recording the preferences of PwDs over a longer period of time; for example, in clinical practice, the recording of an advance directive at the time of diagnosis may be combined with the application of delayed consent, to extend the autonomy of PwDs without the need for substituted consent. Similarly, consent of PwDs in clinical research obtained by rolling informed consent may be combined with data obtained with dynamic consent. Combined methods are more likely to reflect the special conditions and needs of PwDs, and may also improve the validity of the informed consent obtained. In general, the development of better consent methods and procedures should be encouraged to achieve the highest ethical standards possible for informed consent from PwDs.

It is the responsibility of the researcher(s) to assess whether the PwD's competency has changed during the research study and to conduct the research in compliance with the requirements of the *UDBHR* [7]. This should also be reflected in the study design.

It would be advisable to appoint an independent adviser or mediator to support the PwDs and be responsible for the protection of their safety, welfare, and interests during the research study.

ATs do not essentially alter the criteria of informed consent; however, the issues of consent of third parties, partial or full autonomy of ATs, information overload, infinite memory of lifelogs, and safety and security while preserving the usability of ATs for PwDs will need to be investigated further. Similarly, research studies investigating the potential placebo effect of ATs should be established.

Notes

1. The term "assistive technologies" in this chapter is defined as "any item, piece of equipment, or product system, whether acquired commercially, modified, or customized, that is used to increase, maintain, or improve functional capabilities of individuals with disabilities" [1, p. 134]. They are also referred to as digital assistive technologies [2] and welfare technologies [3]. Both terms involve intelligent computing, with elements of pervasiveness and ubiquity, the characteristics of ambient intelligence (AmI) [2, 4, 5]. A subgroup of AmI consists of ambient assisted living (AAL) technologies, which refer to innovative technologies, intelligent systems of assistance

that help elderly people (including PwDs) in all stages of their life in order to extend their stay in their preferred environment, and support systems that maintain people's health and functional capabilities by promoting a healthier lifestyle, allowing active and creative participation in the community, and improving quality of life [6].

2. These safeguards usually extend to circumstances where such research must significantly contribute either to a better understanding of the individual's condition or to the overall knowledge about that disease or disorder. Furthermore, research without direct benefit must pose only minimal risk and minimal burden to the research participant. Finally, the research participant must provide valid consent for participating in such a study [13].

3. For example, an engineer will understand the information much more easily if it is presented using terminology and metaphors from engineering.

4. For example, MacCAT-CR, where CR means clinical research; and MacCAT-T, where T means treatment.

5. Bowman [22] mentions the "gray hinterland" (e.g., somewhere in between capacity and incapacity), where PwDs may sometimes have decision-making capacity [22, p. 73].

6. A study by Fazel et al. [29] suggested that only 20% of PwDs were competent enough to complete their advance directives, compared with a group of relatively healthy elderly volunteers, whose capacity rate was approximately 78%. They concluded that only a relatively small proportion of diagnosed PwDs are competent enough to complete advance directives (those with higher premorbid intelligence). Moreover, they found that competence was affected by aspects of higher intellectual functioning, which are not fully assessed by the The Mini-Mental State Examination (MMSE) or Folstein test [29].

7. http://www.alzheimer-europe.org

8. Vorm and Rikkert [25] advise that PwDs who are incompetent most of the time should not be included in research.

9. For example, Phase I studies in particular involve the administration of investigational medication to participants in increasing dosages in order to test the drug's toxicity. Although these drugs may carry a potential for benefit (recognition for researchers, profit for drug companies, etc.), the participants receive no direct health benefit (beyond the fulfillment of their altruistic motivations [33]).

10. Muramoto [38] refers to this as the pure beneficence argument (PBA).

11. Also called the pure autonomy argument (PAA [38]).

12. A similar discussion occurred between the philosophers Dworkin [40], Dresser [41], and Shiffrin [42].

13. The protocol of the NICE Study [46] in the intensive care unit environment allows the possibility of a form of retrospective consent (i.e., delayed consent) where the respondents who provided delayed consent were less likely to delegate the decision making to another person or an organization [45]. However, the NICE Study [46] did not focus on PwDs.

14. EnCoRe—Ensuring Consent & Revocation Project: http://www.hpl.hp.com/breweb/encoreproject/index.html (visited on September 30, 2015). The details of the process

are described in deliverable D2.3 Third EnCoRe Technical Architecture: http:// www.hpl.hp.com/breweb/encoreproject/deliverables_material/D2_3_EnCoRe_ Architecture_V1.0.pdf (visited on September 30, 2015).

15. Achieving this may be challenging because of the possible forgetfulness of PwDs. For this reason, authentication by fingerprint reading or voice or face recognition may be preferable.

16. Lifelogs are a form of pervasive computing, which consist of unified, digital records [57].

17. For example, most of the systems were affected by the security exploit FREAK (Factoring RSA Export Keys): https://freakattack.com (visited on October 28, 2015).

18. Such automatic upgrade, with minimal need for user input, has been recently advertised: http://www.forbes.com/sites/gordonkelly/2015/10/30/windows-10-upgrades-now-automatic/ (visited on October 30, 2015).

References

1. Appleyard, Richard. 2005. Disability Informatics. In *Consumer Health Informatics*, ed. Deborah Lewis, Gunther Eysenbach, Rita Kukafka, P. Zoë Stavri, and Holly B. Jimison, 129–142. Springer New York.

2. Francis, Peter, Sandrine Balbo, and Lucy Firth. 2009. Towards co-design with users who have autism spectrum disorders. *Universal Access in the Information Society* 8: 123–135.

3. Hofmann, Bjørn. 2012. Ethical challenges with welfare technology: A review of the literature. *Science and Engineering Ethics* 19: 389–406.

4. Cook, Diane J., Juan C. Augusto, and Vikramaditya R. Jakkula. 2009. Ambient intelligence: Technologies, applications, and opportunities. *Pervasive and Mobile Computing* 5: 277–298.

5. Zaad, Lambert, and Somaya Ben Allouch. 2008. The influence of control on the acceptance of ambient intelligence by elderly people: An explorative study. In *Ambient Intelligence*, ed. Emile Aarts, James L. Crowley, Boris de Ruyter, Heinz Gerhäuser, Alexander Pflaum, Janina Schmidt, and Reiner Wichert, 5355: 58–74. Springer Berlin/Heidelberg.

6. Broek, Ger van den, Filippo Cavallo, and Christian Wehrmann, eds. 2010. *AALIANCE Ambient Assisted Living Roadmap 6*.

7. UNESCO. 2005. *Universal Declaration on Bioethics and Human Rights*. Records of the General Conference, 33rd session, Paris, 3–21 October 2005. https://unesdoc.unesco. org/ark:/48223/pf0000142825.page=80

8. United Nations. 1948. The Universal Declaration of Human Rights. *UN General Assembly*. https://www.un.org/en/universal-declaration-human-rights/index.html

9. Kollek, Regine. 2009. Article 6: Consent. In *The UNESCO Universal Declaration on Bioethics and Human Rights: Background, Principles and Application*, ed. Henk A. M. J. ten Have, Michèle S. Jean, and Michael Kirby, 123–138. UNESCO Publishing.

10. Vollmann, Jochen, and Rolf Winau. 1996. Informed consent in human experimentation before the Nuremberg code. *BMJ* 313: 1445–1447.

11. The Nuremberg Code (1947). 1996. *BMJ* 313: 1448.

12. Rickham PP. 1964. Human Experimentation. Code of Ethics of The World Medical Association. Declaration of Helsinki. *British Medical Journal.* 2(5402): 177. doi:10.1136/bmj.2.5402.177. PubMed PMID: 14150898; PubMed Central PMCID: PMC1816102.

13. Gefenas, Eugenijus, and Egle Tuzaite. 2014. Persons without the capacity to consent. In *Handbook of Global Bioethics*, ed. Henk A. M. J. ten Have and Bert Gordijn. Chapter 7, pp. 85–103, doi:10.1007/978-94-007-2512-6_70. Springer.

14. Council for International Organizations of Medical Sciences. 2002. *International Ethical Guidelines for Biomedical Research Involving Human Subjects. Bulletin of Medical Ethics,* (182), p. 17. https://cioms.ch/wp-content/uploads/2016/08/International_Ethical_Guidelines_for_Biomedical_Research_Involving_Human_Subjects.pdf

15. Council of Europe. 1997. *Convention for the Protection of Human Rights and Dignity of the Human Being with Regard to the Application of Biology and Medicine: Convention on Human Rights and Biomedicine. European Treaty Series,* 4(164). https://rm.coe.int/CoERMPublicCommonSearchServices/DisplayDCTMContent?documentId=090000168007cf98

16. Beauchamp, Tom L., and James F. Childress. 2009. *Principles of Biomedical Ethics.* Oxford University Press.

17. Wallace, Jonathan, Maurice D. Mulvenna, Suzanne Martin, Sharon Stephens, and William Burns. 2010. ICT interface design for ageing people and people with dementia. In *Supporting People with Dementia Using Pervasive Health Technologies,* ed. Maurice D. Mulvenna and Chris D. Nugent. Chapter 11, pp. 165–188. Springer London.

18. Stanton-Jean, Michèle, Hubert Doucet, and Thérèse Leroux. 2014. Informed consent. In *Handbook of Global Bioethics*, ed. Henk A. M. J. ten Have and Bert Gordijn. Chapter 43, pp. 737–753. Springer.

19. Árnason, Viljhámur, Hongwen Li, and Yali Cong. 2011. Informed consent. In *The SAGE Handbook of Health Care Ethics*, ed. Ruth Chadwick, Henk ten Have, and Eric M. Meslin. Chapter 10, pp. 106–116. SAGE Publication.

20. International Bioethics Committee. 2008. *Report of the International Bioethics Committee of UNESCO (IBC) On Consent.* UNESCO.

21. UNESCO. 2005. Explanatory Memorandum on the Elaboration of the Preliminary Draft Declaration on Universal Norms on Bioethics. First Intergovernmental Meeting of Experts Aimed at Finalizing a Draft Declaration on Universal Norms on Bioethics (21 February 2005, Paris). http://unesdoc.unesco.org/images/0013/001390/139024e.pdf

22. Bowman, Deborah. 2008. Who decides who decides? Ethical perspectives on capacity and decision making. In *Competence Assessment in Dementia*, ed. European Dementia Consensus Network and Gabriela Stoppe. Chapter 5, pp. 51–60. Springer.

23. Fountoulakis, Konstantinos N., and Katerina Despos. 2008. Testamentary and financial competence issues in dementia. In *Competence Assessment in Dementia*, ed. European Dementia Consensus Network and Gabriela Stoppe. Chapter 7, pp. 71–76. Springer.

24. Martin, Jean F. 2009. Article 7: Persons Without the Capacity to Consent. In *The UNESCO Universal Declaration on Bioethics and Human Rights: Background, Principles and Application*, ed. Henk A. M. J. ten Have, Michèle S. Jean, and Michael Kirby, 139–154. UNESCO Publishing.

25. Vorm, Anco van Der, and Marcel G. M. Olde Rikkert. 2008. Informed consent in dementia research. In *Competence Assessment in Dementia*, ed. European Dementia Consensus Network and Gabriela Stoppe. Chapter 9, pp. 85–92. Springer.

26. Appelbaum, Paul S., and Thomas Grisso. 1995. The MacArthur Treatment Competence Study. I: Mental illness and competence to consent to treatment. *Law and Human Behavior* 19: 105–126.

27. Grisso, Thomas, Paul S. Appelbaum, Edward P. Mulvey, and Kenneth Fletcher. 1995. The MacArthur Treatment Competence Study. II: Measures of abilities related to competence to consent to treatment. *Law and Human Behavior* 19: 127–148.

28. Grisso, Thomas, and Paul S. Appelbaum. 1995. The MacArthur Treatment Competence Study. III: Abilities of patients to consent to psychiatric and medical treatments. *Law and Human Behavior* 19: 149–174.

29. Fazel, Seena, Tony Hope, and Robin Jacoby. 1999. Dementia, intelligence, and the competence to complete advance directives. *Lancet* 354: 48.

30. Caulfield, Timothy, Ross Upshur, and Abdallah Daar. 2003. DNA databanks and consent: A suggested policy option involving an authorization model. *BMC Medical Ethics* 4: 1.

31. Stoppe, G. 2007. Competence assessment in dementia. *Springer Science & Business Media*. ISBN 978-3-211-72368-5. doi:https://doi.org/10.1007/978-3-211-72369-2.

32. Council of Europe. 2005. *Additional Protocol to the Convention on Human Rights and Biomedicine, concerning Biomedical Research*. CETS No.195. Strasbourg, 25/01/2005. https://rm.coe.int/CoERMPublicCommonSearchServices/DisplayDCTMContent? documentId=090000168008371a

33. Groves, Kashina. 2006. Justified paternalism: The nature of beneficence in the care of dementia patients. *Penn Bioethics Journal* 2: 17–20.

34. Ashcroft, Richard Edmund, Angus Dawson, Heather Draper, and John R. McMillan, eds. 2007. *Principles of Health Care Ethics*. John Wiley & Sons. ISBN: 978-0-470-02713-4.

35. World Medical Association. 2013. World Medical Association Declaration of Helsinki. *Journal of American Medical Association* 310: 2191–2194.

36. Novitzky, Peter, Alan F. Smeaton, Cynthia Chen, Kate Irving, Tim Jacquemard, Fiachra O'Brolcháin, Dónal O'Mathúna, and Bert Gordijn. 2015. A review of contemporary work on the ethics of ambient assisted living technologies for people with dementia. *Science and Engineering Ethics* 21: 707–765.

37. Astell, Arlene, Norman Alm, Gary Gowans, Maggie Ellis, Richard Dye, and Phillip Vaughan. 2009. Involving older people with dementia and their carers in designing computer based support systems: Some methodological considerations. *Universal Access in the Information Society* 8: 49–58.

38. Muramoto, Osamu. 2011. Socially and temporally extended end-of-life decision-making process for dementia patients. *Journal of Medical Ethics* 37: 339–343.

39. Holm, Søren. 2001. Autonomy, authenticity, or best interest: Everyday decision-making and persons with dementia. *Medicine, Health Care and Philosophy* 4: 153–159.

40. Dworkin, Ronald. 1993. *Life's Dominion: An Argument About Abortion, Euthanasia, and Individual Freedom*. Knopf.

41. Dresser, Rebecca. 1995. Dworkin on dementia: Elegant theory, questionable policy. *Hastings Center Report* 25: 32–38.

42. Shiffrin, Seana Valentine. 2004. Autonomy, beneficence, and the permanently demented. In *Ronald Dworkin and His Critics*, ed. Justin Burley.

43. Huxtable, Richard. 2012. *Law, Ethics and Compromise at the Limits of Life: To Treat or not to Treat?* Taylor & Francis.
44. Honeybul, Stephen, Grant R. Gillett, Kwok M. Ho, Courtney Janzen, and Kate Kruger. 2014. Long-term survival with unfavourable outcome: A qualitative and ethical analysis. *Journal of Medical Ethics.* 41: 963–969. doi:http://dx.doi.org/10.1136/medethics-2013-101960
45. Potter, J. E., S. McKinley, and A. Delaney. 2013. Research participants' opinions of delayed consent for a randomised controlled trial of glucose control in intensive care. *Intensive Care Medicine* 39: 472–480.
46. *Normoglycaemia in Intensive Care Evaluation.* 2004. Australia and New Zealand Intensive Care Society Clinical Trials Group, Canadian Critical Care Trials Group (CCCTG) and The George Institute for International Health.
47. Kaye, Jane, Edgar A. Whitley, David Lund, Michael Morrison, Harriet Teare, and Karen Melham. 2015. Dynamic consent: A patient interface for twenty-first century research networks. *European Journal of Human Genetics* 23(2): 141. doi:10.1038/ejhg.2014.71
48. Kelly, Paul, Simon J. Marshall, Hannah Badland, Jacqueline Kerr, Melody Oliver, Aiden R. Doherty, and Charlie Foster. 2013. An ethical framework for automated, wearable cameras in health behavior research. *American Journal of Preventive Medicine* 44: 314–319.
49. van Hoof, Joost, H. S. M. Kort, P. Markopoulos, and M. Soede. 2007. Ambient intelligence, ethics and privacy. *Gerontechnology* 6: 155–163. doi:10.4017/gt.2007.06.03.005.00
50. van Hoof, J., H. S. M. Kort, P. G. S. Rutten, and M. S. H. Duijnstee. 2011. Ageing-in-place with the use of ambient intelligence technology: Perspectives of older users. *International Journal of Medical Informatics* 80: 310–331. doi:https://doi.org/10.1016/j.ijmedinf.2011.02.010
51. Portet, François, Michel Vacher, Caroline Golanski, Camille Roux, and Brigitte Meillon. 2011. Design and evaluation of a smart home voice interface for the elderly: acceptability and objection aspects. *Personal and Ubiquitous Computing* 17(1): 127–144. doi:https://doi.org/10.1007/s00779-011-0470-5
52. Duquenoy, Penny, and Diane Whitehouse. 2006. A 21st century ethical debate: Pursuing perspectives on ambient intelligence. In *The Information Society: Emerging Landscapes,* ed. Chris Zielinski, Penny Duquenoy, and Kai Kimppa, 195:293–314. Springer, Boston, MA. doi:https://doi.org/10.1007/0-387-31168-8_18.
53. Kang, Hyun Gu, Diane F. Mahoney, Helen Hoenig, Victor A. Hirth, Paolo Bonato, Ihab Hajjar, and Lewis A. Lipsitz. 2010. In situ monitoring of health in older adults: Technologies and issues. *Journal of the American Geriatrics Society* 58: 1579–1586.
54. Ploug, Thomas, and Søren Holm. 2015. Routinisation of informed consent in online health care systems. *International Journal of Medical Informatics* 84: 229–236.
55. Ploug, Thomas, and Søren Holm. 2013. Informed consent and routinisation. *Journal of Medical Ethics* 39: 214–218.
56. Ploug, Thomas, and Søren Holm. 2014. Agreeing in ignorance: Mapping the routinisation of consent in ICT-services. *Science and Engineering Ethics* 20: 1097–1110.

57. Jacquemard, Tim, Peter Novitzky, Fiachra O'Brolcháin, Alan F. Smeaton, and Bert Gordijn. 2014. Challenges and opportunities of lifelog technologies: A literature review and critical analysis. *Science and Engineering Ethics* 20: 379–409.
58. Louhiala, Pekka, and R. Puustinen. 2008. Rethinking the placebo effect. *Medical Humanities* 34: 107–109.
59. Miller, Franklin G., and Luana Colloca. 2011. The placebo phenomenon and medical ethics: Rethinking the relationship between informed consent and risk-benefit assessment. *Theoretical Medicine and Bioethics* 32: 229–243.
60. Burton, Adrian. 2013. Dolphins, dogs, and robot seals for the treatment of neurological disease. *Lancet Neurology* 12: 851–852.

11

Personal Identity, Neuroprosthetics, and Alzheimer's Disease

Fabrice Jotterand

Introduction

Alzheimer's disease (AD) is one of the most dreaded diseases among people 55 years old and over (Chiong 2013). The main reason is that the condition affects not only the motor skills of individuals but also their identity. It is not uncommon to hear patients in the early stages of AD speaking of their selves "disintegrating," stating that "I feel like I cannot find myself," or complaining that "I am no longer me" (Leadbeater 2015; Chiong 2013). Changes in personal identity are not a unique phenomenon limited to the devastating effects of AD on people. Traumatic insult to brain structure (e.g., Phineas Gage), the purposive manipulation of brain structure (e.g., lobotomy—procedure abandoned in the mid-1950s with the advent of psychopharmacology) to attenuate psychiatric symptoms, the use of psychotropic drugs (e.g., Prozac), and the use of neurostimulation technologies (e.g., deep brain stimulation) can affect personal identity (Jotterand and Giordano 2011). What is disconcerting with AD is the way it impacts people. As Charles Leadbeater points out:

> Dementia is troubling because, at the same time as it erodes someone's memory, it also eats away at th[e] capacity to create shared meaning. If someone cannot remember not just where the milk bottle goes, but what a milk bottle is for, then the shared pre-suppositions on which communication, meaning and identity depend become badly strained. (Leadbeater 2015)

Various approaches are under development to counteract the effects of AD, including neurotechnologies that include deep brain stimulation (DBS) and the use of an artificial hippocampus. In this chapter, I explore the implications of the use of neuroprosthetics on questions pertaining to personal identity and meaning making. I examine the implications of the use of artificial hippocampi for our understanding of personal identity in patients with AD: first, regarding a conceptualization of personal identity based on psychological continuity (memory), and second, according to a conceptualization of personal identity based on psychological continuity (memory) *and* embodiment. In a nutshell, this chapter focuses on how the use of an artificial hippocampus could limit our definition of personal identity if we confine our understanding of self to psychological continuity.

In what follows, first, I provide an overview of the various stages of AD, including how the disorder impacts people's memory capabilities and personality and generates behavioral changes. The next section focuses on neuroprosthetics (i.e., artificial hippocampus) as a technique to help patients in the early stages of AD to compensate for lost neural functionality and cognitive abilities. The use of an artificial hippocampus raises questions about the intended goals of the intervention, either to restore and preserve identity integrity or to allow the creation of a new identity regardless of past events and personal history. The next two sections critically examine the concept of personal identity through the work of John Locke (1690/1999) and Derek Parfit (1984, 1995) (psychological continuity) and provide an alternative account (bio-psycho-somatic unity) to capture the fullness of the human experience. The last section of the chapter offers an ethical framework for the care of patients with AD who experience identity loss that includes the preservation or restoration of psychological continuity, the acknowledgment of an embodied identity, and the necessity of a relational narrative.

Stages of AD and Its Impact on Memory

Typically, AD progresses in three stages: mild (early stage), moderate (middle stage), and severe (late stage). A more refined description of the disease progression was developed by Dr. Barry Reisberg, clinical director of New York University's Aging and Dementia Research Center. He outlines seven major clinical stages of AD. Stage 1 (no impairment) includes individuals with no memory problems for which there is no evidence that any symptoms can be diagnosed by healthcare professionals. Stage 2 (very mild cognitive decline—normal cognitive decline related to age or early signs of AD) includes persons who may experience memory lapses but which cannot be detected by a medical examination. Stage 3 (mild cognitive impairment) can be diagnosed in some individuals, while Stage 4 (moderate cognitive impairment) can be detected due to clear deficiencies in remembering recent events and a decreased ability to perform complex tasks. More important, in the context of this chapter, in Stage 4, individuals experience reduced memory of personal history (more on this point later in the chapter). In Stage 5 (moderately severe cognitive impairment), persons have major cognitive deficits and need help with some everyday activities. Stage 6 (severe cognitive decline) is characterized by a worsening of cognitive decline but also by personality changes and the inability to recount their personal history with exactitude. In the final stage, Stage 7 (very severe cognitive decline), people suffering from AD lose their ability to interact with their environment and to speak appropriately. Changes in personality and behavior can also occur (alz.org). With end-stage AD, patients are totally dependent on other people for their care. It is estimated that following diagnosis, the average individual suffering from AD will live an additional 8 to 10 years; however, some persons have survived up to 20 years (Blass 2009).

In the initial stages, AD alters short-term memory because the disorder first affects the hippocampus, where memories are stored. When short-term memories are not transformed into long-term memories, they are lost indefinitely. For this reason, individuals suffering from AD will be able to remember events from childhood or events in early adulthood (long-term memory) but will very often forget what occurred a few hours ago (short-term memory). In the next phase of the progression of the disease, the temporal lobe is affected— the structure of the brain where speech, sound, and words are processed. As the disease continues its damage to the brain, the prefrontal cortex will eventually be affected, which is responsible for decision making and judgments. Ultimately, the neurological impact of the disorder is so severe that patients might experience hallucinations resulting in the inability to care for themselves (Schmid 2016).

Neuroprosthetics: Artificial Hippocampus

It is important to keep in mind that, as the disorder progresses, AD affects personality and behavior significantly. Therefore, efforts to address AD ought not to be limited to cognition but also to other dimensions such as decision-making capacity and speech, sound, and words processing. Whether technology to compensate for the failings of the prefrontal cortex or the temporal lobe is possible remains an open question that is beyond the scope of this analysis.

That said, various efforts have been made to address the deleterious effects of the disorder on brain integrity and functionality. Currently there is no cure and no preventive measures to slow down the progression of AD. The US Food and Drug Administration (FDA), however, has approved five prescription drugs (Aricept—donepezil, Razadyne—galantamine, Namenda—memantine, Exelon—rivastigmine, and Namzaric—donepezil and memantine) to treat the symptoms of AD in relation to thinking, learning, language, judgment, and memory. As with many other areas in medicine, when psychopharmacology does not provide solutions, the alternative is to look at devices or neurotechnologies (interestingly, lobotomies were rendered obsolete when the FDA approved the drug Thorazine in the 1950s). Researchers are developing techniques for neuromodulation (DBS) or for substituting damaged brain functions through neuroprosthetics (i.e., artificial hippocampus—implantation of a chip in the brain attached to the nervous system that would replace or compensate for lost cognitive functions such as memory) to help patients improve their cognitive functions. A 2012 study examined the effects of DBS on the entorhinal cortex (the gateway to the hippocampus involved in memory and learning) on seven subjects with pharmacoresistant epilepsy to determine whether the procedure would enhance memory (Suthana et al. 2012). After testing, the data demonstrated that entorhinal stimulation positively affects memory. More recently, a team of neuroscientists at the University of Pennsylvania developed a technique to compensate for the failings of the hippocampus through electrical stimulation of the hippocampus (Ezzyat et al. 2017). The process consists of stimulating the brain when lapses of memory encoding occurred. As Micheal Kahana, psychologist and principal investigator of the project, explained, "when electrical stimulation arrives during periods of effective memory, memory worsens. . . . But when the electrical stimulation arrives at time of poor function, memory is significantly improved" (cited in Baillie and Berger 2017). This procedure is still in the experimental stage, and more testing is needed before therapeutic applications. The point here, however, is not to evaluate the safety and efficacy of the procedure but to illustrate that, in principle, neurostimulation or the use of neuroprostheses could provide a means to compensate for memory lapses in the early stages of AD. The evidence indicates that improved memory function of the human brain is possible by electrically stimulating brain regions associated with memory consolidation or implanting a cortical neural prosthesis (Berger et al. 2011).

These technologies, if they become a standard of care, could help patients in the early stages of AD when only the hippocampus is affected by the disorder. The question remains, however, concerning how to care for this patient population as the disorder progresses and affects other areas of the brain such as the temporal lobe and the prefrontal cortex, which are crucial for speech, decision making, and judgment. Will other types of brain stimulation techniques or neuroprosthetics provide the support to compensate for lost neural functionality and cognitive abilities? While these are important considerations, this chapter is more limited in scope. In particular, as stated in the introductory comments, I examine how the use of an artificial hippocampus could limit our definition of personal identity if we confine our understanding of self to psychological continuity. The development of an artificial hippocampus will not restore lost memories between the onset of the disorder (when there is actual loss of memory) and the current condition of the patient. The technology will help consolidate current short-term memory, and therefore, it is essential to ask whether any technology should aim at helping regain *identity integrity* (in response to the issue of the "disintegrating self") or whether brain interventions, through technological means, should aim at *creating a new identity regardless of past history* (in response to "I am no longer me"). Identity integrity refers to a continuity in identity and memory that includes cognitive and physical memory. The creation of a new identity implies that following the implant of an artificial hippocampus, there is no attempt to use the technology to allow the "new person" to reconnect with past events that occurred when memory failed.

The Case of Mr. Jones

To illustrate the scope of issues I wish to address, let's assume the technology (artificial hippocampus) is proven to be safe and improve memory, or compensates for memory lapses in the early stage of AD. In addition, let's use the case of Mr. Jones:

> Peter Jones is a 75-year old man with the diagnosis of Alzheimer disease (AD). There is no history of dementia in Mr. Jones's family. He has no history of substance abuse. Before the onset of his illness, Mr. Jones had no history of psychiatric symptoms or treatment. For the first time, at age 71, Mr. Jones began having difficulty with his memory. . . . His wife noticed that he would occasionally repeat a question just 5 to 10 minutes after asking it and would have no memory of asking it the first time. . . . He started to make subtle language errors, substituting pencil for pen and table for desk. . . . He would begin home-improvement projects . . . and then leave them uncompleted. . . . Eventually, Mrs. Jones took Mr. Jones to see a neurologist. . . . They spent the first 10 minutes "talking about the old days," and Mr. Jones remembered details from 40 years ago flawlessly. . . . Memory-enhancing medications prescribed by the neurologist were only minimally helpful and were ultimately discontinued. . . . At one point, Mr. Jones developed the belief that someone was hiding the wallet and keys from him. . . . Two years after his official diagnosis, Mr. Jones was admitted to the hospital for treatment of hyperglycemia. . . . Later, he did not remember why he was in the hospital or what the problem was that led to the hospitalization. (Blass 2009, 50–52)

Mr. Jones is an excellent case to illustrate the use of an artificial hippocampus for a patient with early-stage AD. As the previous account outlines, Mr. Jones displays the symptoms of an individual whose memory is faulty. His short-term memory is affected, as are his cognitive functions such as language and behavior. Remarkably, however, he remembers perfectly events that happened 40 years ago.

We can confidently state that Mr. Jones does not indicate any radical changes of personality but a continuous transformation occurring as the result of the effects of AD and life in general. He has, as the disorder progresses, a "diminished self," but we are not dealing with a "different person, in the strong sense." His "identity change[s], in the psychological sense, but [he is] the same person, diminished and changed" (Perry 2009, 149). Would the implant of neuroprosthetics challenge this claim? This is what I intend to investigate in what follows.

Personal Identity

In their book *Personal Identity and Fractured Selves*, Mathews, Bok, and Rabins (2009) conclude that based on the consensus gathered from the analysis of a multidisciplinary team, the definition of personal identity is characterized by (a) "an ability to express a self-narrative that recognizes the presence of an acting individual (a self or identity)" and (b) "a constructed narrative that demonstrates intentionality, reasoned choice, and coherence" (193). This definition, however, does not capture the fullness of the human experience. For instance, it fails to include various groups of individuals who do not or never did have these abilities, such as severely handicapped persons, infants, people who lost their capacity to express a self-narrative or to make rational choices due to brain damage, or individuals suffering from AD in the latter stages. Their account assumes a functionalist approach that reduces personal identity to psychological or cognitive capacities. In the case of individuals with AD, it would mean that they have a "shattered" personal identity. The gap in memory, particularly short-term memory, results in a lack of psychological continuity, which can be considered problematic for the construct of personal identity. For instance, John Locke (*An Essay on Human Understanding*, 1690/1999) and Derek Parfit (*Reasons and Persons*, 1984) argue that gaps in memory result in a shattered self. For Locke, memory is central to the definition of personal identity, and consciousness is what allows an individual to connect the past to the present self to create personal identity. As he points out:

> Consciousness alone unites actions into the same person. . . . Self depends on consciousness. . . . Self is that conscious thinking thing . . . which is . . . capable of happiness or misery, and so is concerned for itself, as far as that consciousness extends. . . . Person is the name for this self. . . . This personality extends itself beyond present existence to what is past only by consciousness. . . . [I]n this alone consists personal identity, i.e. the sameness of a rational being: and as far as this consciousness can be extended backwards to any past action or thought. (Locke, Book II, Chap. 27, 9, 17, 26)

Parfit espouses views similar to those of Locke. Parfit starts his discussion about the nature of persons and personal identity exploring three fundamental issues: (a) the nature of persons, (b) the factors that make a person the same (numerically identical) at two different times, and (c) the elements that ensure "continued existence" of a person over time. He then outlines three criteria that can be used to define personal identity: (a) the physical criterion, that is, the physical continuity of a living person's brain and body over time; (b) the psychological criterion #1, which involves the continued existence "of a purely mental entity, or thing—a soul, or spiritual substance"; and (c) the psychological criterion #2, which focuses on the continuity of memory (Parfit 1984, 199–217). While Parfit favors the psychological criterion based on the continuity of memory, in his view, personal identity is not what matters. What *really* matters, as his essay entitled "The Unimportance of Identity" suggests, is not how we conceptualize the notion of personal identity, but rather what he calls the *Relation R*: psychological connectedness and/or continuity, that is, the connectedness of intentions, memories, desires, and other psychological features (Parfit 1984, 1995). The logical conclusion of Parfit's position on the conceptualization of personal identity is that the body does not play any role in defining and constructing one's self. Hypothetically, one's psychological makeup could be transferred onto a computational substrate and the person would be the same, if there are no memory gaps and there is psychological continuity. In short, Parfit contends that personal identity is closely related to one's ability to create a coherent and organized whole based on a continuum of life experience events that describe one's identity.

Bio-Psycho-Somatic Unity

Contrary to approaches such as the ones offered by Locke or Parfit, I argue that the notion of embodiment should be included in our definition to provide a more robust understanding of personal identity. "Being in the world," to refer to Merleau-Ponty (1945/1962), cannot be limited to memory (cognitive memory), as suggested by Parfit. The body is the medium through which one makes memory and shared meaning in relation to others. Hence, continuing the development of memories could certainly include the help of an artificial hippocampus, but it needs to incorporate the process by which one enters into relation with others as a source of narration to rebuild lost memory—assuming the artificial hippocampus transforms short-term memories into long-term memories. This point is important in the context of the care of patients with AD because memory is an issue of not only mental impressions stored in the brain (hippocampus) but also how the body provides the medium through which mental impressions are perceived, interpreted, and recorded. In other words, if short-term memory is affected by AD and if identity is defined by the continuous stream of memories (cognitive memory) without the input of the body (physical memory—e.g., the scar on the hand that reminds someone of a specific event in space and time), this means that individuals suffering from AD are trapped in a body that is foreign to them. In short, the corporeal experience does not provide any sensory input to provide a sense of self, personal identity, or shared memories. The justification of the use of many technologies—and neuroprostheses are no exception—reflects an adoption of the type of dualism I just described. There is an assumption that the body does not provide any framework for personal identity. The body is simply a canvas that experts in biotechnologies and biomedical sciences can shape at will without restriction as long as there is a strong enough justification (on utilitarian grounds) to transcend its limitations. The body (the whole body) is not considered as part of the essence of human identity or the generator of identity, only the brain, aka psychological continuity.

Contrary to these perspectives, I argue that human identity cannot be reduced to the brain or mental states (i.e., neuroessentialism; for a critique of neuroessentialism see Jotterand 2016). In this regard, psychiatrist John Sadler is helpful. He defines personal self as a "heuristic concept" that "is personal, autobiographical, and permeated with purposes, conditions, and the primordial experiences of an 'I.' A 'personal self' . . . provides a meaningful orientation to the world. . . . [It] is 'owned' by an individual subject" (Sadler 2007, 114). This orientation toward the world is constituted by five elements: (a) agency—the ability to act in the world as an agent; (b) identity—the recognition of oneself as different from others; (c) trajectory—a sense of purpose; (d) history—the temporal dimension that provides a sense of the past, the present, and the future to the "I"; and (e) perspective—a unique outlook and experience of the surrounding world (Sadler 2007). These five elements locate the personal self in space and time with a unique status *within* the world, a unique relation *to* the world, a unique history and destiny *in* the world, and a unique perspective *about* the world (Jotterand 2010).

In light of these considerations, a more robust definition of personal identity can be suggested. The previous analysis demonstrates that, contra Locke and Parfit, personal identity includes two interrelated dimensions of human existence: psychological and biological aspects. On the one hand, psychological aspects correspond to mental abilities and character traits that allow individuals to reason, use language to communicate, make decisions and act as moral agents, and so forth. However, as human beings, we don't live in a virtual world totally detached from our bodily realities in the material world. Human agency consists of biological aspects. The body is a biological organism that allows humans to experience and interpret space and time. French philosopher Merleau-Ponty, in *Phenomenology of Perception* (1945/1962), states that "being-toward-the-thing through the intermediary of the body" is an essential condition for humans to develop a sense of self or personal identity based on the notions of spatiality and temporality. He writes:

> Consciousness is being-toward-the-thing through the intermediary of the body. A movement is learned when the body has understood it, that is, when it has incorporated it into its "world," and to move one's body is to aim at things through it; it is to allow oneself to respond to their call, which is made up independently of any representation. In order that we may be able to move our body toward an object, the object must first exist for it, our body must not belong to the realm of the "in-itself." . . . The space and time which I inhabit are always in their different ways indeterminate horizons which contain other points of view. The synthesis of both time and space is a task that always has to be performed afresh. Our bodily experience of movement is not a particular case of knowledge; it provides us a way of access to the world and the object. (160–162)

The body is the means by which humans inhabit the world, engage with it, and make sense of it through the interpretation of the various stimuli (touch, sight, smell, taste, hearing) available. Our psychological (mental) states are conditioned by what we experience through the body, and consequently we can rightly support the definition provided by Jennifer Radden (1996) that human beings are an "embodied repository of integrated psychological states" (11).

Identity Loss and Meaning Making

The idea that a human being is an integrated, embodied psychological entity constitutes a crucial concept for how we should assess the impact of AD on the personal identity of patients. When an AD patient is unable to engage with the surrounding world and interact with persons, the use of an artificial hippocampus might be of limited use without a broader understanding of personal identity formation that includes the assertions of others. The earlier distinction between *identity integrity* and *creation of a new identity* becomes the key question about this type of technology. In other words, it is not clear what the boundaries are regarding the applications of devices that would, hypothetically, compensate for loss of memory functions but without the ability to recall a segment of the life of the individuals for which there are no recollections. Two options are available. Either the patient decides to allow the use of the devices to help the individual functions based on what he or she recalls (creation of a new identity regardless of past history) or the device should be used to help the patient reconstruct the old self as much as possible. If the latter option is the plan of action, it means that clinical interventions should aim at restoring personal identity and avoid a detachment from the past as much as possible. In everyday life, it means that others—family, friends, and caregivers—play an important role in the re-formation (i.e., providing a narrative or facts) of these memories that give meaning to these individuals suffering from AD.[1] Identity is not just how one is able to construct a sense of self but also how others continue to recognize and shape the identity of the demented patient. As Bullington remarks, "The lived body is to be understood as someone's lived relationship to the world. It is an ambiguous unity, both subject and object, both mind and body, intertwined, understood in terms of levels, or planes of signification rather than mutually exclusive categories of being" (Bullington 2013, 30).

But what exactly is the nature of this relationship to the world if ability to recall biographical events is impaired? Persons suffering from AD don't recognize close relatives and cannot remember how to use certain objects or devices. This breakdown occurs on two levels: first, at the functional level—that is, the disorder limits the ability of a demented person to function in the world independently; and second, at the cognitive level—that is, the surrounding people of a person with AD can become strangers. Combined, these two dimensions lead to the breakdown of the integrity of the self or the emergence of a self negatively affected by illness.

Meaning Making

To address the question of the relationship between personal identity, embodiment, and meaning making, it is worth exploring the perspective defended by Francoise Baylis called the "relational narrative account of personal identity" (Baylis 2012, 2017). In her account of personal identity, she outlined a relational and socially oriented position that values personal embodiment and "the social, political, and cultural embeddedness and interdependence of persons" (Baylis 2017, 215). This means that personal identity is shaped by past and present interactions that occurred or are occurring in the private and public sphere. It is through this synergic exchange with others that meaning and belonging are developed and cultivated. Formation of the personal identity occurs not only through an autobiographical story but also through the lived experience in relation to others. It is this dual dimension of inner (self-ascription) and outer (ascription by others) input that ultimately assigns our place in the world and ascribes us an identity. As Baylis (2012) remarks, the ongoing "(more or less conscious) interpretations of our values, memories, actions, experiences, and so on as well as the (more or less conscious) interpretations of these same characteristics by others" leads to the formation of one's personal identity, character traits, memories, meaning, and so forth (117).

The formation of one's identity, in the relational narrative identity account, cannot be limited to memories or inner life, contrary, as we have seen, to Locke and Parfit. It is in relationship to others that an individual is recognized, affirmed, and embraced throughout one's life span. While sources of meaning making include an ability to engage with the world, interact with objects, and communicate with individuals (Widdershoven and Berghmans 2006), it is crucial, in the context of this chapter, to stress that personal identity is also a fact of how others shape one's biographical narrative. The inability of an AD patient to recall short-term events underscores the necessity of the inner circles of relatives and friends to be agents of meaning making and identity recognition and affirmation, recognizing that ultimately the patient interprets facts and ideas and reconstructs meaning.

This relational posture is echoed by philosopher Alasdair MacIntyre, who stated that "what [an] agent is able to do and say intelligibly as an actor is deeply affected by the fact that we are never more (and sometimes less) than the co-authors of our own narratives . . . each of us being a main character in his own drama [who] plays subordinate parts in the dramas of others, and each drama constraints the others" (MacIntyre 1984, 213, quoted in Baylis 2017, 216). Regardless of mental state, cognitive abilities, or lack of communication, it is through the encounter of the other that identities are affirmed, recognized, and valued.

Identity Integrity

Another aspect to take into consideration is how human agency is constituted within what Charles Taylor calls *frameworks* in his discussion about moral life (Taylor 1989). In what follows, I would like to make an analogy between moral identity and personal identity. In the context of his discussion of the self in moral space, Taylor notes that frameworks provide the background in which our moral judgments take place. One's ability to outline a framework provides a justification of his or her moral response. In other words, these frameworks provide a moral identity to individuals according to "horizons within which [they] live [their] lives" and make sense insofar as they include "qualitative discriminations" (Taylor 1989, 27).[2] These frameworks provide identity and integrity. Outside these boundaries, Taylor points out, the integrity of human agency is compromised. As he points out, "the claim is that living within such strongly qualified horizons is constitutive of human agency, that stepping outside these limits would be tantamount to stepping outside what we would recognize as integral, that is, undamaged human personhood" (Taylor 1989, 27). By analogy, the horizon of a patient with AD is constituted by the elements that define the identity of the individual, past and present, mental and corporeal. These elements form the "frameworks" that are intrinsic to a person, regardless of health status, and are constantly shaping the identity of the patient during the progression of the disease (neuroplasticity). To step outside these horizons or boundaries through technological means equates to stepping outside identity integrity.

Ethical Framework

Whether it is moral formation of the self (Taylor) or identity formation of the self, preserving or restoring the self, according to the patient narrative, constitutes a moral imperative. Let's go back to the case of Mr. Jones. Following his admission to the hospital for treatment of hyperglycemia, Mr. Jones "did not remember why he was in the hospital or what the problem was that led to the hospitalization." Granted, this is a somewhat trivial example, but it illustrates how people surrounding him play an integral part in shaping his narrative and identity. The fact that Mr. Jones has high blood sugar (hyperglycemia) is an important piece of information, clinically speaking. In addition, this medical condition confers a special identity to him that requires special attention. Only in relation to others will Mr. Jones be able to acknowledge, even for a short period of time, that he is diabetic and that this is part of his biographical narrative. There would of course be less serious elements in Mr. Jones's life that could be omitted because they might not have the same potential outcomes on his health. However, preserving or restoring the integrity of personal identity is a moral imperative. Each element of the narrative of the life of Mr. Jones is part of this "horizon within which he lives his life," and therefore dismissing some aspects deemed unimportant is tantamount to a lack of integrity of the (damaged or diminished) self. The care of individuals suffering from AD (by caregivers, family, and friends) and the use of an artificial hippocampus for treatment of this population of patients (ideally) require more than addressing the symptoms of AD. A neural prosthesis is certainly an extraordinary means to enhance the quality of life of these individuals, but restoring the identity as much as possible according to patients' framework is an essential task for their care. This undertaking will include the preservation or restoration of psychological continuity, the acknowledgment of an embodied identity, and the necessity of a relational narrative.

Concluding Remarks

Recent developments in neuroscience and neurotechnologies have increased our knowledge about brain functions, how various diseases can disrupt neural functionality, and how structures and functions of the brain can be manipulated and/or replaced. This progress challenges some of the assumptions held concerning personal identity and the role of embodiment in determining it. This chapter demonstrates that the implementation of neuroprostheses in the clinical context for the treatment of AD must protect, or aim at restoring, the integrity of the self, regardless of the patient's cognitive abilities, and recognize the role of the relational dimension in the care of this population of patients. Memory is at the core of personal identity. When it fails, levels of both functionality and competence are affected to a point where an individual feels his or her self is disintegrating. The use of an artificial hippocampus could be a promising option to help individuals with AD to regain a sense of wholeness and purpose. However, it is imperative to provide an environment where patients are recognized and affirmed in their identity, past and present. To bypass the boundaries (frameworks) in which individuals constructed themselves throughout their lives would damage further their personhood already affected by the horrendous effects of AD. Only by being attentive to their cognitive, emotional, psychological, spiritual, and physical needs and their dignity will we provide the care they need.[3]

Notes

1. Of course, there is the risk that people may impose a narrative on persons with AD, hence the importance of creating an environment in which these technologies will not be abused and patients will be respected.
2. Taylor (1989) defines "frameworks" as follows: "Frameworks provide the background, explicit or implicit, for our moral judgments, intuitions, or reactions in any of the three dimensions. To articulate a framework is to explicate what makes sense of our moral responses. That is, when we try to spell out what it is that we presuppose when we judge that a certain form of life is truly worthwhile, or place our dignity in a certain achievement or status, or define our moral obligations in a certain manner, we find ourselves articulating inter alia what I have been calling here 'frameworks'" (26).
3. I want to thank two external reviewers for the helpful comments on a previous draft of this chapter.

References

1. Baillie U, Berger W. Penn Researchers Show Brain Stimulation Restores Memory During Lapses. *Penn News.* 2017.
2. Baylis F. Still Gloria: Personal Identity and Dementia. *International Journal of Feminist Approaches to Bioethics.* 2017; 10(1): 210–224.
3. Baylis F. The Self In Situ: A Relational Account of Personal Identity. In: J Downie and J Llewellyn (Eds.), *Relational Theory and Health Law and Policy.* University of British Columbia Press; 2012: 109–131.
4. Berger TW, Hampson RE, Song D, Goonawardena A, Marmarelis VZ, Deadwyler SA. A Cortical Neural Prosthesis for Restoring and Enhancing Memory. *Journal of Neural Engineering.* 2011; 8(4): 046017.
5. Blass M. Case Studies. In: DJH Mathews, H Bok, and PV Rabins (Eds.), *Personal Identity and Fractured Selves.* Johns Hopkins University Press; 2009: 50–62.
6. Bullington J. *The Expression of the Psychosomatic Body from a Phenomenological Perspective.* Springer; 2013.
7. Chiong W. Dementia and Personal Identity: Implications for Decision-Making. In: JL Bernat and R Beresford (Eds.), *Handbook of Clinical Neurology.* Elsevier; 2013: 409–418.
8. Ezzyat Y, Kragel J, Burke J, et al. Direct Brain Stimulation Modulates Encoding States and Memory Performance in Humans. *Current Biology.* 2017; 27(9): 1251–1258.
9. Jotterand F, Giordano J. Transcranial Magnetic Stimulation, Deep Brain Stimulation and Personal Identity: Ethical Questions, and Neuroethical Approaches for Medical Practice. *International Review of Psychiatry.* 2011; 23(5): 476–485.
10. Jotterand F. Human Dignity and Transhumanism: Do Anthro-Technological Devices Have Moral Status? *American Journal of Bioethics.* 2010; 10(7): 45–52.
11. Jotterand F. Moral Enhancement, Neuroessentialism, and Moral Content. In: F Jotterand and V Dubljevic (Eds.), *Cognitive Enhancement: Ethical and Policy Implications in International Perspectives.* Oxford University Press; 2016: 42–56.
12. Leadbeater C. The Disremembered. Aeon 2015. Available online: https://aeon.co/essays/if-your-memory-fails-are-you-still-the-same-person
13. Locke J. *An Essay on Human Understanding.* Pennsylvania State University; 1690/1999.
14. MacIntyre A. *After Virtue.* University of Notre Dame Press; 1984.
15. Mathews DJH, Bok H, and Rabins PV. *Personal Identity and Fractured Selves.* Johns Hopkins University Press; 2009.
16. Merleau-Ponty M. *Phenomenology of Perception.* Routledge & Kegan Paul; 1945/1962.
17. Parfit D. *Reasons and Persons.* Oxford University Press; 1984.
18. Parfit D. The Unimportance of Identity. In: H Harris (Ed.), *Identity.* Oxford University Press; 1995: 13–45.
19. Perry J. Diminished and Fractured Selves. In: DJH Mathews, H Bok, and PV Rabins (Eds.), *Personal Identity and Fractured Selves.* Johns Hopkins University Press; 2009: 129–162.
20. Radden J. *Divided Minds and Successive Selves: Ethical Issues in Disorders of Identity and Personality.* MIT Press; 1996.
21. Sadler JZ. The Psychiatric Significance of the Personal Self. *Psychiatry.* 2007; 70(2): 113–129.

22. Schmid J. The Alzheimer's Brain. 2016. Available online: http://www.best-alzheimers-products.com/category/alzheimers-disease-2/what-is-alzheimers-disease

23. Suthana N, Haneef Z, Stern J, Mukamel R, Behnke E, Knowlton B, Fried I. Memory Enhancement and Deep-Brain Stimulation of the Entorhinal Area. *New England Journal of Medicine.* 2012; 366: 502–510.

24. Taylor C. *Sources of the Self.* Harvard University Press; 1989.

25. Widdershoven GAM and Berghmans RLP. Meaning-Making in Dementia: A Hermeneutic Perspective. In: Julian C. Hughes, Stephen J. Louw and Steven R. Sabat (Eds.), *Dementia: Mind, Meaning, and the Person.* Oxford University Press; 2006.

12

Developing Assistive Technologies for Persons with Alzheimer's Disease and Their Carers

The Ethics of Doing Good, Not Harm

Diane Feeney Mahoney

Introduction

As this compendium indicates, there is a growing interest worldwide in the role of technology in the care spectrum of services for older adults with dementia and their carers. Over time, societal expectations have influenced the approach to persons with dementia from stigmatization and social exclusion to inclusion and empowerment (1). Globally, contemporary advocates seek to enable and better support both the person with the disease and his or her carers (2). Among the innovations in dementia caregiving, certain approaches, such as wireless sensor technologies for monitoring daily activities at home, are controversial. Home is personal space, typically filled with objects that offer meaning and symbolism. It offers a sense of comfort from being surrounded by the known, the experienced, and the familiar. Critics contend that installing assistive technologies disrupts the sense of place and replaces human relationships and refocuses attention on computer interactions rather than personal ones (3). Moreover, others claim that technology causes a loss of autonomy as it takes over the directing and/or reporting of activities (4). The "big brother" surveillance attributed to monitoring technologies is seen as reducing privacy and negatively substituting for human carers (5). The presumption is that this reduces human interactions and leads to increased social isolation of older adults: "high tech" at the loss of "high touch." Yet Lawton, a prominent gerontologist who studied the environments of older adults and their activities of daily living over several decades, embraced the potential of new technologies as a means for fortifying fading function in his later years (6).

Indeed, the idea of developing assistive technologies as cognitive orthotics to help remind, cue, sustain, and oversee the safety of a person with dementia has been actuated. As an example, Huschilt and Clune report, in their review of the literature on socially assistive robots (SARs), that the studies to date demonstrate that persons with dementia and their caregivers particularly like the prompting, reminding, and serving as cowalking companions that SARs can provide (7). The critics, however, propose multiple adverse effects such as diminished autonomy through device dependence, inappropriate emotional attachment to the device, and replacement of human service professionals and human interactions by these machines (8, 9). Similarly, Landau et al. conducted a review of families' and professional caregivers' views of using GPSs to locate people with dementia who wander away. Caregiving users embraced GPS as a means to promote safety and avoid the harms associated with persons with dementia becoming lost, typically injury and death (10). GPS opponents view this technology as a negative form of "big brother" tracking surveillance, one that impinges on human dignity, freedom, and privacy (11). The technologizing of the self by a hypercognitive society is seen as devaluing people with dementia (3). Alternatively, Essen's study of frail older users of technology found that they perceived electronic surveillance as freeing and protecting their privacy because it enabled them to continue to stay at home instead of having to move to a nursing home (12). Given the plethora of articles detailing the potential harms of technology, proportional evidence based on in situ data is not found in the research literature to support the numerous proposed adverse outcomes (13).

Gerontechnology cross-fertilizes the fields of gerontology (scientific study of aging) and technology (engineering sciences) and originated in the 1990s as an interdisciplinary field to link existing and developing technologies to the aspirations and needs of aging adults to enhance their quality of life (14). As gerontechnology research and related literature matures, data from actual end-users about the positive effects of technology on their lives is growing. Harm can occur if persons with dementia or their carers are denied the opportunity to participate in technology trials and thus miss being able to give input about their wants, needs, and preferences or to gain any benefits from the experience. Widdershowen supports using technology to overcome person- and environmental-determined disabilities but calls for a better integration of ethics and technology (15). Consequently, the development of systems that are inclusive of, acceptable to, and ethically supportive of persons with dementia and their carers warrants current attention.

The scope of this chapter is not to replicate the significant body of ethical literature or reviews on ambient assistive technologies for older adults. Readers interested in general philosophical ethical debates about technology and aging are referred to the comprehensive reviews by Novitzky et al. (16), Queirós et al. (17), Marziali et al. (18), and Ni Scanaill et al. (8) and related content in this book. Instead, this chapter seeks to provide a unique perspective, a discussion focused on the ethical guidelines for in-home monitoring of older adults with Alzheimer's disease (AD) (19) applying findings from our series of in situ "real world" research studies of persons with dementia and/or their carers. Contrary to the literature promulgating dehumanizing harms from technology usage, our research findings do not support these negative outcomes but identify benefits reported by end-users.

Challenges and Opportunities for Dementia Technology Interventions

There is no single technology solution or standard approach to developing dementia interventions because of the progressive fluctuating aspects of the disease. In the early stage, the person with dementia will experience intermittent to increasingly common forgetfulness. Home safety–type sensors initially become useful such as smoke, stove left on, and temperature detection along with intrusion alerts. Personal emergency response systems can be added and monitored from off-site locations to contact the user to see if help is needed when an alarm is triggered. Virtual visits connecting to family or friends through smartphones, tablets, and computers can be offered to maintain visual connections using Skype, FaceTime, and other emerging programs for less cost than traditional long-distance calling. By the late early through the middle stages of dementia, a constellation of symptoms can occur including daily fluctuations in a person's level of awareness, mood swings, energy levels, interest, and affect. Attention span decreases; distractibility increases; and understanding, executive functioning, and long-term memory progressively decline. Excessive stimuli or performance expectations that exceed the person's processing capability can cognitively overload and upset the person with dementia. During these stages, the connected home technologies that passively link a variety of motion, door, bed, chair, and bathroom sensors to a computer system that monitors and alerts carers when major variants in daily activities occur become relevant to support safer aging in place (20).

However, uniformity and standardization are critical technology elements. Scalability relies on standardized approaches. Algorithms demand it. Data generation loves it. Monitoring systems send alerts to report deviances, but they can't have too many options because intricate branching patterns are too difficult to debug and operate reliably. Machine learning algorithmic designs are gaining in popularity, but they require consistent patterns to distinguish deviances from normal routines, inform predictions, and direct meaningful responses. Persons with dementia, however, are not reliably consistent! According to Wherton and Monk, the design challenge is to provide flexible prompting systems that are sensitive to the intentions, capabilities, and values of their users (21). To attain that flexibility, my team waited for the maturing of context-aware affective/ambient intelligent technologies in order to develop custom applications for persons with dementia. We knew participants could not meaningfully interact with current technologies that require consistent, accurate, and predictable input from end-users. We adapted the affective technologies to develop the first prototype for an automated coaching aid for persons experiencing dementia-related dressing problems, one that could be tailored to their dressing habits and preferences (22).

Why did we wait? A technology–user mismatch occurs when devices are developed that exceed the cognitive capacity of the persons with dementia for the stage they are currently experiencing. Unfortunately, this is a common technology design error. At a recent conference, technologists presented their wayfinding GPS public transportation aid for persons in the middle stage of dementia. In their design, the user had to remember to take and carry the device on the bus/train, recall how to activate it, tap on the correct screen, interpret the guidance, and correctly follow the directions. Although it would have been fine for a user in the early stage to overcome intermittent memory losses, it was not a good match for those in the middle stage given the high probability that either the device or how to use it would be forgotten. Similarly, a food preparation prompting guide was presented for those needing intensive help to turn on a stove and boil water. However, at that stage, you would worry about cognitively impaired users burning themselves. An automated stove safety shutoff to avoid setting a fire, should the person wander away and become distracted elsewhere, would offer a lower-tech but more realistic and economical application. The mismatch to the end-users' needs could have been avoided in both these applications by including people experienced with AD from the clinical, social, personal, and/or caregiving perspectives at the preliminary design stage.

Additionally, these critical questions remain: How do we develop assistive technologies that respect users' fluctuating abilities by tailoring to their personalized needs? How do we do this while being mindful that we don't take away opportunities that enable the person to maintain his or her dignity and personhood? Overall, what are the benchmarks to ensure ethical technology research, development, and usage with persons with dementia? These questions will be answered throughout the remainder of this chapter.

Given the complex interplay of end-users' and technology design challenges, and the related ethical concerns, an interdisciplinary international working group of gerontechnologists collaborated with an ethicist to establish a humanistic-focused model and guidelines for home monitoring of persons with dementia (19). The following section discusses their key ethical principles now informed by examples from our technology development and program of caregiving research with persons with AD and their family, or significant others, as informal (unpaid) carers.

Key Ethical Principles

Respect for Persons

The principle of respect for persons directs us to ask for the opinion of our end-users, to offer them details about all the known information, and to disclose the anticipated benefits and the associated risks to technology usage. For persons with AD, we accomplish this by assessing and adjusting to the person's cognitive capabilities and, if this is not possible, including their legal surrogate decision maker to increase mutual understanding. Gerontechnology developers have a unique opportunity to design and develop applications that demonstrate respect for persons by fortifying their fading abilities. As detailed in the literature, carers attempt throughout the stages of dementia to preserve and protect the personhood or individuality of their care recipient/loved one (23). As they face increasing difficulties with their care recipient's cognition, emotional responses, and functional abilities, technology-based supports may be enabling. At the same time, the care recipient will probably experience fluctuations in cognition, sometimes having moments of lucidity where they can do the activities of daily living on their own. Adapting systems to respond to situational variations, by encouraging autonomy and avoiding a one-size-fits-all system approach, is the key technological challenge but critical to demonstrating respect for the person. We always start our projects using a qualitative focus group perspective to give voice to and gain the perspectives of our potential end-users. In our "Sensors for Seniors" project, the stakeholder focus groups held in three independent living facilities resulted in a model of "connected disconnections" reflecting deviances in care service expectations among residents, families, and staff (24). Subsequently, we designed a home monitoring system to address the tension points and quantitatively assessed outcomes (20). Similarly, a qualitative study of dementia-related dressing difficulties in phase 1 of the DRESS project also resulted in a model labeled the "preservation of self" (23). Participants emphasized the high importance of respecting the personhood of the person with dementia. In response, we proposed an assistive device to prompt dressing as a means to support the self-esteem and independence of the user. Given the participants' affirmation, the follow-up focus groups critiqued the mockup and they particularly liked the personalized dialogues and the way the system would adapt the type of support depending on the user's specific response (22).

In the mild or the early phases of AD, persons with dementia can understand and critique visual and video technology prototypes or simple mockups. Soliciting their opinions and providing opportunities for them to make choices about operations and features demonstrates respect for them as persons. In the early middle stage, full form factor developed prototypes that provide a "concrete" tangible example may enable responses. Thereafter, we have found that the cognitive ability to understand a mockup prototype and apply its usage in the abstract to one's personal situation is typically not achievable. For the latter and advanced stages, the involvement of the carer as a proxy will help to provide end-users' input. Family members, who are also the carers, are usually aware of the preferences and behavioral patterns of their relative over his or her lifetime, before and after acquiring AD. Knowing this history, as well as providing current help with care, knowledgeable carers/legal guardians can be asked to convey what they believe the affected person would reasonably self-determine to be in her or his best interest. As Baldwin indicates, the final best design is the one that best reflects the values and interests of those involved in that design. Moreover, he recommends including universal design elements to enhance technology usage across disabled and able-bodied populations, thus avoiding stigmatizing those with dementia (3).

Autonomy and Consent

Those with a presumptive diagnosis of neurocognitive impairment need to be screened to determine whether they have the capacity to understand and provide informed consent to participate in gerontechnology studies. Competency to consent remains with mild cognitive impairment and usually through the early stages of AD. Thereafter, those who are found not to have legal decision-making capacity may be able to assent at the moment to identify their wishes or have their surrogate decision makers provide this input. There may be cultural differences affecting the consent process. For example, in tribal societies the head of a village may need to consent. In the United States, federal regulations require that all parties directly involved in a study need to be informed about the study protocol and then given the opportunity to individually consent (25). At minimum, our studies involving a person with dementia and his or her carer require dual consents. Additional consents may be needed if other informal or professional carers are involved.

Potential participants, however, can be deferentially vulnerable when they are able to consent but are subject to the authority of others who might have biased interests in whether they agree to enroll in a research study. In our Elder Care project we experienced recruitment sabotage from the geriatric case managers, who, despite assurances otherwise, believed their union leaders, who insisted that the telephone interactive voice response (IVR) technology being tested to help monitor their waiting list of cases would be used to eliminate their jobs. The study had to be moved to a nonunionized home care agency with case managers open to technology testing. The research outcomes not only supported the value of the IVR system in helping case managers to identify and prioritize older adults in need of home visits but also identified the role aspects performed by case managers that this technology was not able to substitute for (26). Paradoxically, the technology complemented the case managers' work but could not replace them as was feared. In two of our other studies, agency staff refused to let us post or leave brochures for their clients to see in their offices because of "ethical concerns." When queried about the concerns, they focused on their personal anti-technology beliefs and noted they were "doing good" by protecting their patients from technology's perceived harm. We find that study recruitment becomes quite challenging if it is dependent on technophobic gatekeepers to disseminate study recruitment information. If persons are technology skeptics, they either do not refer potential participants to technology studies or do not volunteer if they are potential participants. Those who do volunteer to participate have a clear reason to do so and see the value of the technology to address an unmet need. Professionals using their gatekeeping position to not inform caregivers and competent patients about opportunities to participate in studies is ethically problematic due to paternalism. Prejudging and eliminating competent people's ability to make a choice disrespects their autonomous decision-making capacity and personal values.

As a workaround to gatekeepers' blockades, our recruitment activities include numerous presentations to geriatric consumer groups. We post notices online, distribute local flyers and brochures, place ads in newsletters, and have letters sent by our hospital's research registry staff to persons who have enrolled and given permission to be notified about study opportunities in their area of interest. To ensure easy-to-understand, unbiased, and noncoercive information, all recruitment materials are stringently reviewed and approved by our organization's Institutional Review Board (IRB) for human studies research prior to usage.

Typically family carers of potential participants contact us and then the carer and person with dementia are screened for eligibility. One aspect of the screening is an assessment of the cognitive status to determine the person's capacity to legally consent or assent or the need to obtain consents from their legal guardian. Nonconsenters cannot enroll in a study and have a technology "forced" on them. Moreover, given the progressive nature of the disease, we revisit the consent process prior to system installation and during interim home visits to remind the end-users and carers of their option to withdraw from the study without any loss of supportive services or other recriminations. The annual continuing study

review by the IRB ensures ongoing oversight of the consent process, study enrollment, participant safety, and adverse event monitoring.

Beneficence (Do Good)

Beneficence guides us to maximize possible benefits (do good) and minimize
possible harms. In the gerontechnology model of technology adoption, it arises
from the category of perceived value (27). Doing good addresses a need that the
end-users value. The offering is designed based on a need that resonates with
the end-users. This is not the realm of developing an innovative technology and
pushing the technology for technology's sake—that is, we have this great technology and were wondering if you could help us figure out how we can promote this to the Alzheimer's and geriatric marketplace? A technology solution
in search of a problem is not the optimal starting point. As companies develop
a greater appreciation for the marketplace for cognitive assistive devices, their
rush to claim this product space increases the risk of producing products that
won't match to the consumer's needs.

One way we address this gap in understanding, and foster doing good, is to
conduct team-building experiential learning simulations (28). The aim is to
sensitize technology developers to the practical real-world constraints found
in the home or other target settings (small space, limited outlets, and no Wi-
Fi) and provide carers' reactions to the proposed application (e.g., too difficult).
Developers benefit from the inclusion of not only the end-users and/or their
proxies but also other interprofessional team and family members who together
will help technologists avoid mismatching devices and capabilities. Healthcare
clinicians, for example, will be able to provide the generalized expectations for
abilities and inabilities per functional stage. Rehabilitation clinicians such as occupational, speech, and neurocognitive therapists can provide specialty in-depth
task assessments. Social and behavioral scientists assess the user friendliness and
human factor issues while promoting an intuitive empathetic end-user experience that can be rigorously evaluated through qualitative and quantitative outcome results.

Nonmalfeasance (Do No Harm)

Intrusiveness of technology is another common concern and refers to the extent
to which the living environment must be changed to support the use of a technology. It is critical to understand that changing routines and the home environment may provoke stress-related agitated behaviors in persons with dementia.

To do no harm means integrating into the person's rituals and daily habits as much as possible. For carers, we minimize the demands on their time to care for the technology. Requiring caregivers to perform complicated system checks and maintenance, we believe, disrespects the value of their personal and caregiving time. Information overload has been reported as particularly burdensome for end-users who are sent too frequent biometric, medication, and activity reports or false alarms (29, 30). Do no harm directs the thoughtful developer to know what product-generated information is and is not needed and wanted by end-users. What is nice to know, necessary to know, and critical to know should be thoughtfully identified to initiate the appropriate level of alert action, such as none, routine check-in, or immediate action, to avoid alarm fatigue and harm from missed alerts.

Obtrusiveness is a related concern that refers to installing undesirably prominent and noticeable parts such as computer components, monitors, and cameras or making other changes that only support the technology (31). To avoid this, we hide base stations/computers in a closet or behind furniture. Sensors can be blended in with busy wallpaper designs or other fixtures or retrofitted onto home appliances or dressers. Everything is pretested by us on our own dressers and walls to ensure removal will not cause residual damage. Our installers are trained on how to communicate with cognitively impaired persons and to minimally disrupt the home environment and routines during installations. Should the installer and/or family member believe it would be less stressful for the person if he or she was distracted and redirected to other activities, then our Alzheimer's nurse specialist accompanies the installer. Design considerations must endeavor to minimize and conceal system parts as much as possible to visually and symbolically avoid taking over the person's space and reducing the familiarity and comfort of home (32).

Exaggerated performance claims or vague wording can also cause harm. In the realm of monitoring, end-users may believe that the technology is more robust and encompassing and includes more features than it actually does offer. Harm can arise if an untested or known unreliable technology is substituted for reliable safeguards. Hence, clear delineation of the technology offering is critical, as are statements of its limitations. Due to liability and user satisfaction concerns, commercial products usually advise that backup provisions be made for power outages, Internet loss, and battery and component failures. Other more subtle issues may arise that affect usage. For example, in the AT EASE project conducted in several independent living residences, we did systematic signal checks for strength and interference prior to deploying our wireless activity monitoring system (20). During testing in an empty apartment, we picked up numerous unexpected signals and queried the neighbors to determine the sources. One resident who used a personal emergency response system (PERS) mentioned that every time she used her microwave while wearing her PERS pendent, she would be contacted by the company's call center to confirm her emergency. To avoid these calls, she stopped wearing her pendent in the kitchen and admitted that she frequently forgot to put it back on. This situation raised the possibility of harm from a fall or fainting episode that was assumed to be under PERS monitoring when it was not. Under the "do no harm" premise, we resolved the errant signal interference before installing our system to avoid false alerts and reduce the potential for harm from a similar workaround.

Safety concerns are prominent among technology critics and members of IRBs. Many technologists have expressed dismay at the unscientific interpretations of improbable low-voltage safety issues raised by many reviewers (19). In another situation, our proposal to test device development using off-the-shelf standard components in a new configuration received an "ethical concern for human safety" despite not including any intervention testing with human subjects. The reviewer commented that given the likelihood of (presumed) technology harm when used with vulnerable older adults, safety provisions needed to be included. In the revised proposal, the requested information was added, but the new reviewers critiqued it for being unnecessary. In the United States, the gold standard for research ethical guidance is found in the Belmont Report, which notes that the ethical imperative to "do no harm" does not mean the elimination of every and all harms, but the minimization of them using accepted practices (33). We intentionally used certified off-the-shelf technology components that met the accepted practices for safety standards.

Other critics claim that major harms will result from technologies that erode intimate human relationships (3). They assert that remote monitoring increases users' social isolation by eliminating in-person visits, thus reducing the social interactions that enhance elders' quality of life. We tested this assertion across several of our studies, and notably, the participants did not validate these concerns (27). Instead, the value to the older adult was not in the number of human contacts that occurred per day, but in the type and quality of the social interactions (27). In the WIN project, we investigated the effect of providing working carers an employer-supported computer link to remotely monitor their at-risk homebound older relatives left alone during the workday (34). The first enrollee, Mr. G., previously received three brief telephone calls daily from his son at work querying whether he ate and took his pills at breakfast, lunch, and dinner. Mr. G. usually forgot at least one of those events and received a chastising comment from his son. He would get angry and yell at his son to "stop treating me like a child." With the WIN application, the son could check online and see whether those activities had happened. This allowed the father and son to have a more enjoyable telephone conversation in which they discussed the grandson's baseball game from the night before and shared in the excitement of the child's first home run. The father and son gladly made the trade-off between three short nagging calls to one longer pleasant conversation that conveyed parental respect and reinforced the grandparent role (35).

A monitoring system can also prevent harm from human neglect by sending alerts to the designated contacts reporting missed visits and care activities. For example, a hired helper reported that she visited daily, but she did not. She claimed that the older person forgot and did not remember due to dementia. She could not, however, explain how she comes and leaves without triggering the door sensor! In this type of situation, technology, rather than eroding personal contacts, can help to ensure them and prevent abuse and elder neglect.

Justice and Distributional Fairness

The principle of justice and distributional fairness in scientific research has historical roots in the exploitation of vulnerable groups, frequently the institutionalized, who were disproportionally made to bear the burdens of research for the benefit of society (33). There should be fairness not only in the bearing of research burdens but also in the receipt of benefits. The technology field tends to disproportionally offer applications that benefit the young, well-educated, higher-income, and healthy segments of our society. In response, the gerontechnology field gained impetus to offset the lack of attention to older adults' issues and to provide older adults with equitable access to contemporary technologies.

Additionally, some critics have challenged the development of technology-based carer interventions as an unnecessary societal expense since family and friends provide "free help." Yet the research literature indicates that family caregivers shoulder the majority of the financial burden for dementia care, providing an economic value to society ranging between $40,000 and $60,000 per caregiver per year in the United States, and approximately $142 billion worldwide (36–38). One of the DRESS focus group participants (39) mentioned

> outsiders (those who have never done intensive caregiving) have this romantic notion that it is my mom and I in this fulfilling relationship. It's not! It's frustrating, difficult, fatiguing, and the majority of the time I am at my wit's end. I do it because I love her and owe her for my wonderful upbringing. I have been caring for her for 8 years but I don't know how much longer I can go on. I need to take care of myself too, for my children and husband.

She would get up at 5 a.m., ready herself, and drive to her mother's home to get her washed and dressed and to make her breakfast and lunch. She would then drive back to her home to make her children's lunches and take them to school after her husband supervised their dressing and was leaving for his job. After the school drop-off, she would go to work. After work she would visit her mom, frequently finding her lunch still in the refrigerator. She would prepare her mom's dinner and make sure that she ate, then get her washed, in her pajamas, and ready for bed. But her mom was becoming more resistive. She would lock the doors so her mom did not wander outside during the night. She would then drive back to her house to put her children to bed. She always felt guilty for not spending enough time with her children or her husband or attending to her own health needs. Research indicates that caregivers have a significantly higher mortality than noncaregivers (40). The Alzheimer's Association reports that one-fifth of carers cut back on their own medical visits, one-third reduce or quit their jobs, and one-half reduce personal expenses to afford dementia-related care (41). Applying the principle of distributional fairness, it does not appear fair that carers experience all the stressors while society gains the economic benefits from their contributed labor. Tax and pension credits and/or financial reimbursement for evidence-based technologies and interventions shown to reduce caregiver stressors would help to offset societal exploitation of this vulnerable group.

Nonabandonment

Some suggest that technology usage leads to overreliance and dependency among users that will result in harm when it is removed (16). From the research perspective, interventions usually stop when the grant funding ends. Responsible investigators make prior plans to transfer services or bridge to other forms of support for participants. Similarly, technology trials need to consider what may assist the participants to maintain any positive momentum. Given the iterative phases of developing new technologies, often the participants desire to be kept involved and participate in future focus groups and/or related trials; others ask to consult with the team experts as issues arise or for assistance in obtaining caregiving services. Informing the participants about the study results, linking them to other sources of support, and being available for consultation afterward help to mitigate a sense of abandonment by those projects that need to withdraw technologies upon project completion.

Affordability

New first-generation innovative technologies are quite expensive, and usually only the more affluent sectors of society can afford to purchase them. We make a point to query our end-users about their perceptions of affordability and willingness to pay should the system they are currently testing becomes commercially available. We find that high user satisfaction levels correlate with a higher level of willingness to pay. Moderate-income participants favor monthly fees and/or outright system purchase at costs similar to their Internet, TV, and telephone bundle fees (34). In our current DRESS study with lower-income Hispanic participants, focus group members suggested lower cost rental options, equipment trades, and/or return credits to enable access. Cross-cultural studies and comparisons offer important insights (42). We consciously strive as we move from our first system version through the third iteration and onto maturity to reduce the final costs to foster affordable marketplace options. I have resisted the premature calls for cost-effectiveness studies on first-generation systems, knowing they will be negatively biased toward high costs. Realistic cost estimates can only be made in the later iterations, with full system maturity, taking advantage of Moore's law, which has accurately predicted major cost reductions in new technologies with increasing capabilities over short periods of time (43).

Privacy and Confidentiality

In the United States, technology researchers are expected to develop a data safety plan and meet stringent governmental privacy standards if their applications exchange any personally identifiable health information (44). Besides the legal mandate, ethically there is a duty to preserve privacy and respect the confidentiality of our research participants. Good practices involve separating personal identifiers from the data, always using encrypted devices, working behind firewalls, using dual-level passwords, and proactively monitoring for attempted intrusions. Given the worldwide experiences of nefarious hacking into commercial, healthcare, and governmental systems, developers are charged with installing and updating the most rigorous data and privacy safeguards.

From the home monitoring perspective, developers need to recognize the rights of users to control whether and how their data are shared. We repeatedly found across our home activity monitoring studies that the participants were very willing to trade off their privacy to gain the ability to remain at home (27). Their carers greatly valued the "peace of mind" that came from knowing that the person with dementia is safe at home. Safety trumps privacy concerns. However, we attempt to mitigate privacy loss by giving the end-users the ability to control when the system is or is not in use and offering a selection of monitoring options they can select according to their personal privacy preferences. As gerontechnologists strive to protect personal privacy, however, the public is increasingly disclosing their private information and seeking publicity on social media (45). How society addresses this privacy-publicity paradox in the future remains to be seen.

Ethical Model for Gerontechnology: Putting Technology into Perspective

In the ethical model for gerontechnology research and development there are three concentric circles (Figure 12.1) (19). The core inner circle purposely reflects the central focus on humanistic concerns, which are surrounded by research needs, and technology offerings are at the periphery. Conspicuously, technology development is not at the center. Rather, the humanistic or person-centered approaches are the central core aspects encircled by the other domains.

As mentioned previously, tension arises between the desire to personalize and respect the end-users' wishes and the technological need to standardize applications for widespread scalability. This model suggests developing integrative applications, balancing personalization and standardization. For example, the REACH project offered a computer-mediated automated telephone conversation that engaged persons with dementia by talking about their personal favorite memories, including playing their favorite song (46). The system was standardized to administer a core conversation with subroutines to embed the individualized components. Participants whose caregivers had stopped their telephone usage due to their inability to initiate and have a conversation once again were able to independently have a pleasant personalized conversation. One man who had stopped talking the previous year, after several "listening only" calls,

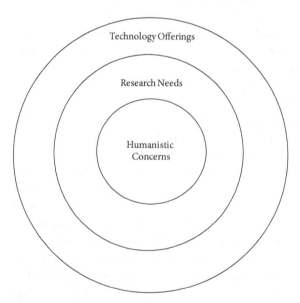

Figure 12.1 Ethical model for technology research and development.
© R. Purtilo. Used with permission.

started to sing along to his favorite song. His wife was thrilled to hear his voice once again! Carers used this conversation period in two ways; first, as a mini-respite break to accomplish other tasks while their loved ones were safely occupied for 20 to 40 minutes on the telephone, and second, as a diversionary tool that helped the users reduce their increasing agitation through pleasant memories. This operationalizes the ethical model by placing the person's humanistic need for personally meaningful conversation in the center, with research findings informing the dialogue development, and the technology creating the secured structural means to convey this discourse at any time through any telephone.

The research circle highlights the needs and concerns about end-users' privacy and considerations to ensure data confidentiality. It also emphasizes causing the least disruption to the person and home by minimizing installation hassles and product invasiveness. The outer technology realm expands ethical considerations beyond the direct end-users to a larger societal context. Justice and distributional fairness call for crafting new technologies from inception with a consideration of how, if they are successful, they may scale to benefit affected populations nationally and worldwide. Truthfulness calls for disclosure of sponsorship, especially commercial; whether intervention intentions are met; and if the findings yielded expected and/or unexpected outcomes. A disclosure of positive and negative findings helps to advance implementation science and aids society and potential end-users to distinguish between marketing hyperbole and product reality to minimize the potential for harm.

Conclusions

This chapter reports that the egregious proposed harms raised by technology critics have not occurred in the significant body of technology-based intervention research studies we have conducted. Technology is neither inherently harmful nor beneficial. Humans maintain the responsibility for developing applications that respect the personhood and dignity of those experiencing cognitive declines. To foster that, the discussion reviewed the ethical principles that underpin gerontechnology system development for older adults and their carers, aiming to respect their rights and personal values. The need for thoughtful consideration of the right technology fit for the right stage of dementia was stressed. Paternalistically dismissing opportunities for older adults to influence or use technologies can be seen as a new form of ageism, a technoageaphobia, an unwarranted and harmful generalization that older adults fear, do not want, and need to be protected from technology offerings. Harm can occur by usurping potential end-users' opportunities to critique and improve assistive technologies to better meet their personal needs for optimal well-being.

Acknowledgment

Support for this paper was funded in part through the US National Institutes of Health National Institute of Nursing Research grant #R21NR013471, and the MGH Institute of Health Professions' Jacque Mohr Research endowment. Gratitude is extended to my numerous collaborators who have been part of my research teams and especially to the persons with AD and their carers who enrolled in the gerontechnology studies and shared their valuable insights.

References

1. World Health Organization. Dementia: A public health priority. Dementia [Internet]. 2012;112. Available from: http://whqlibdoc.who.int/publications/2012/9789241564458_eng.pdf
2. Fortinsky RH, Downs M. Optimizing person-centered transitions in the dementia journey: A comparison of national dementia strategies. Health Aff. 2014;33(4):566–73.
3. Baldwin C. Technology, dementia, and ethics: Rethinking the issues. Disabil Stud Q. 2005;25(3):1–29.
4. Kenner AM. Securing the elderly body: Dementia, surveillance, and the politics of "aging in place." Surveill Soc. 2008;5(3):252–69.
5. Percival J, Hanson J. Big brother or brave new world? Telecare and its implications for older people's independence and social inclusion. Crit Soc Policy. 2006;26(4):888–909.
6. Lawton MP. Future society and technology. In Graafmans J, Taipale V, Charness N, editors. Studies in Health Technology Informatics. 48th ed. IOS Press; 1998;48:12–22.
7. Huschilt J, Clune L. The use of socially assistive robots for dementia care. J Gerontol Nurs. 2012;38(10):15–19.
8. Ni Scanaill C, Carew S, Barralon P, Noury N, Lyons D, Lyons GM, et al. A review of approaches to mobility telemonitoring of the elderly in their living environment. Ann Biomed Eng. 2006;34(4):547–63.
9. Sparrow R, Sparrow L. In the hands of machines? The future of aged care. Minds Mach. 2006;16(2):141–61.
10. Landau R, Auslander GK, Werner S, Shoval N, Heinik J. Families' and professional caregivers' views of using advanced technology to track people with dementia. Qual Health Res. 2010;20(3):409–19.
11. Welsh S, Hassiotis A, O'Mahoney G, Deahl M. Big brother is watching you—the ethical implications of electronic surveillance measures in the elderly with dementia and in adults with learning difficulties. Aging Ment Health. 2003;7(5):372–75.
12. Essén A. The two facets of electronic care surveillance: An exploration of the views of older people who live with monitoring devices. Soc Sci Med. 2008;67:128–36.
13. Zwijsen SA, Depla MFIA, Niemeijer AR, Francke AL, Hertogh CMPM. Surveillance technology: An alternative to physical restraints? A qualitative study among professionals working in nursing homes for people with dementia. Int J Nurs Stud. 2012;49(2):212–19.

14. van Bronswijk JEMH, Bouma H, Fozard JL, Kearns WD, Davison GC, Tuan P-C. Defining gerontechnology for R&D purposes [References]. Gerontechnology. 2009;8(1):3–10.

15. Widdershoven GAM. Ethics and Gerontechnology: A Plea for Integration. In: Graafmans J, Taipale V, Charness N, editors. Studies in Health Technology Informatics. 48th ed. IOS Press; 1998;48: 105–11.

16. Novitzky P, Smeaton AF, Chen C, Irving K, Jacquemard T, O'Brolcháin F, et al. A review of contemporary work on the ethics of ambient assisted living technologies for people with dementia. Sci Eng Ethics. 2015;21(3):707–65.

17. Queirós A, Silva A, Alvarelhão J, Rocha NP, Teixeira A. Usability, accessibility and ambient-assisted living: A systematic literature review. Univers Access Inf Soc. 2015;14(1):57–66.

18. Marziali E, Serafini JMD, McCleary L. A systematic review of practice standards and research ethics in technology-based home health care intervention programs for older adults. J Aging Health. 2005;17(6):679–96.

19. Mahoney DF, Purtilo RB, Webbe FM, Alwan M, Bharucha AJ, Adlam TD, et al. In-home monitoring of persons with dementia: Ethical guidelines for technology research and development. Alzheimers Dement. 2007;3(3):217–26.

20. Mahoney DF, Mahoney EL, Liss E. AT EASE: Automated Technology for Elder Assessment, Safety, and Environmental monitoring. Gerontechnology. 2009;8(1):11–25.

21. Wherton JP, Monk AF. Technological opportunities for supporting people with dementia who are living at home. Int J Hum Comput Stud. 2008;66(8):571–86.

22. Mahoney DF, Burleson W, Lozano C, Mahoney EL. Prototype Development of a Responsive Emotive Sensing System (DRESS) to aid older persons with dementia to dress independently. Gerontechnology. 2015;13(3):345–58.

23. Mahoney DF, LaRose S, Mahoney EL. Family caregivers' perspectives on dementia-related dressing difficulties at home: The preservation of self model. Dementia. 2015;14(4):494–512.

24. Mahoney DF, Goc K. Tensions in independent living facilities for elders: A model of connected disconnections. J Hous Elderly. 2009;23(3):166–84.

25. Protection of Human Subjects. 45 CFR 46 2009 [Internet]. Available from: http://www.hhs.gov/ohrp/humansubjects/guidance/45cfr46.html

26. Mahoney D, Tennstedt S, Friedman R, Heeren T. An automated telephone system for monitoring the functional status of community-residing elders. Gerontologist. 1999;39(2):229–34.

27. Mahoney DF. An evidence-based adoption of technology model for remote monitoring of elders' daily activities. Ageing Int. 2010;36(1):66–81.

28. Mahoney DF. From nursing simulation lab to engineering lab: Experiential training aiding robotic design. Gerontechnology. 2010;9(2):307.

29. Kang HG, Mahoney DF, Hoenig H, Hirth VA, Bonato P, Hajjar I, et al. In situ monitoring of health in older adults: Technologies and issues. J Am Geriatr Soc. 2010;58(8):1579–86.

30. Mahoney DF. The aging nurse workforce and technology. Gerontechnology. 2011;10(1):13–25.

31. Hensel BK, Demiris G, Courtney KL. Defining obtrusiveness in home telehealth technologies: a conceptual framework. J Am Med Inf Assoc. 2006;13(4):428–31.

32. Mahoney DM. Developing technology applications for intervention research: A case study. Comput Nurs. 2000;18(6):260–64.

33. US Department of Health and Human Services. The Belmont Report: Ethical Principles and Guidelines for the Protection of Human Subjects of Research [Internet]. 1979. Available from: http://www.hhs.gov/ohrp/humansubjects/guidance/belmont.html

34. Mahoney DMF, Mutschler PH, Tarlow B, Liss E. Real world implementation lessons and outcomes from the Worker Interactive Networking (WIN) project: Workplace-based online caregiver support and remote monitoring of elders at home. Telemed J E Health. 2008;14(3):224–34.

35. Mahoney DF, Tarlow B. Workplace response to virtual caregiver support and remote home monitoring of elders: The WIN project. Studies in Health Technology Informatics. 2006;122:676–80.

36. Harrow BS, Mahoney DF, Mendelsohn AB, Ory MG, Coon DW, Belle SH, et al. Variation in cost of informal caregiving and formal-service use for people with Alzheimer's disease. Am J Alzheimers Dis Other Demen. 2004;19(5):299–308.

37. Wimo A, Winblad B, Jonsson L. The worldwide societal costs of dementia: Estimates for 2009. Alzheimer's Dement. 2010;6(2):98–103.

38. Hurd MD, Martorell P, Delavande A, Mullen KJ, Langa KM. Monetary costs of dementia in the United States. N Engl J Med. 2013;368(14):1326–34.

39. Mahoney DF, LaRose S, Mahoney EL. Family caregivers' perspectives on dementia-related dressing difficulties at home: The preservation of self model. Dementia. 2015;14(4):494–512.

40. Schulz R, Beach SR. Caregiving as a risk factor for mortality: The Caregiver Health Effects Study. JAMA. 1999;282(23):2215–19.

41. Alzheimer' s Association. 2016 Alzheimer's disease facts and figures. Alzheimer's Dement. 2016;12(4):459–509.

42. Neary SR, Mahoney DF. Dementia caregiving: The experiences of Hispanic/Latino caregivers. J Transcult Nurs. 2005;16(2):163–70.

43. Chien AA, Karamcheti V. Moore's Law: The first ending and a new beginning. Computer (Long Beach Calif). 2013;46(12):48–53.

44. Health Insurance Portability and Accountability Act of 1996. Pub. L. No. 104-191, 110 Stat. 1936 (1996).

45. Taddicken M. The "privacy paradox" in the social web: The impact of privacy concerns, individual characteristics, and the perceived social relevance on different forms of self-disclosure. J Comput Commun. 2014;19(2):248–73.

46. Mahoney DF, Tarlow BJ, Jones RN. Effects of an automated telephone support system on caregiver burden and anxiety: Findings from the REACH for TLC intervention study. Gerontologist. 2003;43(4):556–67.

13

Privacy and Security Issues in Assistive Technologies for Dementia

The Case of Ambient Assisted Living, Wearables, and Service Robotics

Marcello Ienca and Eduard Fosch Villaronga

Introduction

A key functional component of most intelligent assistive technologies (IATs) for dementia is the capacity to sense, track, and monitor patients and their activities. The process of tracking and monitoring adults with dementia and their activities may have various purposes. These include alarming in case of detected abnormalities, conveying or facilitating the supervision or intervention of caregivers, generating data flows useful for diagnostics and therapy, and favoring a more adaptive and personalized interaction with other assistive technologies. Monitoring and tracking tools are primarily instrumental to collecting relevant information for increasing patient safety and enhancing the effective support of users in the completion of activities of daily living (ADLs). The capacity of tracking and monitoring is enabled by sensors, which convert physical parameters (e.g., temperature, blood pressure, CO_2 levels, speed, etc.) into a signal that can be measured electrically. Such electrically measurable signals may contain various types of information about the patients, the most common being behavioral and physiological information. Behavioral monitoring technology collects information about the user's behavior, such as movements, actions, and sounds. In contrast, physiological monitoring systems track and record patient physiological data such as heart rate, breathing rates, blood pressure, electrocardiogram (ECG) and electroencephalography (EEG) signals, and blood chemistry information. Both behavioral and physiological records are likely to contain private and sensitive information. Behavioral records, for example, may contain information about the patient's habits, locations, and daily activities in his or her private sphere. Physiological records, on the other hand, may contain information about physiological correlates of a person's health as well as biometric information. While the collection of such private and sensitive information is critical for the effective development, deployment, and implementation of IATs and for the subsequent effective support of older adults with dementia, it raises privacy and security issues. Having others know intimate details about a person's life such as his or her behavior or medical records may infringe upon that person's right to privacy as well as diminish his or her autonomy.

In this chapter, we will describe and discuss the major privacy implications associated with the use of IATs in the context of dementia care. In particular, we will focus on the three classes of IATs that most largely rely on the monitoring and tracking of personal data: ambient assisted living systems, service robotics, and wearable technology. Both general and class-specific issues will be discussed.

We will proceed as follows. First, we will present the notion of privacy, its role in our current ethical and legal discourse, and its relation to other notions such as medical beneficence and data protection. Second, we will explain how certain classes of IATs may generate novel issues for privacy and data protection. Third, we will discuss the implications of defective privacy protection in the context of IATs and highlight the need for unambiguous privacy standards in IATs for dementia care. Finally, we will conclude by providing preliminary insights into privacy-enhancing solutions.

Informational Privacy, Beneficence, and the Goals of Care

The need to set limits on the public dissemination of information relating to a person's private life was first defended by Warren and Brandeis (1890). In their seminal analysis, the emergence of novel technologies was seen as an increased risk of intrusion into a person's private domain and a potential breach for unintended public disclosure of personal information (Beauchamp and Childress 2001; Warren and Brandeis 1890). The notion of informational privacy, that is, the control over information about oneself, was further developed by authors such as Alan F. Westin (1968). Westin described privacy as the ability to determine for ourselves when, how, and to what extent information about us is communicated to others (Westin 1968). Such an account of privacy became central to the legal discourse after the US Supreme Court explicitly ruled that privacy is a central reason for Fourth Amendment protection. Consequently, to that deliberation, informational privacy has been frequently extended to include the protection against unwarranted searches, eavesdropping, surveillance, and appropriation and misuses of one's communications. With the emergence of digital computers and the Internet, novel debates arose about the privacy and security status of personal records of information. The reason for that stems primarily from the fact that people may not know what information is stored about them or what parties have access to it—a problem that has been recently exacerbated by cloud computing. The possibility for service providers to access and link databases containing personal information, with few controls on how those data are used, shared, or exploited, has hindered individual control over information about oneself in an unprecedented manner.

In the ethics tradition, the notion of privacy has often been attributed moral value based on the argument that it is necessarily associated with certain basic freedoms, personal autonomy, and other moral values. For example, Bloustein (1964) stated that invasion of privacy is best understood, in sum, as an affront to human dignity. In a similar fashion, Allen (1988) has argued that a degree of privacy is required by the liberal ideals of personhood, civil liberty, and the participation of citizens as equals (Allen 1988). In light of the informational privacy account and its interconnectedness to core moral values such as equality, liberty, personhood, and dignity, it becomes questionable to what extent it is legitimate to monitor and track activity from older adults with dementia, and hence to access control of their physiological and behavioral information. To properly appreciate this ethical problem, however, it is necessary to balance privacy with another value in the moral spectrum, that is, the principle of beneficence in biomedical ethics.

Beneficence is the principle of biomedical ethics that requires that any procedure or intervention be provided with the intent of doing what is in the best interest of the patient involved and to promote the patient's welfare (Beauchamp and Childress 2001). Under some circumstances, privacy and beneficence may be in mutual conflict. One common ethical dilemma involving these two values arises when the patient's informational privacy conflicts with the physician's beneficence-based duty to look out for the patient's best interests. For example, the doctor of a patient with mild dementia may gain valuable treatment-related information from monitoring the patient's everyday behavioral habits even without the patient's consent. However, this unauthorized monitoring might represent an intrusion into that patient's privacy. In these situations, the protection of the patient's informational privacy might conflict with the physician's duty of beneficence, and following each principle would lead to different courses of action.

In light of this complex dynamic among potentially conflicting principles, it is clear that the healthcare system and healthcare professionals have an obligation to prevent or mitigate harms, and they must weigh and balance possible benefits against other principles (e.g., privacy and autonomy) as well as against possible risks of an action.

In the context of IATs, some might recognize an obligation to use monitoring and tracking technologies to prevent and mitigate harms as well to promote the health and safety of older users. For example, smoke detectors could employ sensor technology to detect unusually high levels of carbon dioxide in the home environment and send alarms to prevent harms such as intoxication or fire. Analogously, fall detectors could be employed to detect falls and facilitate prompt assistance. However, some specific clauses on the legitimate conditions for the recording, storage, access, and reuse of behavioral and physiological information might hold. A weighed and balanced calibration of the various moral values at stake would likely exclude any account that disproportionally sacrifices one value over the other. For example, renouncing the implementation of monitoring and tracking technology altogether on the grounds of privacy rights would dramatically hamper the quality of care, present an obstacle to improvements to the quality of life of the patient, and delay technological innovation. At the same time, however, allowing the unrestricted collection and dissemination of personal information (e.g., behavioral or physiological) from elders with dementia without their knowledge and consent could result in disproportionately invading the private sphere of these patients and ultimately produce harm and injustice.

Current Legal Coverage on Privacy, Security, and Data Protection

Research shows that IAT systems, if adequately implemented, might determine the following potential benefits for dementia care: (a) extending the time people can live in their preferred environment by increasing their autonomy, self-confidence, and mobility; (b) supporting the preservation of health and functional capabilities of the elderly; (c) promoting a better and healthier lifestyle for individuals at risk; (d) enhancing security, preventing social isolation, and supporting the preservation of the multifunctional network around the individual; (e) supporting carers, families, and care organizations; and (f) increasing the efficiency and productivity of used resources in aging societies (Bharucha et al. 2009b; Ienca et al. 2017a, Ienca et al. 2017b). While the pursuit of these goals should be encouraged, it should also be balanced with the protection of two main fundamental rights: the right to privacy and the right to data protection.

In Europe, there are two legal systems that guarantee the protection of fundamental rights: the European Convention on Human Rights (ECHR), an international agreement between the 47 members of the Council of Europe (CoE), and the European Charter of Fundamental Rights (EUCFR), which became binding and primary law after the Lisbon treaty in 2009 (Art. 6.1 Treaty of the European Union, TEU). Inspired by Article 12 of the Universal Declaration of Human Rights (UDHR) and Article 17 of the International Covenant on Civil and Political Rights (ICCPR), both corpuses protect the "right to respect for his private and family life, his home and his correspondence," so as to say *privacy* (Art. 8 ECHR and Art. 7 EUCFR, respectively). With regard to the processing of personal data, however, and unlike the United States, the European countries have extensively developed another right, the right to data protection. This right has been developed within the CoE through the Convention for the Protection of Individuals with regard to Automatic Processing of Personal Data, also called "Convention 108" (Convention 108 1981), and within the EU through the 95/46/EC Data Protection Directive, recently replaced by the General Data Protection Directive Regulation (EU) 2016/679 (GDPR) made by the European Parliament and the Council of the European Union on the protection of natural persons with regard to the processing of personal data and on the free movement of such data. The GDPR was adopted on April 14, 2016, and implemented on May 25, 2018.

Privacy and data protection are "twins, but not identical" (De Hert and Schreuders 2001): while privacy extends to the entire private dimension of the person, data protection focuses solely on the processing of personal data. From this perspective, privacy is broader than data protection. On the other hand, however, personal data may refer to "any information relating to an identified or identifiable individual" (data subject), which makes it broader than privacy because it may encompass information that does not contravene privacy. Indeed, while processing personal data for a legitimate purpose and after obtaining valid consent would not interfere with the right to data protection, the collection, storage, or disclosure of such data could interfere with a person's right to privacy (Gellert and Gutwirth 2013).

In any case, both rights are not absolute and need to be considered in relation to their function in society (CJEU 2010), and they need to be balanced with other rights (Boillat and Kjaerum 2014). In the case of dementia care, the degree of intrusiveness of a certain IAT should be proportional to its contribution to achieving the goals of good care and promoting the patient's best interest. Furthermore, interferences to these rights could be considered lawful under certain circumstances (e.g., preventing terrorist attacks) if they are "provided for by law and respect the essence of those rights and freedoms [*and*] subject to the principle of proportionality" (Art. 52 EUCFR) (Aquilina 2010).

In dementia care and research, the respect of both rights is of paramount importance because the patient might not be capable of understanding which data are being processed and to what extent they are processed, and, accordingly, might not be able to give appropriate consent (Sachs 1998). Furthermore, the collectable information might be sensitive per se. To this regard, the General Data Protection Regulation aims at reinforcing the current data protection schema by offering easier access to the collected data, the right to data portability, the right to be forgotten, and the right to know when the information has been hacked.[1] Other privacy-related issues such as postmortem privacy (the current data protection directive grants protection "to all persons"; it only includes within its scope "living being[s]" [A29WP Opinion 4/2007]), third uses of data, and mental privacy in neurotechnology applications are still being debated (Harbinja 2017; Ienca and Andorno 2017).

Privacy and Security in Ambient Assisted Living Technologies

Ambient assisted living (AAL) or ambient assistive technologies (AATs) are a family of assistive systems that incorporate pervasive and ubiquitous computing into the design of housing facilities for the elderly as well as for people with physical and cognitive disabilities (Georgieff 2008). These technologies "seek to aid people, particularly the elderly, live independently for a longer time period than would otherwise be possible" (Datteri 2013). A large number of AAL systems have been tested effectively also in the support and assistance of older adults with dementia and their informal caregivers (Rashidi and Mihailidis 2013). AALs are normally focused on the prevention and management of chronic conditions, the preservation of social interaction, the facilitated completion of ADLs, the compensation of specific functional deficits, the delivery of medical and rehabilitative interventions, and the fulfillment of the oft-stated wish of older adults to age in place (Bharucha et al. 2009b). In addition, AALs are often designed to promote active aging (Sixsmith and Gutman 2013) and improve the quality of life of the patients. AALs work on a distributed cloud-of-care basis, allowing smart integrated technology to track, monitor, supervise, guide, and support the elder's behavior in a relatively noninvasive way.

In 2008, a study report of the European Commission addressed a number of general ethical and legal issues linked to e-health (EC Study Report 2008). In 2014, the AALIANCE research group identified a core set of specific ethical and legal issues associated with the implementation and use of AATs (van den Broek, Cavallo, and Wehrmann 2010). In this document, researchers identified the major legal corpuses relevant for AAL and in accordance to which every AAL system should be designed, developed, produced, and implemented. These corpuses include data protection regulation (transparency, legitimate purpose, and proportionality), patient safety and medical device directives (although now there is the Regulation 2017/745 on medical devices) (Regulation on Medical Devices 2017), consumer protection (fair treatment, products that meet acceptable standards and a right of redress if something goes wrong),[2] and legislation regarding services (e-commerce) (Directive eCommerce 2000). In addition, they identified some legislative gaps on a number of regulatory issues including (a) broadband access (addressing the question of whether the access to the Internet should become a right in the near future), (b) data mining and the automatic decision-making process (highlighting responsibility issues after an automatic wrong decision), (c) the integration of new technologies into an AAL system (e.g., mHealth, robots, biometrics, smart homes, and nanotechnologies), (d) the accessibility of different goods and services (Proposal 2015/0278 2015), and (e) the quality of services.

To date, many data protection–related issues associated with the use of AALs remain controversial. These include the intertwinement between the mental capacity of an older person with dementia and the provision of informed consent (Grady 2015) as well as the development of broad consent models in relation to third uses of data (Novitzky et al. 2015b). It also remains unclear where the line between privacy and competing interests should be drawn and by which actor (e.g., the manufacturer vs. the user) or who is the data controller/processor, especially in the case of different service/device providers that need to share information to give a coherent response in AAL. In addition, the collection of nonpersonal data from the AAL could generate personally identifiable information, information about the user's patterns of behavior, and potentially release these data to third parties without the user's consent and awareness, for example, through smart TVs.

Researchers have suggested some prerequisites for promoting privacy protection and user acceptance. These include the use of noninvasive sensors, the implementation of sustainability measures, the possibility of home-based data storage, and the obtainment of informed and dynamic consent. Of course, technical limitations constrain the applicability of such protection. For example, home-based platforms for data management are very expensive and require external access by the manufacturing company in case of system failure. Similarly, dynamic consent is easier to obtain in research contexts than in the context of IAT implementation. More research is needed to explore how dynamic consent could be obtained when implementing in-home technologies for ADLs (Kaye et al. 2015). In addition, from an ethical and legal perspective, privacy-enhancing protections must be balanced to emerging rights such as the right to be forgotten (Art. 17 GDPR) and the right not to know in relation to accidental findings (e.g., if the system detects any disease that could affect one's emotional or psychological integrity). Although the nature of the ecosystem might burden the enforceability of such rights (Villaronga, Kieseberg, and Li 2018), the need for "finding appropriate balances between privacy and multiple competing interests" (CENELEC SmartHouse Code of Practice 2005)[3] still remains as a valid statement.

Privacy protection comes along with security issues. These are related to the physical security of individuals such as preventing any physical breach, allowing authorized access, and removing obstacles to evacuation of the house in case of danger, but also the prevention of falls, external threats (in the event of fire or flood, the system should respond safely), electronic data security, and theft prevention technology. The prevention of other users commanding the house of the person with dementia is of paramount importance. The dwelling of the person should be a "fail safe" environment, and broadband access should always be secured as it is recognized as a human right by the United Nations (La Rue 2011). In any case, any unauthorized access should be prevented. This would go in line with the protection of the physical integrity of the person, although safeguards concerning the mental integrity should also be considered (Ienca and Andorno 2017). Some authors believe that offering perfect transparency and making the user the master are additional goals that need to be pursued. However, dementia patients might not have the capacity to be the master of the AAL system. Therefore, delegation issues and advanced directives might become of crucial importance.

Privacy and Security in Service Robotics: The Case of Teleoperated Robots

Service robots differ from industrial robots because they are designed for nonexpert usage. They perform multiple tasks in unstructured environments and their level of human-robot interaction (HRI) is usually very high. A common type of service robotics is teleoperated robots. In dementia care, teleoperated robots have been used to support doctor-patient interaction through videoconference, but also as autonomous robots providing companionship, handling objects, or exchanging information (Jones, Sung, and Moyle 2015; Moyle et al. 2017; Moyle et al. 2014). Some of them have been used along with AAL technologies.[4]

These robots normally provide a two-way audio and video communication, a user interface, an integrated map, multiple cameras and sensors, and the possibility to autonomously navigate around the house (Desai et al. 2011). They differ from AAL or wearable technology because they enable third users to sense and interact with remote environments, leading to an overall sense of extended agency in that environment. The capacity to sense of these systems, together with their mobile physical appearance, raises privacy concerns in relation to both private and family life and data protection.

Although the processing of sensitive data is lawful for "health security, monitoring and alert purposes, prevention or control of communicable diseases and other serious threats to health" (Recital 52 GDPR) and it is deemed necessary in dementia care, appropriate safeguards need to protect how the collection, transmission, and storage of the patient's sensitive data are carried out.

As recently stated, "if the device is capable of remote operation or transmission of data, it could be a target for a malicious actor" (Cerrato 2016, p. 95). Robots lacking security capabilities provide criminals with opportunities to penetrate the system, steal personal data, transmit data online, or even remotely control the robot, which might in turn result in physical harm to the victim. In fact, "robotics combines . . . the promiscuity of information with the capacity to do physical harm" (Calo 2015, p. 515). Under the new GDPR, the data controller has the obligation to inform both the supervisory authority and the patient if the robot has been hacked or a data breach has occurred (Art. 33–34 GDPR), although it remains unclear if these notifications should be transmitted to the person with dementia or to his or her proxy, as well as what kind of action should be taken (e.g., disposing of the robot or simply modifying the access keys, etc.).

Teleconferences between the patient and the care provider as well as with the patient's relatives or friends should remain private and confidential in any case, as eavesdropping represents an interference with the right to privacy, and they should only be stored in cases where necessary for the monitoring. Access to stored information should be granted to those in charge of the patient after they sign a confidentiality agreement. In teleconference mode, moreover, it should be clear in which cases the pilot (e.g., the doctor) can access the camera and establish a conversation with the patient, as in some cases elderly people prefer to pilot a mobile robotic platform system rather than receiving a visit via the robot system (Kristoffersson, Coradeschi, and Loutfi 2013). Oral contracts or agreements performed through the teleconference system should be subject to the patient's capacity to avoid any abuse. In any case, consent should be unambiguous, clear, and explicit.

In autonomous or companionship mode, the robot will have to process a larger quantity of information, not only to be capable to deal with pitfalls but also because the spontaneous HRI will turn into a lifelong relationship once the robot reaches personal environments and needs to provide company (Borenstein and Arkin 2016). The use of cloud services to process all that information, lighten the weight of the robot, and decrease response time will challenge data protection. Indeed, cloud computing encompasses various deployment models and may involve multiple service layers and service providers, with supply chains that are often opaque (Kuan Hon and Millard 2013). Together with the tangible elements of the robot, such complexity can give rise to significant challenges in relation to control, security, and risk management. The more actors will be involved, the more important the division of roles and responsibilities will be. In this respect, and because the robot will be a *thing* within the Internet of Things, it will be crucial to "examine the terms of the relevant contracts to ascertain who is liable for what" (Millard, Hon, and Singh 2017), especially if the robot behavior can be actuated not only from the cloud but also directly from another *thing* (e.g., a wearable device that tells the robot the person is suffering a heart attack).

This cyber-physical nature of robotic systems may also challenge the right to data portability (Art. 20 GDPR). As the appropriate functioning of the robot depends on both the outsourced computing and its embodiment, the user may be interested in retrieving the data not only in a "commonly used and machine-readable format" but also in a manner in which these can actually translate into safe actions/movements of the robot (Fosch-Villaronga 2017). This will be especially relevant for robotic devices fastened to the body of the user (e.g., lower-limb exoskeletons). Connected to this, if the actions of the robot depend on cloud connectivity, the nonavailability of the service could compromise the (physical, maybe even cognitive) safety of the user. The assumption of responsibility in this case will have to be clear, especially for those robots that will be deployed in private homes (Ienca et al. 2016).

A comprehensive life cycle framework that encompasses the whole ecosystem of (healthcare) service robotics, including rights and obligations of cloud service providers, workers (nurses, physiotherapists, and physicians), users, or the robot itself, is still lacking (Fosch-Villaronga 2017). Currently, the industry has investigated how to transform HRI into a human-robot safe interaction (HRSI) through standardization of the robot's spatial behavior in response to human presence, the robot's noise level for robots in the human environment, the establishment of some generic and some high-priority commands for HRI, gestures across different cultures, and so forth (Lasota, Fong, and Shah 2017). However, this only refers to how to make the interaction "technically" and "physically" safe and disregards other rights like privacy or data protection, which is understandable as "what is often missing in the design of information systems is a way to bridge the abstract idea of privacy protection with the very concrete formulation of techno-rules" (Koops and Leenes 2014). Cognitive HRI and recent uses of emotions in HRI (emotionally intelligent robots, emotional adaptation) nevertheless may challenge this physical-centered approach and even the very basic foundation of the concept of "data," as it is not sure whether "emotions" are mere biometrical data or are considered, in the future, a new category of data. In this respect, recent privacy settings that point out the importance of including ethics in the design process of such machines could shed light in this respect (BS 8611:2016; IEEE Ethically Aligned Design 2017).[5] Yet, the enforceability of such instruments remains in question.

Privacy and Security in Wearable Technology

Wearable systems "are designed to be permanently useful and usable in a wide range of mobile settings" (Lukowicz, Kirstein, and Troster 2004, p. 3). Wearables differ from other types of mobile technology (e.g., smartphones or tablets) because they are not, or are only rarely, handheld and enable direct interaction between the system, the user, and the environment (Lukowicz, Kirstein, and Troster 2004). Wearable computing devices may be worn under, over, or in clothing or may also be themselves clothes, and they are capable of collecting a wide range of information from the user's body (e.g., health status, habits, or mood) and environment (e.g., images, temperature, location, sounds, or even third parties' personal data) (Piwek et al. 2016).

Wearable technology is being increasingly used in neurogeriatric care for various purposes including measuring activity (De Bruin et al. 2008) and providing an assistive tool for caregivers of elders with Alzheimer's (Matthews et al. 2015) or Parkinson disease (Cancela, Pastorino, and Waldmeyer 2018). While there are potential benefits of wearable technology in dementia care and, more generally, healthcare, it can be disruptive and raise privacy concerns (Al Ameen, Liu, and Kwak 2012; Luxton et al. 2015). Indeed, the collection of a massive quantity of data may clash with the principle of data minimization enshrined in data protection regulations. In addition, it raises several related legal issues including information security, consent, data ownership, and data control. While these emerging ethical and legal issues apply also to other categories of IATs such as robots and distributed systems, the permanent usage and friction-free design of wearable devices may elevate these issues to a great order of magnitude. In particular, the high level of integration between the wearable device and the user may reduce the user's awareness of the ongoing data collection and processing (Motti and Caine 2015). In addition, wearables can collect a larger variety of physiological and other health-related data than most other families of IATs, including sensitive data such as heart beat rates, blood pressure, sugar levels, and podometrics. Even more remarkably, neurowearables such as consumer-grade brain-computer interfaces (BCIs) can record brainwaves, another form of privacy-sensitive data (Ienca and Haselager 2016; Ienca, Haselager, and Emanuel 2018). A viable strategy to guarantee privacy and protection of data when implementing wearable technology in dementia care is to carry out a technology-specific impact assessment that can match the particularities of the technology with the different impacts it may have (Fosch-Villaronga 2015). In this case, we propose a "wearable impact assessment" (WIA). This methodology could help proactively identify the precise context of implementation, the appropriate characteristics or capabilities of the device, the target user population, the potential unintended risks involved, and the associated safeguards that go beyond the data protection focus of Art. 33 GDPR. We further suggest introducing privacy-enhancing and data protection safeguards early in the design of wearable assistive devices. Finally, more user-oriented research involving older adults with dementia and their professionals or informal caregivers is highly needed (Ienca, Lipps et al. 2018).

Recommendations

While different in architecture, usability, and functionality, AAL systems, telepresence robots, and wearables have the common denominator of collecting and processing large volumes of data from the user with the purpose of extracting valuable information on their health conditions, monitoring or assisting with their activities, supervising or facilitating the completion of everyday tasks, and enhancing their overall quality of life and quality of care.

Based on our analysis, we argue that eight fundamental privacy-related questions must be addressed in the context of IATs for elderly adults with dementia: (a) what data can be legitimately monitored or tracked, (b) in what volume and variety, (c) what degree of intrusion into a person's privacy is legitimated by the goals of dementia care, (d) from which subjects the data can be collected, (e) where these data are stored, (f) who has ownership over and access to those data, (g) what the appropriate procedures for informed consent are, and (h) what third uses of the collected data should be considered legitimate.

The first three questions are strictly connected. AAL and other distributed systems usually collect behavioral, physiological, and environmental data in a quantity and quality that vary depending on the specific goals of the system. For example, fall-detecting systems collect primarily behavioral data with the purpose of detecting anomalies in the resident's motion to alert caregivers about falls or similar domestic accidents. In contrast, smoke-detecting systems collect primarily environmental data (i.e., CO_2 levels) from the resident's domestic environment with the purpose of detecting anomalies that correlate with an increased risk of fire or suffocation. We argue that the quantity and quality of data collected should be coherent, with the purpose explicitly stated in the system's specifications. Producers should include in the product packaging clear statements about what types of data and in what volume will be collected by the system, as well as motivate the reason for their collection from the perspective of optimal care. Anomalous patterns of data collection should be prevented by design, and users should be informed about anomalies in the data collection process. Circumstances where the system collects volumes and varieties of data that were not explicitly stated in the product packaging should be prevented by specific regulations.

It is important to note, however, that since for most AAL and wearable systems this *monitoring* of activity levels is a continuous process, it may be hard to determine what volume of data is coherent with the assistive goals of the system. In addition, the increasing use of data mining techniques and predictive analytics may benefit from the collection of large volumes of data, which may be utilized not only to automatically generate postevent alerts but also to predict upcoming risk situations. For this reason, we recommend that privacy and data protection regulations in the context of IATs for dementia provide sufficient elasticity for maximizing the benefits of technological progress while minimizing the risks of technology misuse. Excessive regulatory restrictiveness may not only harm current technology-assisted dementia care but also temper future technological innovation.

Issues of data volume and variety are subsumed by the problem of determining the degree of intrusion into a person's privacy that is legitimated by the goals of dementia care. A possible solution to address this problem is the appeal to a special application of the proportionality principle (Wright, Hurles, and Firth 2016). As previously mentioned, the degree of intrusiveness of a certain IAT intervention should be in proportion to its contribution to achieving the goals of good care and promoting the patient's best interest. The patient's best interest, in turn, is determined by the severity of his or her medical condition and his or her specific care needs. This application of the proportionality principle is one viable resolution of the conflict between the bioethical principles of privacy and beneficence presented in the first chapter. As we have already seen, the principle of beneficence states that any procedure or intervention be provided with the intent of being in the best interest of the patient involved and promoting their welfare. Therefore, IAT systems can legitimately intrude into the patient's private domain (e.g., domestic environment and continuous activity levels) if these partial sacrifices of the patient's privacy are in the best interest of the patient. For example, the continuous gait monitoring of a patient with mild to moderate dementia may be justified by the prevention of falls and other mobility-related accidents.

The appeal to the principle of proportionality, however, requires technology producers and manufacturers to make explicit claims about the goals and capabilities of their marketed devices. General goals of IAT systems for dementia care include (a) extending the time people can live in their preferred environment by increasing their autonomy, self-confidence, and mobility; (b) supporting the preservation of health and functional capabilities of the elderly; (c) promoting a better and healthier lifestyle for individuals at risk; (d) enhancing security, preventing social isolation, and supporting the preservation of the multifunctional network around the individual; (e) supporting carers, families, and care organizations; and (f) increasing the efficiency and productivity of used resources in aging societies.[6] The degree of intrusiveness of IAT interventions should be in proportion to their contribution to achieving these goals as well as to promoting the best interest of the patient.

With regard to the subjects whose data can be legitimately collected, specific focus should be diverted to the elder with dementia. Data from third parties should only be collected if the third party explicitly consents to their collection. As we have discussed previously, most jurisdictions allow third-party data processing under specific circumstances. Users should be aware that their data are being processed by third parties and should know for what purposes and by whom. In addition, they need to provide explicit informed consent.

Standards for correct data storage also must be clarified. As AAL systems, telepresence robots, wearable technologies, and other IATs may collect highly sensitive and personally identifiable information, safe and secure storage of that information must be guaranteed. Following the principle of data protection by design and by default (Art. 25 GDPR), we suggest enacting the following safeguards:

(I) The immunity of systems to abusive third-party apps should be secured by design.

(II) Access to the data should be limited and the cloud provider should not (except for exceptional circumstances) retain access.

(III) Cloud storage must be supported by cloud encryption and free support services in case the patient and his or her caregivers or responsible health professionals require additional information or have special needs.

Data ownership in the cloud is a complicated legal issue. In the medical context, elderly adults with dementia should be able to claim ownership over their data. Wherever they can no longer exercise their ownership right due to the progression of their disease, data ownership should be extended by proxy (e.g., to the closest family caregiver). It is also important to establish clear roles and responsibilities between controllers and processors.

As we have seen in multiple occurrences throughout this chapter, issues of a legitimate degree of intrusion into privacy, data access, and storage all presuppose the enforcement of formal procedures for the attainment of informed consent. Informed consent can be obtained from people with dementia in three ways: (a) directly, (b) proactively through advanced directives, and (c) or through proxy decision making. Direct consent can be obtained when the patient explicitly shows competence and cognitive capacity. Advanced directives are (usually written) externalizations of a person's decisions and wishes regarding future medical courses of action. Through these directives, patients in the early stages of Alzheimer's disease or other dementias can spell out decisions about their future choices ahead of time, that is, before the progression of the disease makes them incapable of making autonomous and competent choices. Proxy decision making is when the decision is (partly) made by a person different than the patient (proxy) who was previously appointed by the patient or is relevant to the patient in some significant sense. Alzheimer Europe has produced several recommendations for the obtainment of informed consent from persons with dementia,[7] although more research is needed to fully understand how privacy and data protection play a role within new ways of treating Alzheimer's disease.

When providing information for the purpose of consent during the installation of a certain IAT, healthcare professionals and caregivers should communicate in a manner adapted to the patient, respond to questions, use visual and other aids if necessary, and facilitate the communication of the decision by the patient. If consent is being sought for the purpose of installing and using a robot in the patient's home, it must be ensured that the user understands the basic functionality of the robot and its potential usefulness for daily life.

A crucial requirement of consent among dementia patients is that it should be obtained at various intervals throughout the study, following an iterative model usually described as "ongoing consent." Due to the progressive and mood-changing character of the disease, patients may revoke their initial consent and must be free to withdraw from using the technology at any time. In the institutional setting, health professionals should be attentive to signs of distress linked to technology use and if necessary check with the participants about whether they wish to withdraw from using the specific IAT that caused their distress. In the in-home setting, caregivers should be attentive to signs of distress linked to the use of the IAT or to its presence in the house (as in the case of environmental sensors and distributed systems).

Conclusions

In this chapter, we have described some privacy and security issues associated with the use of IATs in dementia care with a special focus on three major families of assistive applications: ambient assisted living technology, service robots, and wearables. After presenting the philosophical and legal framework on privacy and data protection, we have analyzed in detail each of the three aforementioned technological families and their peculiarities from the perspective of informational privacy and data protection. Based on this analysis, we have outlined some preliminary recommendations aimed at preserving or even enhancing privacy in the context of technology-assisted dementia care. Future research is needed to expand these general recommendations and adapt them to specific case scenarios of IAT use and specific patient populations. In addition, future normative studies are required to explore potential conflicts among competing moral values. While the potential of IATs for improving dementia care is unquestionable, the ethical use and social uptake of these technologies risk being tampered with if privacy protections are not integrated into their life cycle process, from early in the design and development of such assistive applications to their actual implementation.

Notes

1. See http://ec.europa.eu/justice/data-protection/.
2. Cfr. ec.europa.eu/info/strategy/consumers/consumer-protection_en.
3. See https://www.evs.ee/products/cwa-50487-2005.
4. Cfr www.hitech-projects.com/euprojects/florence/ and www.giraffplus.eu.
5. See https://ethicsinaction.ieee.org/.
6. AAL Europe (see http://www.aal-europe.eu/about/objectives/#sthash.j7SyeY8N. dpuf, last accessed February 2, 2016).
7. Cfr. www.alzheimer-europe.org/Ethics/Ethical-issues-in-practice/2011-Ethics-of-dementia-research/Informed-consent-to-dementia-research.

Acknowledgements

This project has been co-funded by the Käthe-Zingg-Schwichtenberg-Fonds of the Swiss Academy of Medical Sciences under award KZS 20/17 and by the LEaDing Fellows Marie Curie COFUND fellowship, a project that has received funding from the European Union's Horizon 2020 research and innovation programme under the Marie Skłodowska-Curie Grant Agreement No. 707404.

References

Al Ameen, M., Liu, J., and Kwak, K. 2012. Security and privacy issues in wireless sensor networks for healthcare applications. *Journal of Medical Systems*, 36, 1, 93–101.

Allen, A.L. 1988. *Uneasy access: Privacy for women in a free society*. Rowman & Littlefield.

Aquilina, K. 2010. Public security versus privacy in technology law: A balancing act? *Computer Law & Security Review*, 26, 2, 130–143.

Beauchamp, T.L., and Childress, J.F. 2001. *Principles of biomedical ethics*. Oxford University Press.

Bharucha, A.J., Anand, V., Forlizzi, J., Dew, M.A., Reynolds, C.F., Stevens, S., and Wactlar, H. 2009. Intelligent assistive technology applications to dementia care: current capabilities, limitations, and future challenges. *American Journal of Geriatric Psychiatry*, 17, 2, 88–104.

Bloustein, E.J. 1964. Privacy as an aspect of human dignity: An answer to Dean Prosser. *NYUL Review*, 39, 962.

Boillat, P., and Kjaerum, M. 2014. *Handbook on European data protection law*. Luxembourg: Publications Office of the European Union.

Borenstein, J., and Arkin, R. 2016. Robotic nudges: the ethics of engineering a more socially just human being. *Science and Engineering Ethics*, 22, 1, 31–46.

Calo, R. 2015. Robotics and the lessons of cyberlaw. *California Law Review*, 103, 513-563.

Cancela, J., Pastorino, M., and Waldmeyer, M.T.A. 2018. Trends and new advances on wearable and mobile technologies for Parkinson's disease monitoring and assessment of motor symptoms: how new technologies can support Parkinson's disease. In

Biomedical engineering: concepts, methodologies, tools, and applications. IGI Global, 1180–1204.

Cerrato, P. 2016. *Protecting patient information: a decision-maker's guide to risk, prevention, and damage control.* Syngress.

Datteri, E. 2013. Predicting the long-term effects of human-robot interaction: A reflection on responsibility in medical robotics. *Science and Engineering Ethics*, 19, 1, 139–160.

De Bruin, E.D., Hartmann, A., Uebelhart, D., Murer, K., and Zijlstra, W. 2008. Wearable systems for monitoring mobility-related activities in older people: a systematic review. *Clinical Rehabilitation*, 22, 10–11, 878–895.

De Hert, P., and Schreuders, E. 2001, November. The relevance of Convention 108. In *Proceedings of the Council of Europe Conference on Data Protection, Warsaw*, 19–20.

Desai, M., Tsui, K.M., Yanco, H.A., and Uhlik, C. 2011. Essential features of telepresence robots. In *2011 IEEE Conference on Technologies for Practical Robot Applications (TePRA)*. IEEE, 15–20.

Fosch-Villaronga, E. 2015. Creation of a care robot impact assessment. WASET. *International Journal of Social, Behavioral, Educational, Economic, Business and Industrial Engineering*, 9, 6.

Fosch Villaronga, E. 2017. *Towards a Legal and Ethical Framework for Personal Care Robots. Analysis of Person Carrier, Physical Assistant and Mobile Servant Robots.* Erasmus Mundus Joint Doctorate in Law, Science and Technology, Doctoral dissertation.

Fosch-Villaronga, E.F., Kieseberg, P., and Li, T. 2018. Humans forget, machines remember: artificial intelligence and the right to be forgotten. *Computer Law & Security Review*, 34, 2, 304–313.

Gellert, R., and Gutwirth, S. 2013. The legal construction of privacy and data protection. *Computer Law & Security Review*, 29, 5, 522–530.

Georgieff, P. 2008. Ambient assisted living. *Marktpotenziale IT-unterstützter Pflege für ein selbstbestimmtes Altern, FAZIT Forschungsbericht*, 17, 9–10.

Grady, C. 2015. Enduring and emerging challenges of informed consent. *New England Journal of Medicine*, 372, 9, 855–862.

Harbinja, E. 2017. Post-mortem privacy 2.0: theory, law, and technology. *International Review of Law, Computers & Technology*, 31, 1, 26–42.

Hon, W.K., and Millard, C. 2013. Cloud technologies and services. In: Millard, C.J. (Ed.). *Cloud Computing Law*. Oxford: Oxford University Press, 3–17.

Ienca, M., and Andorno, R. 2017. Towards new human rights in the age of neuroscience and neurotechnology. *Life Sciences, Society and Policy*, 13, 1, 5.

Ienca, M., and Haselager, P. 2016. Hacking the brain: brain–computer interfacing technology and the ethics of neurosecurity. *Ethics and Information Technology*, 18, 2, 117–129.

Ienca, M., Haselager, P., and Emanuel, E.J. 2018. Brain leaks and consumer neurotechnology. *Nature Biotechnology*, 36, 9, 805–810.

Ienca, M., Jotterand, F., Elger, B., Caon, M., Pappagallo, A.S., Kressig, R.W., and Wangmo, T. 2017a Intelligent assistive technology for Alzheimer's disease and other dementias: a systematic review. *Journal of Alzheimer's Disease*, 56, 4, 1301–1340.

Ienca, M., Jotterand, F., Vică, C., and Elger, B. 2016. Social and assistive robotics in dementia care: ethical recommendations for research and practice. *International Journal of Social Robotics*, 8, 4, 565–573.

Ienca, M., Lipps, M., Wangmo, T., Jotterand, F., Elger, B.S., and Kressig, R.W. 2018. Health professionals' and researchers' views on intelligent assistive technology for psychogeriatric care. *Gerontechnology*, 17, 3, 139–150.

Ienca, M., Wangmo, T., Jotterand, F., Kressig, R.W., and Elger, B. 2017b. Ethical design of intelligent assistive technologies for dementia: a descriptive review. *Science and Engineering Ethics*, 24, 4, 1035–1055.

Jones, C., Sung, B., and Moyle, W. 2015. Assessing engagement in people with dementia: a new approach to assessment using video analysis. *Archives of Psychiatric Nursing*, 29, 6, 377–382.

Kaye, J., Whitley, E.A., Lund, D., Morrison, M., Teare, H., and Melham, K. 2015. Dynamic consent: a patient interface for twenty-first century research networks. *European Journal of Human Genetics*, 23, 2, 141–146.

Koops, B.J., and Leenes, R. 2014. Privacy regulation cannot be hardcoded. A critical comment on the 'privacy by design'provision in data-protection law. *International Review of Law, Computers & Technology*, 28, 2, 159–171.

Kristoffersson, A., Coradeschi, S., and Loutfi, A. 2013. A review of mobile robotic telepresence. *Advances in Human-Computer Interaction*, 3, 1–17.

La Rue, F. 2011. Report of the Special Rapporteur on the promotion and protection of the right to freedom of opinion and expression. A/HRC/17/27 General Assembly, United Nations. Available at: https://www2.ohchr.org/english/bodies/hrcouncil/docs/17session/A.HRC.17.27_en.pdf.

Lasota, P.A., Fong, T., and Shah, J.A. 2017. A survey of methods for safe human-robot interaction. *Foundations and Trends® in Robotics*, 5, 4, 261–349.

Lukowicz, P., Kirstein, T., and Troster, G. 2004. Wearable systems for health care applications. *Methods of Information in Medicine-Methodik der Information in der Medizin*, 43, 3, 232–238.

Luxton, D.D., June, J.D., Sano, A., and Bickmore, T. 2015. Intelligent mobile, wearable, and ambient technologies for behavioral health care. In Luxton, D.D. 2016. *Artificial Intelligence in Behavioral and Mental Health Care*, 137–162.

Matthews, J.T., Lingler, J.H., Campbell, G.B., Hunsaker, A.E., Hu, L., Pires, B.R., Hebert, M., and Schulz, R. 2015. Usability of a wearable camera system for dementia family caregivers. *Journal of Healthcare Engineering*, 6, 2, 213–238.

Millard, C., Hon, W.K., and Singh, J. 2017, April. Internet of Things Ecosystems: Unpacking Legal Relationships and Liabilities. In *2017 IEEE International Conference on Cloud Engineering (IC2E)*, 286–291.

Motti, V.G., and Caine, K. 2015. Users' privacy concerns about wearables. In *Financial cryptography and data security*. Springer, 231–244.

Moyle, W., Arnautovska, U., Ownsworth, T., and Jones, C. 2017. Potential of telepresence robots to enhance social connectedness in older adults with dementia: an integrative review of feasibility. *International Psychogeriatrics*, 29, 12, 1951–1964.

Moyle, W., Jones, C., Cooke, M., O'Dwyer, S., Sung, B., and Drummond, S. 2014. Connecting the person with dementia and family: a feasibility study of a telepresence robot. *BMC Geriatrics*, 14, 1, 7.

Novitzky, P., Smeaton, A.F., Chen, C., Irving, K., Jacquemard, T., O'Brolcháin, F., O'Mathúna, D., and Gordijn, B. 2015b. A review of contemporary work on the ethics of ambient assisted living technologies for people with dementia. *Science and Engineering Ethics*, 21, 3, 707–765.

Piwek, L., Ellis, D.A., Andrews, S., and Joinson, A. 2016. The rise of consumer health wearables: promises and barriers. *PLoS Medicine*, 13, 2, e1001953.

Rashidi, P., and Mihailidis, A. 2013. A survey on ambient-assisted living tools for older adults. *IEEE Journal of Biomedical and Health Informatics*, 17, 3, 579–590.

Regulation (EU) 2017/745 of the European Parliament and of the Council of 5 April 2017 on medical devices, amending Directive 2001/83/EC, Regulation (EC) No 178/2002 and Regulation (EC) No 1223/2009 and repealing Council Directives 90/385/EEC and 93/42/EE.

Sachs, G.A. 1998. Informed consent for research on human subjects with dementia. AGS ethics committee. *Journal of the American Geriatrics Society*, 46, 10, 1308–1310.

Sixsmith, A., and Gutman, G.M. 2013. *Technologies for active aging*. Springer.

van den Broek, G., Cavallo, F., and Wehrmann, C. 2010. *AALIANCE ambient assisted living roadmap*. IOS Press.

Warren, S.D., and Brandeis, L.D. 1890. The right to privacy. *Harvard Law Review*, 4, 5, 193–220.

Westin, A.F. 1968. Privacy and freedom. *Washington and Lee Law Review*, 25, 1, 166.

Wright, C.F., Hurles, M.E., and Firth, H.V. 2016. Principle of proportionality in genomic data sharing. *Nature Reviews Genetics*, 17, 1, 1.

14

Developing Ethical Web- and Mobile-Based Technologies for Dementia

Challenges and Opportunities

Julie M. Robillard and Tanya E. Feng

Web- and Mobile-Based Technologies for Dementia

Information and communication technology (ICT) has redefined how our society engages with all aspects of dementia, from diagnosis to long-care care. The emergence of web- and mobile-based technologies (WMBTs) such as dementia-specific websites and mobile applications, or "apps," has empowered patients, families, and caregivers to take on a more active role in their own health or in the care of their loved ones.

Diagnosis

In the last decade, an increasing number of computerized dementia screening tests have been introduced to clinical settings. The use of computerized batteries may hold several advantages compared to traditional pencil-and-paper tests, including better standardization of administration as well as reduced ceiling and floor effects, as many tests are able to adapt to the examinee's performance (1). These tests may also alleviate the burden on the healthcare system, as they can be administered by trained personnel rather than clinicians (2). A growing number of dementia screening tools are also freely available on the Internet, claiming to provide self-diagnostic information (3,4).

Prevention and Treatment

The amount of freely available information about dementia has soared with the rise of the Internet, spanning a wide range of topics from diagnosis to prognosis (5). Findings from a recent analysis of nearly 300 online articles specifically on the prevention of Alzheimer's disease showed that websites offered a large variety of different recommendations, such as exercise, cognitive stimulation, and nutritional recommendations including complementary and alternative interventions such as consuming supplements or turmeric (6). These recommendations came from a broad range of sources, including health websites, news companies, advocacy groups, and government departments. Access to a wealth of information on the Internet may allow users to become better informed about their own health and more empowered in their health decision making (7).

The emergence of social media has further transformed the way Internet users engage with health information in an increasingly dynamic and interactive online environment. Data show that an extensive conversation about dementia is taking place on various social media platforms (8). In an analysis of dementia-related posts on Twitter, research findings dominated the discourse, supporting the role of social media in science communication (9,10).

The increasing popularity of the Internet as a source of health information has led to a rapid growth in direct-to-consumer advertising on this medium (11). A wide variety of different types of products are advertised online to improve brain function, including pharmaceuticals, neuroimaging services, and natural products, and the presentation of these different types of interventions may differ significantly (12). For example, Racine et al. (12) found that websites selling natural products presented less risk information and were less positive toward the role of healthcare providers than websites selling pharmaceuticals.

Mobile phone applications, or "apps," are another rising trend in dementia-related WMBT. The brain training industry, advertising apps that improve brain health and prevent or delay the onset of dementia (13), has rapidly expanded in recent years (14). Other apps have been developed that focus on empowering users to make lifestyle changes with the goal of reducing their risk of Alzheimer's disease, and include features such as health education material, behavioral self-reporting functions, and personalized feedback (15).

Care

WMBTs are playing an increasingly larger role in dementia care. Applications of new assistive technologies include assisting in the care of individuals with dementia, such as in-home monitoring and tracking devices (16,17). Assistive technologies may also directly help patients maintain their independence and quality of life. For example, apps have been developed to support prospective memory by providing reminders and prompts, as well as retrospective memory, such as by assisting with face recognition, allowing smartphones to be used as memory aids, or "cognitive prosthetics" (18). Pinto-Bruno et al. (19) identified several WMBT solutions designed to improve social participation for those with dementia, such as a technology-supported game to stimulate socialization and interaction in a group setting (20). Finally, some technologies have been developed to deliver nonpharmacological interventions to those with dementia, such as cognitive stimulation and reminiscence therapy (21,22).

Caregiver Support

A variety of web- and app-based WMBTs have been developed to support caregivers (23–26). Some programs focus on education and provide information on dementia, caregiving, and local resources (26–28). Others have been designed to facilitate peer support between caregivers through various platforms including telephone support groups, online communities, and video-conferencing (29–32). These interventions have been demonstrated to improve caregivers' mental health and increase confidence in caregiving skills and competence (33). However, a systematic review found mixed results in the efficacy of these interventions on caregiver burden (34).

Ethical Issues with WMBTs for Dementia

Quality

The magnitude of benefit that WMBTs can provide is critically contingent on their quality. For example, while high-quality information on dementia available online can help empower users to make decisions about their own health or support the health of their loved ones, low-quality information may have a negative impact on their health and well-being. Searching for online information about dementia may increase anxiety for some users (35). Promises of cures or interventions guaranteed to prevent or treat dementia may also result in false hope (36). Furthermore, low-quality advice may lead to physical harm if followed. This is a salient issue with regard to complementary and alternative medicine, as Walji et al. (37) found that one-quarter of websites with information on three popular herbal supplements provided recommendations that, if followed, may directly result in physical harm. As another example, Hainer et al. report a case of a patient with maxillary sinus cancer who died from self-medication with hydrazine sulphate purchased over the Internet (38).

Given the potentially serious implications of online resources for Internet users' health, several tools have been designed to assess the quality of health information available online (39). In general, high-quality articles have the following characteristics: (a) a recent date of creation or last update; (b) the names of the authors of the article and their relevant credentials; (c) use of balanced or cautious vocabulary to support their claims; (d) identifiable scientific studies to support their claims, including randomized controlled trials, clinical trials, and meta-analyses; (e) absence of any conflicts of interest; and (f) support of the patient-physician relationship. Recently, our group developed a tool that encompasses these features (6). Articles are scored according to the previously listed criteria, which are weighted and summed to produce a total score, allowing for the quantitative evaluation of article quality. Applying this tool to online articles on the prevention of Alzheimer's disease, we found that quality scores ranged from very poor to excellent. High-quality articles tended to use more scientific evidence to support their claims and use a more balanced or cautious tone and were less likely to endorse a product or service than low-quality articles. In terms of information content, high-quality articles were more likely to discuss modifiable risk factors for Alzheimer's disease, while low-quality articles were more likely to recommend nutritional interventions and complementary and alternative medicine.

Concerns have also been raised over the quality of self-diagnostic tests available online (40). An assessment of freely available tests of cognitive function indicated that these tests generally lacked the validity and reliability necessary to provide accurate diagnostic information (4). Specifically, a panel of experts found that the tests often did not have appropriate content or breadth to achieve their claims, were not grounded in peer-reviewed evidence, and were likely to score poorly in terms of test-retest reliability. One test in the sample was even shown to produce only one possible negative and alarming result regardless of input data. These tests may pose serious risks to users' health and well-being as false-positive results may cause needless anxiety, while false negatives may delay early interventions when they are medically warranted.

Beyond online resources, WMBT interventions for cognitive engagement should also adhere to strict quality standards. The effectiveness of brain training apps has been called into question by over 70 leading scientists in the fields of cognitive science and neuroscience. The 2014 consensus report states that there is insufficient evidence currently to support any claims that "brain games" will forestall the onset of cognitive decline (41). Lumos Labs, creator of Lumosity, one of the most widely marketed brain training apps currently available at the time of writing, was recently fined $2 million by the U.S. Federal Trade Commission for unfounded claims pertaining to the potential benefits of the apps, including delayed cognitive impairment associated with aging and protection against mild cognitive impairment, Alzheimer's disease, and dementia (42). Misleading marketing is especially worrying with regard to dementia-specific products as research suggests that older adults may be more optimistic about cognitive training than their younger counterparts (43).

The benefit of WMBTs for dementia cannot be assessed in isolation from the perceived usefulness of the technology from the end-users' perspective (44). Perceived usefulness is defined by Davis (45) as "the degree to which a person believes that using a particular system will enhance his or her job performance," or in this case, task performance (46), and is found to be highly correlated with acceptance and use (45,47). Cahill et al. showed that individuals with dementia and their caregivers may differ in their perception of the usefulness of assistive technologies (44).

Accessibility

While WMBTs may serve to overcome traditional barriers to access, such as by providing support services to caregivers in rural areas (48), there still exist disparities in access to these technologies. Although the gap in Internet access is closing, the Internet may still be less accessible for people in rural areas, of low socioeconomic status, of older age, from racial minorities, and living with medical limitations (49,50). Individuals from these demographic groups are also more likely to have lower eHealth literacy, "the ability to seek, find, understand, and appraise health information from electronic sources and apply the knowledge gained to addressing or solving a health problem" (51–53). Furthermore, challenges related to health literacy may be exacerbated by the high readability levels of online health information (54). Compounding the barriers to Internet access, some assistive technologies come with additional financial costs, such as expensive hardware and proprietary software, which can further limit the adoption and use of these technologies.

A second ethical consideration related to accessibility is whether users are able to effectively use the technology once they have access to it. Special consideration should be taken when designing websites for individuals with dementia. Haesner et al. demonstrated that older adults with mild cognitive impairment (MCI) may face more difficulties in terms of orientation and navigation within websites (55). Furthermore, those with MCI may stand to gain as much benefit from procedural training on these web platforms as older adults without MCI.

Usability is an especially crucial factor to be considered in the development of computerized tests of cognitive function. For this application, it is critical to discriminate between errors arising from cognitive impairment and those resulting from challenges in computer interactions such as fatigue. For example, the test interface of online dementia screens should be designed to optimize human-computer interaction, such as by considering the quality of the visual display (4). In addition, it is critical that computerized dementia tests be developed with consideration of cross-cultural differences, as they may affect performance in cognitive testing (56). In an assessment of the usability of a novel computerized cognitive assessment tool, Jacova et al. (57) successfully incorporated participants' recommendations of improved instruction format, being clearer about the task, and practice trials into the iterative development process.

Consent

While commonly discussed in the context of medicine and research ethics, informed consent is also relevant in the context of WMBTs for dementia, and is crucial in ensuring that users fully understand the benefits and risks of the intervention or service in question. However, the process of consenting to the use of various WMBTs is often problematic and frequently involves overly lengthy and complicated text or the absence of meaningful information and choice.

Most freely available dementia screening tests scored poorly on criteria related to consent (4), in stark contrast to the thorough process of informed consent used in clinical dementia screens (58–60). Brain training and other dementia-related apps may also lack opportunities for users to give or deny consent (61).

With regard to the online environment, Bashir et al. highlight that the length and complexity of privacy policies and terms of agreement make them inaccessible to users. As a result, the informational asymmetry between Internet service providers and users threatens the comprehension and voluntariness of informed consent (62). Furthermore, the very same characteristics of these documents may contribute to why the majority of individuals who visit health websites do not read the terms of use or privacy policies (63). Ploug and Holm (63) describe this as the routinization of consent, where the act of consent becomes habitual and unreflective, and far from truly informed.

The process of informed consent warrants even more careful consideration when it involves individuals with varying levels of cognitive impairment. When decisions are to be made regarding the use of technologies to assist in the care of an individual with dementia, the patient should be involved as much as possible (64). In situations where surrogate consent must be obtained, it is crucial to ensure that the best interests of the patient are the utmost priority. This may become more complicated in cases of monitoring and tracking technologies, where a balance must be struck between preserving the patient's autonomy on the one hand, and maintaining the patient's safety and easing caregiver burden on the other (65,66).

Privacy

In the digital era, privacy is a salient issue with forms of WMBTs that collect or require the input of personal information. Before utilizing monitoring or tracking devices with this vulnerable population, risks to individuals' privacy must be carefully considered alongside potential safety benefits (67). Studies of public attitudes toward the use of these devices show that acceptance depends on whether potential end-users hold privacy or safety to be a more critical priority (65,68).

Online dementia screening tools are another form of WMBTs associated with risks to privacy. As these tests were scored poorly by experts on measures of privacy, this draws into question the confidentiality of users' intimate health information (4). In the context of mobile platforms, developers of cognitive training apps may collect a variety of personal data such as demographic and geographic information, sleep, and alcohol use in conjunction with information on cognitive function (69), raising ethical concerns about the privacy of app users (70). Indeed, the privacy of personal information submitted to health apps is a priority for users (71,72), and these concerns are negatively correlated with adoption intention of mobile health services (73).

An analysis of healthcare-related organization websites highlights a discrepancy between what consumers want to know and what is actually discussed in the privacy policies of these organizations (74). Specifically, participants were generally most concerned with the transfer of their data, awareness of how their information will be used, and the storage of their information. In contrast, privacy policies for these resources placed more emphasis on integrity/security, collection, and choice/consent. In addition, the reading grade level of privacy policies of mobile apps may far exceed the reading level of an average user (75,76). Even in an assessment of accredited health apps, only two-thirds included a privacy policy (77). Furthermore, although no apps transmitted information where the privacy policy stated they would not, a majority of apps collected or transmitted data not mentioned in the privacy policy, and some apps handled information completely inconsistently with the statements put forth in the privacy policy. A study of nearly 18,000 health-related apps available in the iOS and Android app stores found that a vast majority (96%) were associated with some degree of potential damage through information security and privacy breaches (78).

A recent review of the literature on security and privacy in mobile health has raised concerns about the currency and relevance of existing laws governing mobile apps in the United States and European Union (79). Furthermore, the US Department of Health and Human Services recently released a report emphasizing that laws protecting health information, such as the Health Insurance Portability and Accountability Act of 1996, do not apply to health information submitted on mobile apps, social media, or the Internet. As a result, McCarthy has identified "large gaps in policies around access, security, and privacy" for WMBT-based resources (80).

Conflicts of Interest

Conflicts of interest, both obvious and insidious, may pose significant ethical risks in dementia-related WMBTs. In recent years, direct-to-consumer advertising (DTCA) has rapidly expanded from traditional media to the online realm, including social media platforms (11,81). Advocates for DTCA claim that it may increase consumers' knowledge (82); however, this may not be the case. Research indicates that DTCA of medications for Alzheimer's disease may only be making older adults feel more knowledgeable about Alzheimer's disease, rather than increasing their factual knowledge (83). Moreover, pharmaceutical companies may use DTCA in more subtle ways, such as through third-party blogs that do not disclose their affiliation (84).

DTCA is used not only in the pharmaceutical industry but also in the sale of supplements, services, and books related to dementia (6,12). For example, results from a study by our group found that nearly one-fifth of the articles we assessed that provided information on the prevention of Alzheimer disease included an endorsement of a product or service within the text of the article. The information in these websites may be biased toward self-promotion and may lead to inappropriate requests for prescription medications, unnecessary financial expenditures on pharmaceutical and nonpharmaceutical products, false hope in the case of treatments and preventative interventions, and direct harm to consumers' health when risks of medication, supplements, and other treatments are understated (12,84–87). Furthermore, DTCA may have a negative impact on the patient-physician relationship depending on factors such as the quality of the information and whether the physician followed the patient's request (88).

Conflicts of interest are also a salient ethical problem for online tests for dementia, as experts generally rated these tests very poorly in terms of the disclosure of these conflicts (4). These issues extend to health-related apps, as pharmaceutical and medical device companies are becoming more involved in the development of these types of WMBTs (89). Krieger draws attention to the lack of discussion of potential conflicts of interest in these apps in both public and academic spheres (90).

Patient-Physician Relationship

As people are increasingly turning to digital resources about dementia (91), it is crucial to carefully consider the consequences of this revolution on the patient-physician relationship. WMBT-based information may bring many benefits to this relationship, such as by encouraging individuals to visit their physician (92) and improving communication and increasing patients' confidence during appointments (93). However, the emergence of WMBTs in the doctor's office may also negatively impact the patient-physician relationship.

While the current literature is mixed, research on the impact of online health information on the patient-physician relationship may suggest a discrepancy between patients' and physicians' perspectives, with patients perceiving that the effects are more positive than physicians (91,93–95). From their experiences, physicians may view online health information as a source of unnecessary concern and anxiety (94,96,97). In addition, while information found online may encourage individuals to see their physician, it may also lead to unnecessary visits and requests for inappropriate tests or treatments (91,98). On the other hand, it may also discourage patients from visiting their physician if they feel that the Internet has satisfied their informational needs (92). Some physicians may find it difficult to discuss patient-sourced information in depth with their patients due to time constraints (91,94), while patients may feel hurried when they bring up information from the Internet to their physicians (93). Other difficulties physicians may face include feeling challenged and devalued by their patients, a loss of control in the clinical relationship, and increased physician burden (94,96,98). Furthermore, online health information may degrade trust in this relationship when patients receive different information from their physician than the information they found online (95).

However, the impact of online health information on the patient-physician relationship also depends on several factors such as the quality of the information (98), the physician's reaction and communication skills (93), the prior relationship (96), and whether patients view the information as complementary to advice from their physician or as more important (95).

Computerized cognitive testing in a clinical setting may also impact the patient-relationship. Research from Werner and Korczyn indicates that older adults may perceive computerized dementia testing as evidence of the degradation of the patient-physician relationship. These findings emphasize the importance of maintaining interaction with healthcare providers during the process (99).

Societal Implications

There are broader ethical implications of WMBTs for society as a whole. Freely available resources on the Internet and social media that are at odds with evidence-based information supported by the scientific community may erode trust in science. The anti-vaccination movement is a quintessential example of how social media allows for the rapid dissemination of misinformation, sparking tension between the public and government authorities (100). Moreover, tactics employed by this movement include mentioning previous scientific errors and associating supports of vaccinations with "big pharma," further propagating mistrust in the medical community (101).

The rise of celebrity doctors promoting low-quality health information may also contribute to the public's loss of trust in medical professionals. For example, doctoroz.com, the popular website of "America's doctor," cardiothoracic surgeon Dr. Mehmet Oz, serves as the "24/7 informational concierge" of the Dr. Oz show (102,103). An assessment of televised medical talk shows including the Dr. Oz Show found that scientific evidence was not found for 39% of the recommendations made on the show and an additional 15% of the recommendations were contradicted by evidence (104); however, the show still has a widespread, tangible impact on viewers' health (105). In another example, at the time of writing, mercola.com, the popular health website of osteopathic physician Dr. Joseph Mercola, makes factually incorrect claims about the causes and cures of Alzheimer's disease (106–108).

The Internet may also play an important role in the hype surrounding new treatments and technologies, exaggerating the benefits of these novel developments while diminishing the limitations and risks (36). These sensationalized representations of health research and novel interventions may lead to negative consequences for public trust in science when these expectations are not met (109).

Finally, dementia prevention and care through technology places a significant economic burden on both individuals, who may need to purchase specific devices, and society in instances where governmental assistance is provided to help cover the costs of these technologies. As such, careful health economic assessments of dementia technology will be required moving forward, as well as a consideration of the financial impact that these technologies may place on already burdened healthcare systems (110).

For a summary of ethical issues and associated potential harms and possible solutions, please see Table 14.1.

Table 14.1 Summary Ethical Issues, Potential Harms & Possible Solutions

Ethical Issue	Key Themes	Potential Harms	Possible Solutions
Quality	• Accuracy • Validity • Reliability • Effectiveness • Usefulness • Alignment with needs	• False hope • Anxiety • Physical harm • Delayed medical interventions • Low adoption • Wasted resources	• Quality assessment • Guidelines for developers and researchers around quality • End-user engagement
Accessibility	• Availability • Usability • Culture	• Inequality • Lack of relevance • Low adoption	• End-user engagement • User testing
Consent	• Capacity • Comprehensibility • Autonomy	• Unawareness of risks • Loss of autonomy • Misuse	• Enhanced consent
Privacy	• Information security • Data sensitivity	• Privacy breach	• Increased legal regulation
Conflict of interest	• Transparency	• Inappropriate requests • Unnecessary financial expenditures • False hope • Physical harm	• Guidelines for developers and researchers around transparency
Patient-physician relationship	• Trust • Patient-centered care	• Mistrust • Inappropriate requests • Increased physician burden • Conflict	• Increased awareness among healthcare professionals
Societal implications	• Reputation of medical community • Hype • Resource allocation	• Mistrust in medical community • False hope • Burden on health care resources	• Public engagement

Design Considerations for Future Development

Ethical Assessment

Structured and unstructured instruments have been developed to assist with the ethical evaluation of health-related technologies. These instruments have been used extensively in the context of health technology assessments. The Socratic approach, which has been applied in practice for technologies such as stem cell transplantation and bariatric surgery, incorporates several branches of ethics (e.g., consequentialism, deontology, principlism) into a set of questions designed to examine value issues (111,112). The Socratic method has been subject to revisions to address certain limitations (113); however, its interpretation and application remain variable. Other initiatives have attempted to integrate ethical evaluation and technology assessment to address the issue of health technology assessment in itself being a value-laden process. For example, the EUnetHTA model is composed of 16 key ethical questions designed to be discussed with a variety of stakeholders at the earliest stage of health technology assessment (114). These types of ethical considerations are critical when evaluating emerging technologies but offer little practical guidance specifically for dementia technology developers and researchers.

In the context of WMBT solutions specifically, practical instruments have been designed to evaluate the quality, and to some extent the ethics, of different types of resources. For online health information, for example, there are four categories of quality assessments available: (a) criteria-based evaluation tools that users can apply to websites (e.g., the DISCERN tool); (b) third-party certifications, or "trust marks" (e.g., the HON [Health on the Net] Code of Conduct [HONcode]); (c) medical search engines that automatically filter for recent and high-quality online content (e.g., Omni); and (d) recommended principles that content creators can use to self-regulate (e.g., E-Health Code of Ethics). As the need to empower end-users to recognize high-quality content and solutions is increasingly being recognized (115), the evaluation and development of user-applied evaluation tools have become a key priority in health literacy. There are currently a number of quality evaluation tools available that range from generic assessments intended for use across multiple domains of health information to assessments targeted to a specific health condition (e.g., Alzheimer's disease), aspects of a condition (e.g., treatment), type of evidence (e.g., systematic review), or audience (e.g., patients, clinicians). Many of the existing quality evaluation tools incorporate some ethical criteria such as the presence of conflict of interest and the balance of the information (6,116–119). When applied in their proper context and for their intended use, these tools are valuable assets in the identification of high-quality online content. However, they are not without limitations. Many tools were originally developed for written materials such as pamphlets and information sheets and may not be applicable in the context of the dynamic, multicontributor online environment. Other drawbacks include limited scope of application (e.g., tool is for a single disease), inaccessibility to the average health information consumer (e.g., tool incorporates academic concepts or language), lengthy application time (e.g., tool has large number of criteria), and lack of quantitative result, which makes it difficult to compare information quality across various sources. Further, few of the existing tools have been evaluated for validity, reliability, and efficacy, and as such their application in a research setting is limited.

In response to these limitations, our group has developed the QUality Evaluation Score Tool (QUEST), a short, 7-item quality evaluation assessment tool that can be easily and rapidly applied to large samples of online health information. Through all of its criteria, QUEST considers key ethical principles in health and science communication such as transparency, balance, the promotion of autonomy, and the support of the patient-healthcare professional relationship. To date, QUEST has been tested for reliability and convergent validity and has been applied to a large sample ($n = 290$) of online articles about the prevention of Alzheimer's disease. Results showed that the quality of these articles varies greatly, allowing for an in-depth comparison of high- and low-quality online articles (6). This study clearly demonstrated the potential of quality evaluation tools as research instruments to characterize the current landscape of online health resources and develop recommendations for best practices moving forward.

Some instruments have also been designed specifically for interactive online resources, such as online health self-assessments (4). In a recent study from our group, an evaluation grid was developed to characterize scientific validity (4 items), human-computer interaction features (5 items), and ethics factors (8 items) for a sample of 16 freely accessible online tests for Alzheimer's disease (4). As described previously, most tests scored poorly on ethics factors such as privacy and conflict of interest, and as such were considered to be potentially harmful by the two panels of experts who reviewed them. These results are particularly problematic in light of evidence about the perceptions of older adults on online health information. In a study exploring credibility issues among older adults seeking online health information, Robertson-Lang et al. found that a majority of participants were uncertain as to how to seek out the credibility of a given online resource, and some believed that the fact that online health information was available online validated its credibility (120). Taken together, our results and that of others highlight two areas of critical need: (a) the development and promotion of resources specifically designed to empower the older adult population to independently assess the quality and ethics of interactive online resources, and (b) the creation and implementation of guidelines for technology developers and researchers.

End-User Engagement

A proposed solution to ensure that WMBTs are ethical and needs driven is to engage end-users from the beginning of the development process. Several models have been put forward to address this goal. One approach draws from the patient engagement revolution in the research context, whereby patients actively participate as partners rather than subjects throughout the process, from agenda setting to the execution and translation of research (121). Not only does patient engagement democratize the research process, but also it brings a wealth of experience and knowledge from the perspectives of patients to the table, resulting in more relevant, higher-quality research (122), or in the case of WMBT development, technology better suited to the needs of users. However, there may exist several unique challenges in implementing patient engagement in dementia research, such as progressive cognitive decline (123). Despite these potential obstacles, we have demonstrated that patient engagement with the dementia community is logistically feasible. In a brief, 15-minute interactive session with members of the patient community and the public, we were able to gather rich data on their perspectives on ethical priorities in dementia clinical research (124).

Another framework that can be utilized to engage end-users in the development of WMBTs is user-centered design (125). In user-centered design, the technology is designed with the needs of the user as a priority. For example, before designing a new prototype for a new memory aid, Inglis et al. (126) conducted focus groups and interviews with individuals with memory impairment to better understand the specific problems faced by the participants. However, in some cases, the actual involvement of the user may only be limited to providing information to researchers by means such as completing surveys, participating in interviews, or performing tasks under observation, and often only occurs in the initial stages of product development (127–129). It is important to ensure continued involvement by the intended end-users such as through evaluations of subsequent prototypes (126).

A third approach is participatory design, where the users play an active, collaborative role throughout all stages of the development process (130). Several groups have successfully implemented these strategies in the development of various technologies for use by individuals with dementia (131–133). For example, Meiland et al. (132) involved individuals with mild dementia and their carers throughout the process of developing an integrated digital prosthetic, through workshops and interviews as well as field testing of the device. From a pragmatic standpoint, participatory design can help ensure that the technology is designed to meet the needs of the individual user, and thus may increase acceptance and tangible benefits to the target population (134). In addition, Carroll and Rosson introduced the moral proposition that end-users should have a voice in the development process of a technology that directly affects them. Furthermore, this act of "democratizing innovation" may foster strong, positive relationships between the patient community, researchers, and industry (135,136). As with patient engagement, it is crucial to keep in mind that traditional participatory

design methods may not be suitable for working with all individuals with dementia for reasons such as cognitive symptoms, heterogeneity of the forms and
severity of dementia, and burden on the participant (137,138). However, conventional methods may be adapted accordingly and furthermore, these challenges
may catalyze the innovation of novel participatory methods.

Despite the significant benefits of involving individuals with dementia in the
process of designing WMBTs, the voices of the end-users still remain underrep-
resented. Span et al. (139) suggest several barriers to explain this underrepresen-
tation: the intention to avoid distress that may be caused by using beta versions
of the technology, progressive cognitive impairment of study participants, and
the stigma associated with dementia.

It is critical that developers of dementia-related WMBTs collaborate with
representatives from the target population to overcome these challenges to ensure that the design of these technologies is driven by user needs and ethical
considerations.

User Testing and Impact Assessment

When designing WMBTs for dementia, it is critical to consider the emotional
impact of technology usage on end-users. Often overlooked, this impact can
have important consequences, both positive and negative, for the experience
of a given technology as well as the adoption of future technologies. In dementia, harmful emotions such as anxiety and acute stress may be worsened by
the use of WMBTs if these are not designed to address affective factors. While
many lines of evidence suggest that online health resources can have a beneficial impact on the well-being of older adults, such as increased feelings of
support (140), others point to a strong relationship between anxiety and online health information seeking and self-monitoring. High levels of health
anxiety are linked with more frequent searches for online health information (141,142). When exploring the converse of that relationship, White and
Horvitz found that while some individuals report a reduction in anxiety as a
result of consulting online resources, others experience a web-based escalation
of concerns (143).

End-users who experience negative consequences as a result of interacting
with WMBTs may decrease their use of these technologies. However, we must
also consider the issue at the other end of the spectrum: that of overadoption.
In recent years, there has been an explosion of behavioral research aimed at
characterizing how to elicit compulsive behaviors with features such as infinite
scrolling and variable rewards. Technology developers should be mindful not

to design WMBTs in ways that engage users beyond what is required and appropriate to derive maximum benefit from the technology.

Moving forward, in addition to the user engagement approaches described previously, the development of WMBTs for dementia should include rigorous user testing to characterize the emotional impact of the technology and incorporate, where possible, computational models of affect to limit potential emotional harms (144).

Conclusion

WMBT solutions hold much promise for the prevention, screening, diagnosis, and treatment of various forms of dementia and for caregiver support. To ensure these solutions deliver maximum benefits for people with dementia and their families and caregivers, it is critical to engage end-users early in technology development. Incorporating the needs, values, and priorities of people with dementia and their caregivers in the process of WMBT development can help ensure that the solutions will be useful and effective for the intended end-users. Further, careful ethical and impact assessments should be conducted to ensure adherence to norms such as meaningful informed consent and disclosure of conflicts of interests and to minimize potential emotional harms. Moving forward, technology developers and researchers would benefit from a set of consensus-driven guidelines that recognizes the challenges of technology development for older adult end-users and provides practical guidance in the application of ethical principles.

Acknowledgments

The authors wish to gratefully acknowledge Jessica Jun, Jen-Ai Lai, Emanuel Cabral, and Monica Ta for conducting research related to the content of this chapter; Dr. Patrick MacDonald for his thoughtful insights on the manuscript; and funding sources: Canadian Consortium on Neurodegeneration in Aging, Canadian Foundation for Innovation, Canadian Institutes for Health Research, and Vancouver Coastal Research Institute.

References

1. Zygouris S, Tsolaki M. Computerized cognitive testing for older adults: a review. Am J Alzheimers Dis Other Demen. 2015;30(1):13–28.

2. Wild K, Howieson D, Webbe F, Seelye A, Kaye J. Status of computerized cognitive testing in aging: a systematic review. Alzheimers Dement. 2008;4(6):428–37.
3. Kluger BM, Saunders LV, Hou W, Garvan CW, Kirli S, Efros DB, et al. A brief computerized self-screen for dementia. J Clin Exp Neuropsychol. 2009 Feb;31(2):234–44.
4. Robillard JM, Illes J, Arcand M, Beattie BL, Hayden S, Lawrence P, et al. Scientific and ethical features of English-language online tests for Alzheimer's disease. Alzheimers Dement Diagn Assess Dis Monit. 2015;1(3):281–88.
5. Dillon WA, Prorok JC, Seitz DP. Content and quality of information provided on Canadian dementia websites. Can Geriatr J CGJ. 2013;16(1):6–15.
6. Robillard JM, Feng TL. Health advice in a digital world: quality and content of online information about the prevention of Alzheimer's disease. J Alzheimers Dis. 2017;55(1):219–29.
7. Forkner-Dunn J. Internet-based patient self-care: the next generation of health care delivery. J Med Internet Res [Internet]. 2003 May 15;5(2). Available from: https://www.ncbi.nlm.nih.gov/pmc/articles/PMC1550561/
8. Mac Mahon C, O'Neill D. Clarity on social media? An appraisal of available information regarding dementia on social media websites. Age Ageing. 2016;45:55.
9. Illes J, Moser MA, McCormick JB, Racine E, Blakeslee S, Caplan A, et al. Neurotalk: improving the communication of neuroscience research. Nat Rev Neurosci. 2010;11(1):61–69.
10. Robillard JM, Johnson TW, Hennessey C, Beattie BL, Illes J. Aging 2.0: health information about dementia on Twitter. PLoS ONE. 2013;8(7):e69861.
11. Mackey TK, Cuomo RE, Liang BA. The rise of digital direct-to-consumer advertising? Comparison of direct-to-consumer advertising expenditure trends from publicly available data sources and global policy implications. BMC Health Serv Res. 2015;15:236.
12. Racine E, Van Der Loos HA, Illes J. Internet marketing of neuroproducts: new practices and healthcare policy challenges. Camb Q Healthc Ethics. 2007;16(02):181–94.
13. Ratner E, Atkinson D. Why cognitive training and brain games will not prevent or forestall dementia. J Am Geriatr Soc. 2015;63(12):2612–14.
14. Executive summary: infographic on the digital brain health market 2012-2020 [Internet]. SharpBrains. 2008 [cited May 4, 2017]. Available from: https://sharpbrains.com/executive-summary/
15. Hartin PJ, Nugent CD, McClean SI, Cleland I, Tschanz JT, Clark CJ, et al. The empowering role of mobile apps in behavior change interventions: the Gray Matters randomized controlled trial. JMIR MHealth UHealth. 2016;4(3):e93.
16. Olsson A, Engström M, Lampic C, Skovdahl K. A passive positioning alarm used by persons with dementia and their spouses—a qualitative intervention study. BMC Geriatr. 2013;13:11.
17. Teipel S, Babiloni C, Hoey J, Kaye J, Kirste T, Burmeister OK. Information and communication technology solutions for outdoor navigation in dementia. Alzheimers Dement. 2016;12(6):695–707.
18. Jamieson M, Cullen B, McGee-Lennon M, Brewster S, Evans JJ. The efficacy of cognitive prosthetic technology for people with memory impairments: a systematic review and meta-analysis. Neuropsychol Rehabil. 2014;24(3-4):419–44.
19. Pinto-Bruno ÁC, Antonio G-C, Emese C, Cristina J-R, Manuel F-M. ICT-based applications to improve social health and social participation in older adults with dementia. A systematic literature review. Aging Ment Health. 2016;21(1):58–65.

20. Nijhof N, van Hoof J, van Rijn H, van Gemert-Pijnen JEWC. The behavioral outcomes of a technology-supported leisure activity in people with dementia. Technol Disabil. 2013;25(4):263–73.

21. Lazar A, Thompson H, Demiris G. A systematic review of the use of technology for reminiscence therapy. Health Educ Behav. 2014;41(1 Suppl):51S–61S.

22. Tárraga L, Boada M, Modinos G, Espinosa A, Diego S, Morera A, et al. A randomised pilot study to assess the efficacy of an interactive, multimedia tool of cognitive stimulation in Alzheimer's disease. J Neurol Neurosurg Psychiatry. 2006;77(10):1116–21.

23. Davis BH, Nies MA, Shehab M, Shenk D. Developing a pilot e-mobile app for dementia caregiver support: lessons learned. Online J Nurs Inform. 2014;18(1):21–28.

24. Lee E. Do technology-based support groups reduce care burden among dementia caregivers? A review. J Evid-Inf Soc Work. 2015;12(5):474–87.

25. Lundberg S. The results from a two-year case study of an information and communication technology support system for family caregivers. Disabil Rehabil Assist Technol. 2014;9(4):353–58.

26. Torp S, Bing-Jonsson PC, Hanson E. Experiences with using information and communication technology to build a multi-municipal support network for informal carers. Inform Health Soc Care. 2013;38(3):265–79.

27. Beauchamp N, Irvine AB, Seeley J, Johnson B. Worksite-based Internet multimedia program for family caregivers of persons with dementia. Gerontologist. 2005;45(6):793–801.

28. van der Roest HG, Meiland FJM, Jonker C, Dröes R-M. User evaluation of the DEMentia-specific Digital Interactive Social Chart (DEM-DISC). A pilot study among informal carers on its impact, user friendliness and, usefulness. Aging Ment Health. 2010;14(4):461–70.

29. Marziali E, Donahue P. Caring for others: Internet video-conferencing group intervention for family caregivers of older adults with neurodegenerative disease. Gerontologist. 2006;46(3):398–403.

30. Marziali E, Garcia LJ. Dementia caregivers' responses to 2 Internet-based intervention programs. Am J Alzheimers Dis Other Demen. 2011;26(1):36–43.

31. Pagán-Ortiz ME, Cortés DE, Rudloff N, Weitzman P, Levkoff S. Use of an online community to provide support to caregivers of people with dementia. J Gerontol Soc Work. 2014;57(6–7):694–709.

32. Winter L, Gitlin LN. Evaluation of a telephone-based support group intervention for female caregivers of community-dwelling individuals with dementia. Am J Alzheimers Dis Other Demen. 2007;21(6):391–97.

33. Godwin KM, Mills WL, Anderson JA, Kunik ME. Technology-driven interventions for caregivers of persons with dementia: a systematic review. Am J Alzheimers Dis Other Demen. 2013;28(3):216–22.

34. Boots LMM, de Vugt ME, van Knippenberg RJM, Kempen GIJM, Verhey FRJ. A systematic review of Internet-based supportive interventions for caregivers of patients with dementia. Int J Geriatr Psychiatry. 2014;29(4):331–44.

35. Singh K, Brown RJ. From headache to tumour: an examination of health anxiety, health-related Internet use and "query escalation." J Health Psychol. 2016;21(9):2008–20.

36. Caulfield T, Condit C. Science and the sources of hype. Public Health Genomics. 2012;15(3–4):209–17.

37. Walji M, Sagaram S, Sagaram D, Meric-Bernstam F, Johnson C, Mirza NQ, et al. Efficacy of quality criteria to identify potentially harmful information: a cross-sectional survey of complementary and alternative medicine web sites. J Med Internet Res. 2004 Jun 29;6(2):e21.

38. Hainer MI, Tsai N, Komura ST, Chiu CL. Fatal hepatorenal failure associated with hydrazine sulfate. Ann Intern Med. 2000;133(11):877–80.

39. Eysenbach G, Powell J, Kuss O, Sa E-R. Empirical studies assessing the quality of health information for consumers on the World Wide Web: a systematic review. JAMA. 2002;287(20):2691–700.

40. Lovett KM, Mackey TK, Liang BA. Evaluating the evidence: direct-to-consumer screening tests advertised online. J Med Screen. 2012;19(3):141–53.

41. Max Planck Institute for Human Development, Stanford Center on Longevity. A consensus on the brain training industry from the scientific community [Internet]. 2014 [cited May 4, 2017]. Available from: http://longevity3.stanford.edu/blog/2014/10/15/the-consensus-on-the-brain-training-industry-from-the-scientific-community-2/

42. Federal Trade Commission. Lumosity to pay $2 million to settle FTC deceptive advertising charges for its "brain training" program [Internet]. 2016 [cited May 8, 2017]. Available from: https://www.ftc.gov/news-events/press-releases/2016/01/lumosity-pay-2-million-settle-ftc-deceptive-advertising-charges

43. Rabipour S, Davidson PSR. Do you believe in brain training? A questionnaire about expectations of computerised cognitive training. Behav Brain Res. 2015;295:64–70.

44. Cahill S, Begley E, Faulkner JP, Hagen I. "It gives me a sense of independence"—findings from Ireland on the use and usefulness of assistive technology for people with dementia. Technol Disabil. 2007;19(2,3):133–42.

45. Davis FD. Perceived usefulness, perceived ease of use, and user acceptance of information technology. MIS Q. 1989;13(3):319–40.

46. Mao H-F, Chang L-H, Yao G, Chen W-Y, Huang W-NW. Indicators of perceived useful dementia care assistive technology: caregivers' perspectives. Geriatr Gerontol Int. 2015;15(8):1049–57.

47. Adams DA, Nelson RR, Todd PA. Perceived usefulness, ease of use, and usage of information technology: a replication. MIS Q. 1992;16(2):227–47.

48. Blusi M, Asplund K, Jong M. Older family carers in rural areas: experiences from using caregiver support services based on information and communication technology (ICT). Eur J Ageing Heidelb. 2013;10(3):191–99.

49. Anderson M. Digital divide persists even as lower-income Americans make gains in tech adoption [Internet]. Pew Research Center. 2017 [cited May 12, 2017]. Available from: http://www.pewresearch.org/fact-tank/2017/03/22/digital-divide-persists-even-as-lower-income-americans-make-gains-in-tech-adoption/

50. Wang J-Y, Bennett K, Probst J. Subdividing the digital divide: differences in Internet access and use among rural residents with medical limitations. J Med Internet Res. 2011;13(1):e25.

51. Norman CD, Skinner HA. eHealth literacy: essential skills for consumer health in a networked world. J Med Internet Res. 2006;8(2):e9.

52. Chesser A, Burke A, Reyes J, Rohrberg T. Navigating the digital divide: a systematic review of eHealth literacy in underserved populations in the United States. Inform Health Soc Care. 2016;41(1):1–19.

53. Neter E, Brainin E. eHealth Literacy: extending the digital divide to the realm of health information. J Med Internet Res. 2012;14(1):e19.

54. Mcinnes N, Haglund BJA. Readability of online health information: implications for health literacy. Inform Health Soc Care. 2011;36(4):173–89.

55. Haesner M, Steinert A, O'Sullivan JL, Steinhagen-Thiessen E. Evaluating an accessible web interface for older adults—the impact of mild cognitive impairment (MCI). J Assist Technol. 2015;9(4):219–32.

56. Bauer RM, Iverson GL, Cernich AN, Binder LM, Ruff RM, Naugle RI. Computerized neuropsychological assessment devices: joint position paper of the American Academy of Clinical Neuropsychology and the National Academy of Neuropsychology. Arch Clin Neuropsychol. 2012;27(3):362–73.

57. Jacova C, McGrenere J, Lee HS, Wang WW, Le Huray S, Corenblith EF, et al. C-TOC (Cognitive Testing on Computer): investigating the usability and validity of a novel self-administered cognitive assessment tool in aging and early dementia. Alzheimer Dis Assoc Disord. 2015;29(3):213–21.

58. Darby DG, Pietrzak RH, Fredrickson J, Woodward M, Moore L, Fredrickson A, et al. Intraindividual cognitive decline using a brief computerized cognitive screening test. Alzheimers Dement. 2012;8(2):95–104.

59. Dwolatzky T, Dimant L, Simon ES, Doniger GM. Validity of a short computerized assessment battery for moderate cognitive impairment and dementia. Int Psychogeriatr. 2010;22(5):795–803.

60. Hammers D, Spurgeon E, Ryan K, Persad C, Barbas N, Heidebrink J, et al. Validity of a brief computerized cognitive screening test in dementia. J Geriatr Psychiatry Neurol. 2012;25(2):89–99.

61. Albrecht U-V, von Jan U, Jungnickel T, Pramann O. App-synopsis—standard reporting for medical apps. Stud Health Technol Inform. 2013;192:1154.

62. Bashir M, Hayes C, Lambert AD, Kesan JP. Online privacy and informed consent: the dilemma of information asymmetry. Proc Assoc Inf Sci Technol. 2015;52(1):1–10.

63. Ploug T, Holm S. Informed consent and routinisation. J Med Ethics. 2013;39(4):214–18.

64. Black BS, Wechsler M, Fogarty L. Decision making for participation in dementia research. Am J Geriatr Psychiatry. 2013;21(4):355–63.

65. Landau R, Auslander GK, Werner S, Shoval N, Heinik J. Families' and professional caregivers' views of using advanced technology to track people with dementia. Qual Health Res. 2010;20(3):409–19.

66. Welsh S, Hassiotis A, O'Mahoney G, Deahl M. Big brother is watching you—the ethical implications of electronic surveillance measures in the elderly with dementia and in adults with learning difficulties. Aging Ment Health. 2003;7(5):372–75.

67. Eltis K. Predicating dignity on autonomy—the need for further inquiry into the ethics of tagging and tracking dementia patients with GPS technology. Elder Law J. 2005;13:387.

68. Landau R, Werner S, Auslander GK, Shoval N, Heinik J. What do cognitively intact older people think about the use of electronic tracking devices for people with dementia? A preliminary analysis. Int Psychogeriatr. 2010;22(8):1301–9.

69. Sternberg DA, Ballard K, Hardy JL, Katz B, Doraiswamy PM, Scanlon M. The largest human cognitive performance dataset reveals insights into the effects of lifestyle factors and aging. Front Hum Neurosci. 2013;7:292.

70. Purcell RH, Rommelfanger KS. Internet-based brain training games, citizen scientists, and big data: ethical issues in unprecedented virtual territories. Neuron. 2015;86(2):356–59.

71. Cocosila M, Archer N. Adoption of mobile ICT for health promotion: an empirical investigation. Electron Mark Heidelb. 2010;20(3-4):241–50.
72. Fife E, Orjuela J. The privacy calculus: mobile apps and user perceptions of privacy and security. Int J Eng Bus Manag. 2012;4:11.
73. Guo X, Zhang X, Sun Y. The privacy–personalization paradox in mHealth services acceptance of different age groups. Electron Commer Res Appl. 2016;16:55–65.
74. Earp JB, Anton AI, Aiman-Smith L, Stufflebeam WH. Examining Internet privacy policies within the context of user privacy values. IEEE Trans Eng Manag. 2005;52(2):227–37.
75. Doak CC, Doak LG, Root JH. Teaching patients with low literacy skills. Philadelphia: Lippincott; 1985, 171 pp.
76. Sunyaev A, Dehling T, Taylor PL, Mandl KD. Availability and quality of mobile health app privacy policies. J Am Med Inform Assoc. 2015;22(1):28–33.
77. Huckvale K, Prieto JT, Tilney M, Benghozi P-J, Car J. Unaddressed privacy risks in accredited health and wellness apps: a cross-sectional systematic assessment. BMC Med. 2015;13:214.
78. Dehling T, Gao F, Schneider S, Sunyaev A. Exploring the far side of mobile health: information security and privacy of mobile health apps on iOS and Android. JMIR MHealth UHealth. 2015;3(1):e8.
79. Martínez-Pérez B, de la Torre-Díez I, López-Coronado M. Privacy and security in mobile health apps: a review and recommendations. J Med Syst. 2014;39(1):1–8.
80. McCarthy M. Federal privacy rules offer scant protection for users of health apps and wearable devices. BMJ. 2016;354:i4115.
81. Liang BA, Mackey TK. Prevalence and global health implications of social media in direct-to-consumer drug advertising. J Med Internet Res. 2011;13(3):64.
82. Holmer AF. Direct-to-consumer advertising—strengthening our health care system. N Engl J Med. 2002;346(7):526–28.
83. Park JS. Direct-to-consumer prescription medicine advertising and seniors' knowledge of Alzheimer's disease. Am J Alzheimers Dis Other Demen. 2016;31(1):40–47.
84. Liang BA, Mackey T. Direct-to-consumer advertising with interactive Internet media: global regulation and public health issues. JAMA. 2011;305(8):824–25.
85. Block AE. Costs and benefits of direct-to-consumer advertising. PharmacoEconomics. 2007;25(6):511–21.
86. Illes J, Kann D, Karetsky K, et al. Advertising, patient decision making, and self-referral for computed tomographic and magnetic resonance imaging. Arch Intern Med. 2004;164(22):2415–19.
87. Palmour N, Vanderbyl BL, Zimmerman E, Gauthier S, Racine E. Alzheimer's disease dietary supplements in websites. HEC Forum. 2013;25(4):361–82.
88. Murray E, Lo B, Pollack L, Donelan K, Lee K. Direct-to-consumer advertising: physicians' views of its effects on quality of care and the doctor-patient relationship. J Am Board Fam Pract. 2003;16(6):513–24.
89. Lupton D, Jutel A. "It's like having a physician in your pocket!" A critical analysis of self-diagnosis smartphone apps. Soc Sci Med. 2015;133:128–35.
90. Krieger WH. Medical apps: public and academic perspectives. Perspect Biol Med. 2013;56(2):259–73.
91. Kim J, Kim S. Physicians' perception of the effects of Internet health information on the doctor–patient relationship. Inform Health Soc Care. 2009;34(3):136–48.

92. Silver MP. Patient perspectives on online health information and communication with doctors: a qualitative study of patients 50 years old and over. J Med Internet Res. 2015;17(1):e19.

93. Murray E, Lo B, Pollack L, Donelan K, Catania J, Lee K, et al. The impact of health information on the Internet on the physician-patient relationship: patient perceptions. Arch Intern Med. 2003;163(14):1727–34.

94. Ahmad F, Hudak PL, Bercovitz K, Hollenberg E, Levinson W. Are physicians ready for patients with Internet-based health information? J Med Internet Res. 2006;8(3):e22.

95. Tan SS-L, Goonawardene N. Internet health information seeking and the patient-physician relationship: a systematic review. J Med Internet Res. 2017;19(1):e9.

96. Ahluwalia S, Murray E, Stevenson F, Kerr C, Burns J. "A heartbeat moment": qualitative study of GP views of patients bringing health information from the internet to a consultation. Br J Gen Pract. 2010;60(571):88–94.

97. van Uden-Kraan CF, Drossaert CHC, Taal E, Smit WM, Seydel ER, van de Laar MAFJ. Experiences and attitudes of Dutch rheumatologists and oncologists with regard to their patients' health-related Internet use. Clin Rheumatol. 2010;29(11):1229–36.

98. Murray E, Lo B, Pollack L, Donelan K, Catania J, Lee K, et al. The impact of health information on the Internet on health care and the physician-patient relationship: national U.S. survey among 1.050 U.S. physicians. J Med Internet Res. 2003;5(3):e17.

99. Werner P, Korczyn AD. Willingness to use computerized systems for the diagnosis of dementia: testing a theoretical model in an Israeli sample. Alzheimer Dis Assoc Disord. 2012;26(2):171–78.

100. Mitra T, Counts S, Pennebaker JW. Understanding anti-vaccination attitudes in social media. In: Proceedings of the 10th International AAAI Conference on Web and Social Media (ICWSM 2016). 2016.

101. Kata A. Anti-vaccine activists, Web 2.0, and the postmodern paradigm—an overview of tactics and tropes used online by the anti-vaccination movement. Vaccine. 2012;30(25):3778–89.

102. Mehmet O. Written testimony of Dr. Mehmet Oz, M.D. Hearing on "Protecting consumers from false and deceptive advertising of weight-loss products." 2014.

103. Specter M. The Operator [Internet]. New Yorker. 2013 [cited May 25, 2017]. Available from: http://www.newyorker.com/magazine/2013/02/04/the-operator

104. Korownyk C, Kolber MR, McCormack J, Lam V, Overbo K, Cotton C, et al. Televised medical talk shows—what they recommend and the evidence to support their recommendations: a prospective observational study. BMJ. 2014;349:g7346.

105. Bootsman N, Blackburn DF, Taylor J. The Oz craze: the effect of pop culture media on health care. Can Pharm J Rev Pharm Can. 2014;147(2):80–82.

106. Mercola J. How can sunscreen cause Alzheimer's disease? [Internet]. Mercola.com. 2012 [cited May 25, 2017]. Available from: http://articles.mercola.com/sites/articles/archive/2012/03/03/sun-screens-cause-alzheimers.aspx

107. Mercola J. How the CDC uses false fears to promote vaccine uptake [Internet]. Mercola.com. 2017 [cited May 25, 2017]. Available from: http://articles.mercola.com/sites/articles/archive/2017/03/07/cdc-uses-false-fears-promote-vaccine-uptake.aspx

108. Mercola J. This Indian herb may potentially cure Alzheimer's disease [Internet]. Mercola.com. 2012 [cited May 25, 2017]. Available from: http://articles.mercola.

com/sites/articles/archive/2012/04/07/ashwaganda-effect-on-alzheimers-disease. aspx

109. Master Z, Resnik DB. Hype and public trust in science. Sci Eng Ethics. 2013;19(2):321–35.

110. Alwin J, Krevers B, Johansson U, Josephsson S, Haraldson U, Boström C, et al. Health economic and process evaluation of AT interventions for persons with dementia and their relatives—a suggested assessment model. Technol Disabil. 2007;19(2/3):61–71.

111. Droste S, Herrmann-Frank A, Scheibler F, Krones T. Ethical issues in autologous stem cell transplantation (ASCT) in advanced breast cancer: a systematic literature review. BMC Med Ethics. 2011;12:6.

112. Hofmann B. Stuck in the middle: the many moral challenges with bariatric surgery. Am J Bioeth. 2010;10(12):3–11.

113. Hofmann B, Droste S, Oortwijn W, Cleemput I, Sacchini D. Harmonization of ethics in health technology assessment: a revision of the Socratic approach. Int J Technol Assess Health Care. 2014;30(1):3–9.

114. Saarni SI, Hofmann B, Lampe K, Lühmann D, Mäkelä M, Velasco-Garrido M, et al. Ethical analysis to improve decision-making on health technologies. Bull World Health Organ. 2008;86(8):617–23.

115. Robillard JM. The online environment: a key variable in the ethical response to complementary and alternative medicine for Alzheimer's disease. J Alzheimers Dis. 2016;51(1):11–13.

116. Charnock D, Shepperd S, Needham G, Gann R. DISCERN: an instrument for judging the quality of written consumer health information on treatment choices. J Epidemiol Community Health. 1999;53(2):105–11.

117. Chumber S, Huber J, Ghezzi P. A methodology to analyze the quality of health information on the Internet: the example of diabetic neuropathy. Diabetes Educ. 2015;41(1):95–105.

118. Seidman JJ, Steinwachs D, Rubin HR. Design and testing of a tool for evaluating the quality of diabetes consumer-information web sites. J Med Internet Res. 2003;5(4):e30.

119. Silberg W, Lundberg G, Musacchio R. Assessing, controlling, and assuring the quality of medical information on the Internet: caveant lector et viewor—let the reader and viewer beware. JAMA. 1997;277(15):1244–45.

120. Robertson-Lang L, Major S, Hemming H. An exploration of search patterns and credibility issues among older adults seeking online health information. Can J Aging Rev Can Vieil. 2011;30(4):631–45.

121. Domecq JP, Prutsky G, Elraiyah T, Wang Z, Nabhan M, Shippee N, et al. Patient engagement in research: a systematic review. BMC Health Serv Res. 2014;14:89.

122. Esmail L, Moore E, Rein A. Evaluating patient and stakeholder engagement in research: moving from theory to practice. J Comp Eff Res. 2015;4(2):133–45.

123. Hubbard G, Downs MG, Tester S. Including older people with dementia in research: challenges and strategies. Aging Ment Health. 2003;7(5):351–62.

124. Robillard JM, Feng TL. When patient engagement and research ethics collide: lessons from a dementia forum. J Alzheimers Dis. 2017;59(1):1–10.

125. Frascara J. Design and the Social Sciences: Making Connections. CRC Press; 2003, 258 pp.

126. Inglis EA, Szymkowiak A, Gregor P, Newell AF, Hine N, Shah P, et al. Issues surrounding the user-centred development of a new interactive memory aid. Univers Access Inf Soc. 2003 Oct 1;2(3):226–34.

127. Carroll JM. Encountering others: reciprocal openings in participatory design and user-centered design. Hum-Comput Interact. 1996;11(3):285–90.

128. Fischer G. Meta-design: beyond user-centered and participatory design. Proc HCI Int. 2003;4:88–92.

129. Sanders EB-N, Stappers PJ. Co-creation and the new landscapes of design. CoDesign. 2008;4(1):5–18.

130. Ellis RD, Kurniawan SH. Increasing the usability of online information for older users: a case study in participatory design. Int J Human–Computer Interact. 2000;12(2):263–76.

131. Hanson E, Magnusson L, Arvidsson H, Claesson A, Keady J, Nolan M. Working together with persons with early stage dementia and their family members to design a user-friendly technology-based support service. Dementia. 2007;6(3):411–34.

132. Meiland FJM, Bouman AIE, Sävenstedt S, Bentvelzen S, Davies RJ, Mulvenna MD, et al. Usability of a new electronic assistive device for community-dwelling persons with mild dementia. Aging Ment Health. 2012;16(5):584–91.

133. Slegers K, Wilkinson A, Hendriks N. Active collaboration in healthcare design: participatory design to develop a dementia care app. In: CHI '13 Extended Abstracts on Human Factors in Computing Systems (CHI EA '13) [Internet]. New York: ACM; 2013, 475–80. Available from: http://doi.acm.org/10.1145/2468356.2468440

134. Carroll JM, Rosson MB. Participatory design in community informatics. Des Stud. 2007;28(3):243–61.

135. Björgvinsson E, Ehn P, Hillgren P-A. Participatory design and "Democratizing innovation." In: Proceedings of the 11th Biennial Participatory Design Conference (PDC '10) [Internet]. New York: ACM; 2010, 41–50. Available from: http://doi.acm.org/10.1145/1900441.1900448

136. von Hippel E. Democratizing innovation. Cambridge, MA: MIT Press; 2005, 204 pp.

137. Hendriks N, Huybrechts L, Wilkinson A, Slegers K. Challenges in doing participatory design with people with dementia. In: Proceedings of the 13th Participatory Design Conference: Short Papers, Industry Cases, Workshop Descriptions, Doctoral Consortium Papers, and Keynote Abstracts—Volume 2 (PDC '14) [Internet]. New York: ACM; 2014, 33–36. Available from: http://doi.acm.org/10.1145/2662155.2662196

138. Hendriks N, Truyen F, Duval E. Designing with dementia: guidelines for participatory design together with persons with dementia. Springer; 2013 [cited Jul 4, 2017], 649–66. Available from: https://hal.inria.fr/hal-01497469/document

139. Span M, Hettinga M, Vernooij-Dassen M, Eefsting J, Smits C. Involving people with dementia in the development of supportive IT applications: a systematic review. Ageing Res Rev. 2013;12(2):535–51.

140. McKechnie V, Barker C, Stott J. The effectiveness of an Internet support forum for carers of people with dementia: a pre-post cohort study. J Med Internet Res. 2014;16(2):e68.

141. Muse K, McManus F, Leung C, Meghreblian B, Williams JMG. Cyberchondriasis: fact or fiction? A preliminary examination of the relationship between health

anxiety and searching for health information on the Internet. J Anxiety Disord. 2012;26(1):189–96.

142. White RW, Horvitz E. Cyberchondria: studies of the escalation of medical concerns in web search. ACM Trans Inf Syst. 2009;27(4):23:1–23:37.

143. White RW, Horvitz E. Experiences with web search on medical concerns and self diagnosis. AMIA Annu Symp Proc. 2009;2009:696–700.

144. Robillard JM, Alhothali A, Varma S, Hoey J. Intelligent and affectively aligned evaluation of online health information for older adults. In: Workshops at the 31st AAAI Conference on Artificial Intelligence [Internet]. 2017 [cited Jul 6, 2017]. Available from: https://www.aaai.org/ocs/index.php/WS/AAAIW17/paper/view/15078

15

Dementia and the Regulation of Gerontechnology

James Beauregard

Introduction

Three Diversities

The purpose of this chapter is to provide an overview of the regulation of gerontechnology in its various aspects. Regulatory systems can vary markedly from country to country; some frameworks are more centralized, some more distributed. The current regulatory situation in the United States can be captured by the word "patchwork." There is no single regulatory body with authority over gerontechnology, which is not surprising given the diversity of technological interventions available, including smart homes and technology to enhance communication, monitor safety, and assist with household tasks. There are current and historical reasons for this, resulting in practical diversity of regulatory bodies and activities. I would suggest three diversities operative in the field of gerontechnology regulation:

1. The diversity of government structure. The American political system is based on a separation of powers, both within the federal government (executive, legislative, and judicial) and between the federal government and the states (each state having its own executive, legislative, and judiciary branches). So it is not an exaggeration to say that with regard to technology, the United States has, at minimum, 51 regulatory bodies: the federal government and the 50 state governments. Within each of these there are multiple agencies tasked with the assessment, approval, and ongoing oversight of technology. This is a recipe for fragmentation when coherence is needed. Other countries have fundamentally different frameworks. There are supra-national bodies, such as the United Nations and the European Union, that address issues of healthcare and technology with which gerontechnologists will need to interact. In addition to these governmental structures, there are numerous professional associations that address elder care and dementia, and the STEM disciplines in academia have their own regulatory bodies (e.g., Institutional Review Boards, professional associations, and the realities of grant funding) that impact the development of new technologies.

The US regulatory situation is not universal. Berridge et al. (2014) compared the United States, the United Kingdom, and Scandinavia in terms of regulation and financial support for home care services, and found the United States occupied a middle ground of regulation compared to centralized regulation in the United Kingdom and strongly decentralized regulation in Scandinavia. In addition, the level of government support for formal care was low in the United States, where families share care activities and costs with the market sector and nonprofit organizations. In contrast, Scandinavian governments provide a high level of formal care, with much less family support compared to the United States. The situation in the United Kingdom is similar to that of the United States (reliance on family, nonprofit organizations, and the market sector).

2. *The diversity of gerontechnology.* Technology that can assist elders comes in many forms and addresses many issues including stay-at-home technology (e.g., smart homes), healthcare monitoring and service delivery, communication, mobility, and safety. Sophisticated robotics technology is a new player in the gerontechnology field that is finding its way into smart homes and other settings to assist elders in maintaining independence and provide medical and safety monitoring. Smart cars, for example, may provide a means for individuals with dementia to reach places beyond the home when they have retired from driving (see Table 15.1)

3. *The diversity of dementia.* Dementia is a general descriptive term that refers to a decline in some aspect of an individual's cognition, affect, or functioning (activities of daily living [ADLs], instrumental activities of daily living [IADLs], work, social activity, recreation). A dementia diagnosis must include documentation of decline, as well as a specific, or at least suspected, cause of the decline, even at the mild cognitive impairment stage. The most common neurodegenerative illnesses that cause dementia include Alzheimer's disease and vascular dementia, while declines in cognition, affective functioning, and behavior can also result from such conditions as Parkinson's disease, Lewy body dementia, frontotemporal dementia, and a variety of metabolic conditions.[1] As a consequence, there is no single, universal "dementia profile"—individuals vary greatly in clinical presentation from one type of dementia to another, within a given type of dementia, and over the course of a dementing illness as well. Consequently, the safety and care needs of individuals with dementia will vary greatly. No one technology type or model will suffice. Care needs must be individually assessed, and technological options chosen based on the results of such assessment.

An example that illustrates this point is the comparison between two individuals with dementia, one with Alzheimer's disease affecting the temporal and parietal lobes that causes a decrease in acetylcholinesterase production,

Table 15.1 Gerontechnology Domains

Medical	Monitoring/Safety	Mobility	Communication	Robotics
Medications	Biomedical	Wheelchairs	Internet	Cleaning
Devices	Activity trackers	Exoskeletons	Email	Emotion support/
Telehealth	Video monitoring	Self-driving cars	Computers	companion robots, e.g.,
Medication alerts	Motion sensors	Wheelchairs	Smartphones	Paro seal robot
Lighting	Webcams	Scooters	Social media	Emotion recognition tech
Cochlear implants	Virtual environment	Smart walkers	Skype/FaceTime	Smart homes
Lens implants	Location technology	Navigation tools	Tablets	BCI
Pill dispensers	Motion recognition	Lift chairs	Watches	Muscle assist
Hearing aids	Smart homes	Smart homes	E-shopping	Artificial intelligence and
E-med records	Fitbit	BCI	Video links (medical and social)	ambient assisted living
Wearable technology	Remote patient monitoring	Smart cars	E-banking	Robotic shelf system
Aware technology	Emergency call	Smart floors	Voice recognition software	Vocal command
(open doors, etc.)	Sensor mats—bed		Talk to text	technology
BCI			Smart homes	Biomimetics
Biosensors			BCI	Nursing care robots
Infrared sensors				Patient transfer robots
Video cameras				Telepresence robots
Microphones				
Ultrasonic sensors				
Biosensors				
Physiology sensors				
AAL field				
Smart chairs				
Exercise equipment				
Telehealth				
Patient transfer robots				

and one with dementia in the context of Parkinson's disease, with pathology originating in the dopamine-producing neurons of the substantia nigra and spreading in time to cortical structures involved in cognition. An individual with Alzheimer's experiences prominent short-term memory loss that can raise safety issues in medication compliance and kitchen safety and decision making, and the visuospatial deficits common in Alzheimer's can preclude safe driving sooner rather than later. Such an individual would benefit from monitoring technologies to prevent wandering and to guard against fires in the kitchen, from an electronic pill dispenser to ensure accurate medication compliance, from oversight for complex financial or medical decision making, and so forth. An individual with Parkinson's dementia will be contending from early on with a movement disorder involving gait disturbance, bradykinesia, and rigidity, and some with Parkinson's will later face cognitive deficits including bradyphrenia, deficits in attention and executive skills. These individuals would benefit from in-home monitoring and assistance of movement that would provide alerts for falls, as well as instruments to assist with medication compliance and the monitoring of vital signs.[2] Both might benefit from self-driving vehicles to provide transportation and increase opportunities for socialization.

Chapter Overview

To address this complexity, the plan of this chapter is as follows: First, I will review the gerontechnology currently available to address the numerous safety and living concerns that arise in dementia. Second, I will look at the current regulatory framework for gerontechnology and dementia. Finally, I will conclude with an assessment of the current gerontechnology regulatory situation and recommendations to address current and emerging technologies.

Gerontechnology and Dementia

What Are the Gerontechnologies?

Gerontechnology is diverse, so it is not surprising that any country with no central or overarching regulatory system would look to multiple agencies when it comes to the oversight of new technologies. In this section I want to briefly review some of the many technologies that are available for elder care for individuals with dementia. I will group them under five broad headings of medical, monitoring, mobility, communication, and robotics. The robotics category will have overlaps with the others; I have included it as a separate category due to its novelty and its implications for dementia care.

Medical and monitoring technologies are diverse in the context of dementia. They can include specific medications to address cognitive, psychiatric, and functional issues (acetylcholinesterase inhibitors, Namenda, and the four classes of psychiatric drugs: antianxiety agents, antidepressants, medications for bipolar disorder, and antipsychotics). Telehealth technology coupled with biosensor technology can provide monitoring, assessment, and intervention in the home. Information technology such as electronic medical records enables healthcare providers to access information about individual patients from multiple locations to provide care. Pill dispensers can assist with medication compliance. Lens and cochlear implants can markedly improve the sensorium of individuals with dementia. Lighting technology can enhance vision, help reduce fall risk, and diminish behavior problems. Smart chairs and patient transfer robots can assist with movement, reduce fall risk, and reduce rates of healthcare provider injuries. Motion sensors and motion recognition technology in the home can alert healthcare providers and family of falls, and monitor overall activity levels during the day and at night. Video technology can provide a view into the home of an individual with dementia.

Technological developments can also assist individuals with dementia who experience movement difficulties, including motorized wheelchairs, scooters, smart walkers, lift chairs and assistive stair technology, self-driving cars, navigation tools, exoskeletons, and smart floors.

For individuals with dementia who are homebound, communication technologies can help them communicate with the outside world while simultaneously providing opportunities for monitoring. Such technologies include computers, Internet, email, smart phones, social media, Skype/FaceTime, electronic banking and shopping, tablets, voice recognition software, and watches that monitor and communicate health status.

Robotics is a rapidly developing field whose potential for dementia care is under investigation and development, and can include cleaning robots, emotional support and companion robots (e.g., the Paro seal robot), emotional recognition technology, muscle assist robotics, robotic shelf systems, biomimetics, nursing care robots, patient transfer robots, and telepresence robots.

Special Considerations in Dementia and Technology

There are special issues specific to dementia that can impact the adoption and use of gerontechnology. Normally aging individuals retain their cognitive capacities across the life span, experiencing only minor cognitive changes in the context of normal aging that do not typically impact decision making, independent living, self-care, or independent ADLs (e.g., driving, cooking, medication compliance, financial management, and medical decision making). All of these may undergo change over the course of a dementing illness, raising these special concerns.

Capacity/competence. All of the technologies noted previously require the consent of the user and the capacity to use the technology. Many dementias impair cognitive function in varied ways, including memory, executive skills, visuospatial skills, and language. Individuals with dementia may progressively lose decision-making capacity. In many cases, family members acting as healthcare proxies or guardians will be making decisions about the purchase and use of gerontechnology. For example, an individual who has Alzheimer's disease and who presents with short-term memory impairment, poor decision-making skills, and poor insight into his or her deficits may have a healthcare proxy activated or may have a guardian. It is this person who will interact with the patient's healthcare providers and make medical decisions, and who may oversee the patient's finances as well. In such cases, it is the proxy or guardian who will determine, based on medical recommendations, what technologies are feasible and affordable to adopt for the person in his or her care in the wider context of the patient's healthcare status, financial resources, and care planning.

Dementia and adaptation of new technologies. Individuals with dementia experiencing cognitive impairment typically have difficulty adopting any new technology as their dementia progresses. Families frequently report, for example, that an individual with dementia cannot learn to use a new television remote, microwave, or remote control. This will place limits on the use of technologies that require the individual with dementia to operate independently. As the same time, monitoring technologies can come to the fore in these types of situations. A related issue is the cohort differences in the aging population and their attitudes toward new technologies in general (impacting their willingness to try newly available technologies). For example, individuals born during the interwar period of the 20th century are often more hesitant to try new technologies, while those born in the baby boom generation or subsequently, who grew up with technologies now considered common, like computers, the Internet, cell phones, and so forth, are often more willing to—and more interested in—learning about and adopting new technologies.

Socialization. Individuals with dementia need social activity, and lots of it, to help them maintain brain health and their highest possible level of functioning. This immediately becomes an issue for an individual who retires from driving due to dementia. In this case, family typically steps up to the plate (when they are local) to assist with transportation needs, and can also work with healthcare providers to access public transport when available. Self-driving cars may be able to facilitate opportunities for social interaction by bringing elders to senior centers, religious services, and day programs if the person with dementia lives beyond the boundaries for which a program provides transportation.[3]

Cost.   Many elders live on fixed incomes, and any new technology raises the question "Who will pay for it?" Medicare and Medicaid are the two major government health programs providing medical care for the elderly, and whether or not they approve any particular in-home technology for individuals with dementia will have a major impact on whether or not such technologies come into widespread use. Limited financial resources, even with family support, may preclude the introduction of new technologies for many elders.

While these factors may seem daunting, they do not automatically preclude the adoption of a variety of technologies to ensure health and safety for an individual with dementia acting with the assistance of family or a guardian. A critical factor will be the development of strong clinical evidence that a particular technology does have a positive impact for individuals with dementia. The clinical research process will need to walk hand in hand with technology development to demonstrate efficacy and cost containment.

Regulation of Gerontechnology in Dementia

In considering the framework of regulation, I will be using the following working definition of the field of gerontechnology developed by Graafmans (2017, 7):

> The field is defined as the development and adaptation of technology toward the goals and ambitions of aging and aged peoples and it is application oriented in nature. The fundamental concepts underlying gerontechnology comprise: (a) four research and application areas of technology, (b) five domains of life activity to which technology is applicable, (c) the changing dynamics of person-environment interactions over time, and (d) the identification of a multidisciplinary knowledge base.[4]

The *four research and application areas* (a), derived from the field of public health, include primary, secondary, and tertiary prevention, and fourth, the impact of these on overall quality-of-life improvement.

The *five domains of activity* (b) are health and self-esteem, housing and everyday functioning, communication, transportation and mobility, and work and leisure.

The *changing dynamics of* interaction refer to both the aging process as it affects individual abilities and the differences in age cohorts.

The *multidisciplinary knowledge base* Graafmans identifies is broad and includes the STEM disciplines as well as biology and the behavioral sciences (to which I would add the field of medicine—research and practice—including the specialty areas of geriatric internal medicine, geriatric psychiatry and neurology, and rehabilitation medicine).[5] (Graafmans, 2017)

As the preceding sections make clear, gerontechnology is both varied and distinct in terms of what is studied and the development nature of individual products and their use. On the American scene, the practical implication is that the regulation of these technologies will never fall under one single regulatory body. Some technologies are more explicitly medical, some are functional in the sense of physical medicine and rehabilitation interventions, some provide transportation, and some consist of communication outside an explicitly medical context.

Historically, different regulatory agencies were created at different times and for different purposes to oversee specific types of technology. In the United Sates, these include the Department of Health and Human Services (HHS), the Food and Drug Administration (FDA), the General Accounting Office (GAO), the Federal Trade Commission (FTC), and the specific federal regulatory bodies for the Medicare and Medicaid Programs (which are themselves under the umbrella of HHS). In terms of elder care, the Veteran's Administration is a large-scale healthcare provider of medical, hospital, and long-term care. There are also additional private entities that will touch on dementia care. I will review each of these agencies in terms of their missions and the types of technology they regulate (see Table 15.2 for an overview).

Table 15.2 Special Issues to Consider in Dementia Technology

Cognitive	Affective	Behavioral	Autonomy	Capacity/ Competence/ Consent	Caregivers
Attention	Depression	Agitation	Independence	Clinical/legal	Resources
Language	Anxiety	Aggression	Safety	Power of	Burden
Visuospatial	Psychosis	Apathy	Driving	attorney	Education
Memory		Compliance	Assisted Living	Guardianship	
Executive		Incontinence	Long Term	Issues of	
Motor		Wandering	Care	-Insight	
				-Judgment	
				-Reasoning	
				-Decision	
				making	

Department of Health and Human Services

The HHS is an obvious place to begin, though it is only one of many federal agencies of interest to those who address the health and safety problems of dementia. The department's mission is to "enhance and protect the health and well-being of all Americans. We fulfill that mission by providing effective health and human services and fostering advances in medicine, public health, and social services."[6] The department is involved in health insurance and the protection of healthcare information through the Health Insurance Portability and Accountability Act (HIPAA). It is also the government agency that oversees the Affordable Care Act (ACA), Medicare, Medicaid, the Children's Health Insurance Program (CHIP), and various social service programs. Thus, many aspects of this agency will touch directly on healthcare for the elderly in general and for individuals with dementia in particular (see later for specifics of programs that relate to dementia care).

Food and Drug Administration[7]

The FDA is a large and multifaceted government regulatory body tasked with the regulation and oversight of numerous types of technologies including medications, medical devices, general wellness technologies, and medical apps. Each of these aspects of the agency's mission will impact the development and regulation of gerontechnology. I will consider each of these areas as they relate to gerontechnology regulation. Specific bodies within the FDA have specific regulatory provinces including medications, medical devices, general wellness products and low-risk devices, and mobile medical apps.

Medications

Drugs for the treatment of medical conditions in human beings are regulated by the FDA's Center for Drug Evaluation and Research (CDER). For a medication to reach the market for prescribing by healthcare professionals, it must undergo a rigorous testing process to demonstrate both safety and efficacy, typically through multisite double-blind, placebo-controlled trials. The FDA regulates these trials, and when both safety and efficacy are demonstrated, it will approve a medication for clinical use. Approved uses are typically specified, for example, acetylcholinesterase inhibitors (e.g. Aricept/donepezil for the preservation of memory functioning in Alzheimer's disease, or Risperdal/risperidone for the treatment of psychosis). Many medications also come to be used in "off label" prescribing when found to have some efficacy in treating medical and psychiatric conditions.[8] Medications approved by the FDA are used in geriatrics to treat a wide variety of conditions (e.g., for cardiac conditions, diabetes, stroke prevention, psychiatric symptoms, etc.).

Medical Devices

In addition to medications, many types of devices employed in medical care are regulated. The FDA defines medical devices as follows:

Medical devices range from simple tongue depressors and bedpans to complex programmable pacemakers with micro-chip technology and laser surgical devices. In addition, medical devices include in vitro diagnostic products, such as general purpose lab equipment, reagents, and test kits, which may include monoclonal antibody technology. Certain electronic radiation emitting products with medical application and claims meet the definition of medical device. Examples include diagnostic ultrasound products, x-ray machines and medical lasers. If a product is labeled, promoted or used in a manner that meets the following definition in section 201(h) of the Federal Food Drug & Cosmetic (FD&C) Act it will be regulated by the Food and Drug Administration (FDA) as a medical device and is subject to premarketing and post marketing regulatory controls. A device is:

- an instrument, apparatus, implement, machine, contrivance, implant, in vitro reagent, or other similar or related article, including a component part, or accessory which is:
- recognized in the official National Formulary, or the United States Pharmacopoeia, or any supplement to them,
- intended for use in the diagnosis of disease or other conditions, or in the cure, mitigation, treatment, or prevention of disease, in man or other animals, or
- intended to affect the structure or any function of the body of man or other animals, and which does not achieve its primary intended purposes through chemical action within or on the body of man or other animals and which is not dependent upon being metabolized for the achievement of any of its primary intended purposes.[9]

General Wellness Products and Low-Risk Devices

The FDA defines a general wellness product as one that

has (1) an intended use that relates to maintaining or encouraging a general state of health or a healthy activity, or (2) an intended use that relates the role of healthy lifestyle with helping to reduce the risk or impact of certain chronic diseases or conditions and where it is well understood and accepted that healthy lifestyle choices may play an important role in health outcomes for the disease or condition.[10]

In addition:

> General wellness products may include exercise equipment, audio recordings, video games, software programs4 and other products that are commonly, though not exclusively, available from retail establishments (including online retailers and distributors that offer software to be directly downloaded), when consistent with the two factors above.

The FDA divides general wellness products into several categories, first products that maintain general health outside of specific disease diagnoses:

The first category of general wellness intended uses involve claims about sustaining or offering general improvement to functions associated with a general state of health that **do not make any reference to diseases or conditions**. For the purposes of this guidance, this first category of general wellness claims relate to:

- weight management,
- physical fitness, including products intended for recreational use,
- relaxation or stress management,
- mental acuity,
- self-esteem (e.g., devices with a cosmetic function that make claims related only to self-esteem),
- sleep management, or
- sexual function.

The following are examples of this category of general wellness claims:

- Claims to promote or maintain a healthy weight, encourage healthy eating, or assist with weight loss goals;
- Claims to promote relaxation or manage stress;
- Claims to increase, improve, or enhance the flow of qi "energy";
- Claims to improve mental acuity, instruction following, concentration, problem solving, multitasking, resource management, decision making, logic, pattern recognition, or eye-hand coordination[11];
- Claims to enhance learning capacity;
- Claims to promote physical fitness, such as to help log, track, or trend exercise activity, measure aerobic fitness, improve physical fitness, develop or improve endurance, strength, or coordination, or improve energy;

- Claims to promote sleep management, such as to track sleep trends;
- Claims to promote self-esteem, such as to boost self-esteem;
- Claims that address a specific body structure or function, such as to increase or improve muscle size or body tone, tone or firm the body or muscle, or enhance or improve sexual performance;
- Claims to improve general mobility or to assist individuals who are mobility impaired in a recreational activity (e.g., sport wheelchairs, beach access wheelchairs); and
- Claims to enhance an individual's participation in recreational activities by monitoring the consequences of participating in such activities, such as to monitor heart rate or monitor frequency or impact of collisions.

Claims that do not fall into the category of general wellness, according to the agency, include claims that a product can diagnose or treat obesity and products that claim to treat eating disorders or anxiety disorders, claims that a particular computer game can diagnose or treat autism, or products that claim to "restore" function that has been lost due to injury or disease.

The second category of general wellness products regulated by the agency includes products whose "intended uses relate to sustaining or offering general improvement to functions associated with a general state of health while **making reference to diseases or conditions**. For the purposes of this guidance, this second category of general wellness claims is comprised of two subcategories:

1) intended uses to promote, track, and/or encourage choice(s), which, as part of a healthy lifestyle, **may help to reduce the risk of** certain chronic diseases or conditions; and
2) intended uses to promote, track, and/or encourage choice(s), which, as part of a healthy lifestyle, **may help living well with** certain chronic diseases or conditions.

Both subcategories of disease-related general wellness claims should only be based on references where it is well understood that healthy lifestyle choices may reduce the risk or impact of a chronic disease or medical condition. That is, the claim that the healthy lifestyle choices may play an important role in health outcomes should be generally accepted; such associations are described in peer-reviewed scientific publications or official statements made by healthcare professional organizations. Examples of chronic diseases for which a healthy lifestyle is associated with risk reduction or help in living well with that disease include heart disease, high blood pressure, and type 2 diabetes.

The following are examples of this category of disease-related general wellness claims:

- Software product U coaches breathing techniques and relaxation skills, which, as part of a healthy lifestyle, may help living well with migraine headaches.
- Software product V tracks and records your sleep, work, and exercise routine, which, as part of a healthy lifestyle, may help living well with anxiety.

Also included in this category are the following: "Products intended to restore a structure or function impaired due to a disease might be regulated by the FDA as devices. For example, an artificial limb prosthesis intended to provide disabled persons the ability to walk might be regulated under 21 CFR 890.3420 or 21 CFR 890.3500. By organizations we mean associations and colleges such as the American Medical Association (AMA), American Heart Association (AHA), American Association of Clinical Endocrinologists (AACE), American College of Rheumatology, and so forth.

Mobile Medical Apps

The fourth category of medical devices regulated by the FDA reflect the increasingly widespread adoption and use of mobile technologies, which can open new and innovative ways to improve health and healthcare delivery.[12] The FDA defines mobile medical apps as

> software programs that run on smartphones and other mobile communication devices. They can also be accessories that attach to a smartphone or other mobile communication devices, or a combination of accessories and software. Mobile medical apps are medical devices that are mobile apps, meet the definition of a medical device and are an accessory to a regulated medical device or transform a mobile platform into a regulated medical device. Consumers can use both mobile medical apps and mobile apps to manage their own health and wellness, such as to monitor their caloric intake for healthy weight maintenance.

The agency gives the following specific examples of devices that qualify as mobile medical apps:

> The National Institutes of Health's LactMed app provides nursing mothers with information about the effects of medicines on breast milk and nursing infants. Other apps aim to help health care professionals improve and facilitate patient care. The Radiation Emergency Medical Management (REMM) app gives health care providers guidance on diagnosing and treating radiation injuries. Some mobile medical apps can diagnose cancer or heart rhythm abnormalities,

or function as the "central command" for a glucose meter used by an insulin-dependent diabetic patient.[13]

To classify which devices will be considered mobile medical apps, the FDA provides fairly extensive guidelines related to the definition of medical devices:

The FDA is taking a tailored, risk-based approach that focuses on the small subset of mobile apps that meet the regulatory definition of "device" and that:

- are intended to be used as an accessory to a regulated medical device, or
- transform a mobile platform into a regulated medical device.

Mobile apps span a wide range of health functions. While many mobile apps carry minimal risk, those that can pose a greater risk to patients will require FDA review.

Some devices will be exempt from the regulatory process:

For many mobile apps that meet the regulatory definition of a "device" but pose minimal risk to patients and consumers, the FDA will exercise enforcement discretions and will not expect manufacturers to submit premarket review applications or to register and list their apps with the FDA. This includes mobile medical apps that:

- Help patients/users self-manage their disease or condition without providing specific treatment suggestions;
- Provide patients with simple tools to organize and track their health information;
- Provide easy access to information related to health conditions or treatments;
- Help patients document, show or communicate potential medical conditions to health care providers;
- Automate simple tasks for health care providers; or
- Enable patients or providers to interact with Personal Health Records (PHR) or Electronic Health Record (EHR) systems.[14]

Federal Trade Commission

The third major government regulatory organ that will impact gerontechnology is the FTC, whose federal authority covers aspects of business practice and consumer protection in a twofold way:

1. Protect consumers: Prevent fraud, deception, and unfair business practices in the marketplace.
2. Maintain competition: Prevent anticompetitive mergers and other anti-competitive business practices in the marketplace.[15]

With regard to the first point, the FTC's consumer protection role is geared toward

> stopping unfair, deceptive or fraudulent practices in the marketplace. We conduct investigations, sue companies and people that violate the law, develop rules to ensure a vibrant marketplace, and educate consumers and businesses about their rights and responsibilities. We collect complaints about hundreds of issues from data security and deceptive advertising to identity theft and Do Not Call violations, and make them available to law enforcement agencies worldwide for follow-up.[16]

Example: The Case of Lumosity

One goal of the agency is to prevent consumers from being taken advantage of through deceptive marketing and advertising. In terms of consumer protection, the agency gives a detailed example in its litigation against Lumosity; at the conclusion of the investigation/litigation, Lumosity paid a $2 million settlement to the government over its advertising claims for its brain training computer program, claims that were deemed overreaching and lacking empirical evidence. I cite this particular example because of its direct connection to gerontechnology and the issue of vulnerable elders, including those with dementia. On January 5, 2016, the FTC announced that

> the creators and marketers of the Lumosity "brain training" program have agreed to settle Federal Trade Commission charges alleging that they deceived consumers with unfounded claims that Lumosity games can help users perform better at work and in school, and reduce or delay cognitive impairment associated with age and other serious health conditions.[17]

The FTC's investigation concluded that "Lumosity preyed on consumers' fears about age-related cognitive decline, suggesting their games could stave off memory loss, dementia, and even Alzheimer's disease." The computer program was widely marketed across the media (television, radio, email, social media, and on the company website, Lumosity.com) and charged a monthly membership rate of $14.95 or a lifetime membership for $299.95. The FTC noted that Lumosity claimed that the computer program would

> 1) improve performance on everyday tasks, in school, at work, and in athletics; 2) delay age-related cognitive decline and protect against mild cognitive

Table 15.3 Regulatory Agencies

Federal	State	Academic	Professional	The Market (Pseudo Regulation)
FDA	Medicare	Institutional review boards	AMA	Advertising
FTC	Medicaid	Federal grants	American Psychiatric Association	Marketing
GAO	Private health insurance	Industry		
Medicare		InternationalSociety for Gerontology	American Psychology Association	
Medicaid		SocNeruosci	AAN	
VA		INS	AAGP	
			IEEE	

impairment, dementia, and Alzheimer's disease; and 3) reduce cognitive impairment associated with health conditions, including stroke, traumatic brain injury, PTSD, ADHD, the side effects of chemotherapy, and Turner syndrome, and that scientific studies proved these benefits.[18]

It was also charged that Lumosity failed to "disclose that some consumer testimonials featured on the website had been solicited through contests that promised significant prizes, including a free iPad, a lifetime Lumosity subscription, and a round-trip to San Francisco."[19]

Dementia of many types can cause cognitive decline in executive skills (insight, reasoning, judgment, decision making) that can leave elders vulnerable to undue influence and marketing fraud, even at the mild cognitive impairment stage, resulting in their spending potentially large amounts of money on products that claim health or cognitive benefits without sufficient empirical clinical evidence to back up those claims (see Table 15.3).[20]

General Accounting Office and Information Technology

The GAO is a federal agency that provides useful information about the broad range of information technologies and the federal departments that oversee many aspects of healthcare. In 2008, the GAO published "Information Technology: Federal Laws, Regulations, and Mandatory Standards for Securing Private Sector Information Technology Systems and Data in Critical Infrastructure Sectors."[21] These infrastructures are described in the document as "critical to the nations' security, economy, public health, and safety."[22] The document acknowledges from the outset that many of the industries or aspects of an industry are privately owned and operated, and encourages cooperation between the public and private sector. The federal government "uses both voluntary partnerships with private industry and requirements in federal laws, regulations, and mandatory standards to assist in the security of privately owned information technology (IT) systems and data within critical infrastructure sectors."[23]

The agency works toward its goal of information security through "(1) federal laws, regulations, and mandatory standards that pertain to securing that sector's privately owned IT systems and data and (2) identify[ing] enforcement mechanisms for each of the above laws, regulations, and mandatory standards."[24] There are numerous government departments involved in the full spectrum of information technology. In addition to specific government agencies, healthcare security includes oversight from the Department of Homeland Security for emergency medical services and oversight of government facilities, and the use of nuclear materials in medicine. HHS is involved in the oversight of healthcare facilities.[25] With regard to the protection of healthcare information, the GAO notes federal regulations that include enforcement measures of criminal monetary penalties and imprisonment, and gives the following example: "a person who knowingly discloses individually identifiable health information, which is a violation of the underlying statute, may be fined up to $50,000, imprisoned for up to 1 year, or both" (see Figure 15.1).[26]

Medicare, Medicaid, and the Affordable Care Act (or Its Replacement)[27]

A question raised earlier was *who pays* for new gerontechnologies, given that many elders are on fixed incomes (e.g., social security, pensions). The answer in many cases is health insurance, and this exerts a de facto influence on what new technology products will be developed and paid for by insurance companies. In the United States, Medicare and Medicaid are the two federal programs that provide health insurance for the elderly (the latter primarily for individuals with few financial resources). In addition, the ACA enacted by Congress during the Obama administration has provided health insurance to millions of people who had been previously uninsured. While these agencies do not regulate gerontechnology directly in terms of its research and development, they do exert direct influence on which technologies they will or will not pay for.

Medicare is the general government health plan for the elderly.[28] It provides funds for skilled nursing care, long-term care, prescription medications, and some aspects of in-home care, this last being an area in which gerontechnology is greatly interested in terms of helping elders to age in place. Medicaid is the

	Agriculture and food	Banking and finance	Chemical	Commercial facilities	Critical manufacturing	Dams	Defense industrial base	Drinking water and water treatment systems	Emergency services	Energy	Government facilities	Information technology	National monuments and icons	Nuclear reactors, materials, and waste	Postal and shipping	Public health and healthcare	Telecommunications	Transportation systems	Total
Number of applicable laws[a]							1												1
Number of applicable regulations	1	17	1						1	1				1		1	2		25
Number of applicable mandatory standards					8				8										8[b]

Total 34

None apply ☐   Number that apply ▨

Figure 15.1 Summary of federal legal requirements for securing privately owned it systems and data within critical infrastructure sectors.

Source: General Accounting Office, http://www.gao.gov/new.items/d081075r.pdf. The GAO website states, "This is a work of the U.S. government and is not subject to copyright protection in the United States. The published product may be reproduced and distributed in its entirety without further permission from GAO."

comparable federal government health program for low-income individuals. These programs, administered by the Centers for Medicare and Medicaid Services (CMS), are part of HHS.[29]

Veteran's Administration

There is yet another national healthcare entity in the United States that provides health services to the elderly, the Veteran's Administration (VA). The VA provides lifelong care to former members of the military, operating the nation's largest integrated healthcare system, responsible for over 1,700 hospitals, clinics, community living centers, domiciliaries, and counseling centers, covering medication and medical supply costs for retired veterans.[30] The document's stated goal is the protection of information systems, be they public or private. The agency identifies 18 "infrastructure sectors" as being critical to "the nation's security, economy, public health and safety." Public health and healthcare is identified as one of the important infrastructures, but the list includes other areas touching on healthcare practice, including government facilities; information technology; nuclear reactors, materials, and waste; telecommunications; and transportations systems, all of which can be involved in the provision of healthcare services.

Other Healthcare Providers

Private health insurance and nongovernmental healthcare agencies (e.g., privately owned hospitals) are common in America.[31] In addition to Medicare, many elders have secondary private insurance (e.g., obtained as part of their retirement through their former employers or VA benefits for retired military). The private for-profit insurance companies (e.g., Aetna, Anthem, Blue Cross, Cigna, Humana, Wellpoint, etc.) will also be stakeholders in financial matters vis-à-vis funding the purchase of technologies for elder healthcare.[32]

There are many organizations, many of them religion based, that provide healthcare as part of their mission. In the United States, the Roman Catholic Church is the largest provider of healthcare services outside the federal government, and many other religious denominations (e.g., Protestant, Jewish) have founded and continue to oversee hospitals and other healthcare entities. As healthcare providers for older individuals, they will all act to diagnose and treat healthcare problems, and treatment will involve the use of available technologies.

In summary, the current state of oversight and regulation with regard to gerontechnology is multiple rather than unified, existing across many federal agencies, which can be helpful to individuals with dementia. This situation is

Table 15.4 Robotics Gerontechnology

Medical	Monitoring	Mobility	Communication	Safety: Smart Homes
Biosensors	Activity	Wheelchairs		Motion detectors
Physiology sensors	Sleep	Walkers		Smart stoves
	Gait	Stair tech		Smart thermostats
		Cars		Gait sensors

unlikely to change, so anyone working to develop technology will often come under the aegis of one or more agencies depending on the nature of the technology under development (e.g., home robotics technologies that collect, store, and transmit medical information for health and safety monitoring of individuals with dementia—see Table 15.4).

Consequently, the development and regulation of gerontechnology will continue to involve multiple stakeholders—federal, private, and corporate—across multiple domains including academia, healthcare, business, and government. In light of this situation, I would like to offer several suggestions about how this situation can be negotiated in the service of bringing new technologies into elder care for individuals with dementia. They involve education, assessment, integration, and communication and touch on issues both theoretical and practical.

Conclusions and Recommendations

There are many stakeholders in geriatric healthcare and gerontechnology, each having an impact on the process of conceiving, developing, and implementing new technologies. These include:

- Older individuals and their families
- The healthcare professions
- Academia
- Business and industry setting in which gerontechnology is developed
- The media through which these products are marketed
- Federal regulatory agencies that approve, oversee, license, and regulate technologies
- Health insurance companies
- Nongovernmental healthcare organizations

To think through how to deal with this already complex situation, I would first like to return to the three diversities that began this chapter (government, gerontechnology, dementia) and to consider how the federal regulation of technology impacts each.

1. The diversity of government structure. The federal regulation of technology is split among several large organizations that oversee the development, safety, and efficacy of current and emerging gerontechnologies. In many cases, these agencies are the ultimate arbiters of whether any new technology with the potential to improve the lives of older individuals will reach the market and become available for widespread use. Those who develop new technologies in any of these areas, including those in academia and industry, will be dealing with one or more government agencies in the process of bringing their products to market. It will fall to these entities to demonstrate with solid empirical evidence that any new technology they develop is safe, effective, and useful to older individuals, and to make new gerontechnologies attractive to the different aging cohorts. Familiarity with these agencies and their policies will speed the process of new technologies becoming available to the general public.

2. The diversity of gerontechnology. I have identified five broad areas under which gerontechnology might be grouped: medical, monitoring and safety, mobility, communication, and robotics. This means that there is a vast array of current and emerging technology that can positively impact the health and quality of life for older individuals, making it possible for them to remain in their homes much longer than would otherwise be the case due to physical, medical, and cognitive changes associated with the normal aging process in general and with dementia in particular. The diversity of technologies exists within the reality of multiple governmental agencies that will regulate them, and with various payers who will determine whether or not any particular new technology will be funded and thus available for use. It is perhaps in the area of robotics that the biggest obstacles will be met in patient trust and acceptance.

3. The diversity of dementia. There are many illnesses that cause dementia, and no one person goes through the process of dementia the same as another will, depending on myriad factors that include premorbid abilities, medication efficacy (when available for a particular dementia type), and lifestyle changes that are aimed at maintaining optimal health in the context of dementia (e.g., frequent socialization, exercise, healthy diet). In addition, different dementia types cause different patterns of cognitive change and decline. Individuals with Alzheimer's disease and vascular dementia can both experience prominent memory difficulties, while individuals with frontotemporal dementia typically see an early decline of executive skills while memory is relatively preserved. Individuals with Parkinson's disease can, later in the course of their illness, experience dementia, while those with Parkinson-plus syndromes experience movement and dementia symptoms of simultaneous onset. In short, the clinical needs of any given individual that might be served by gerontechnology will vary greatly, both by the particular dementia type and by the individual course any dementia takes in a given individual.

Recommendations

Can there be any overarching, systematic body of knowledge that can inform a clinical and regulatory situation of such diversity, with so many different stakeholders, that can inform the conception, development, and implementation of new gerontechnologies? I would suggest that there can. For guidance, we can look to the definition of the field of gerontechnology outlined earlier. Graafmans (2017) defined the field of gerontechnology as "the development and adaptation of technology toward the goals and ambitions of aging and aged peoples and it is application oriented in nature."

For gerontechnology, there is a core body of knowledge that should be available to individuals operating in any of the entities involved in the development and regulation of gerontechnology, even when greater depth of knowledge will differ by the specific context or discipline. I will conclude with several recommendations for bringing some commonality and uniformity to the field of gerontechnology regulation.

Who Needs to Know?

Individuals involved in any aspect of gerontechnology need a common core body of knowledge in geriatrics and technology to create safe and effective new technologies for older individuals. This includes:

- The three branches government: executive, legislative, and judiciary
- Federal regulatory agency staff: FDA, FTC, VA, Medicare, and Medicaid
- State governments that oversee the distribution of healthcare resources, for example, Medicaid
- Engineers, scientists, and computer specialists involved in the development of gerontechnology
- The healthcare professions, including:
  - Physicians and nurse practitioners (especially in geriatric primary care, psychiatry, and neurology)
  - All healthcare providers working in geriatrics (e.g., nursing, occupational therapists, physical therapists, social work)
  - Inpatient hospital staff
  - Outpatient healthcare providers
  - Staff of assisted living facilities
  - Staff of nursing homes

- Mental healthcare providers
- Visiting nurses
- Elder law attorneys
- Hospice care staff
- Families of individuals diagnosed with dementia
- Individuals with dementia, insofar as their cognitive capacities allow them to participate in education and decision making
- Professionals in academia dedicated to the development of new gerontechnologies
- The business and marketing communities
- Insurance companies: these should be included in outreach about new technologies and their benefits, given the financial role they hold in the availability of new technologies to consumers
- The automotive industry
- Bioethicists

How Can They Come to Know It?

Many healthcare professionals who have been in the field for several decades had little or no geriatric training during their clinical education. This information can be provided through continuing education requirements, including online education. Today, geriatric education can be built into undergraduate and graduate training programs across disciplines so that new professionals enter the field with a good knowledge of geriatrics.

What Needs to Be Known?

There is a core body of knowledge in geriatrics that can be useful to anyone working in the field of gerontechnology, knowledge necessary for anyone involved in technology development because it points to likely technological needs of an aging population:

- Normal aging: what it is and what it isn't, as to its impact on biology, cognition, affective functioning, mobility, sensation, and potential impact of any of these on daily functioning (ADLs and IADLs)
- Mild cognitive impairment
- Reliable early warning signs of dementia
- Major dementia types and their characteristic clinical profiles
- Common safety risks that arise in the context of dementing illnesses to help target new technologies

- Technologies that are already available for the care of individuals with dementia, and technologies that are under development

Assessment

Age is the greatest risk factor for most dementias, including Alzheimer's disease. Medicare now requires a cognitive screening at annual wellness visits to promote early identification of cognitive difficulties. Currently there is no standardization regarding the nature of this assessment; developing common practices in the assessment of normal aging individuals in the primary care setting and elsewhere could assist technology development through research documentation of the most common cognitive changes experienced by those in the normal aging process and in dementia.[33]

Communication

Gerontechnology by its very nature includes individuals from numerous professions and spheres, from healthcare to academic, from business to local communities. Facilitating communication across disciplines will be vital in expanding the common core of knowledge needed for gerontechnology and for stimulating creativity and technology development.

Integration

The more the different disciplines of gerontechnology interact, the more likely will be the cross-fertilization of information and ideas that can promote technology development. One way this might occur is through dedicated sessions at national and international academic organizations such as the International Society for Gerontechnology, the Society for Neuroscience, and the International Neuroethics Society, as well as professional engineering organizations and computer science conferences.

Summary

The federal regulation of gerontechnology in the United States is a complex and diverse issue involving numerous federal agencies. Furthermore, gerontechnology itself is not a unified area, but covers multiple types of technology that can help with medical care, safety monitoring, communication, and mobility, most recently through advances in robotics. This chapter reviews the major federal agencies involved in the regulation of technology, including the FDA, which exerts widespread influence over the adoption of new technologies; the VA; Medicare and Medicaid; and others. Furthermore, there are many different stakeholders with regard to gerontechnology and dementia, from elderly patients to their caregivers, federal regulators, and healthcare professionals. Based on the examinations of these issues, I concluded by offering several recommendations, including who needs to be familiar with gerontechnology regulation, ways in which stakeholders can become educated about the numerous issues involved in technology regulation, the content with which the stakeholders need to be familiar, issues of assessment in individuals with dementia directly impacting technology choices, and, lastly, the need for cross-fertilization of knowledge across the different areas, including, STEM, healthcare, and federal agencies, to bring needed services to elders with dementia.

Notes

1. See American Psychiatric Association, *Diagnostic and Statistical Manual of Mental Disorders*, 5th ed. (DSM V) (Washington, DC: American Psychiatric Publishing, 2013). Cognitive difficulties among the elderly are currently classified as either mild or major neurocognitive disorders and require reference to a specific underlying condition such as Alzheimer's disease, frontotemporal lobar degeneration, Lewy body disease, vascular disease, traumatic brain injury, HIV infection, Prion disease, Huntington's disease, etc.

2. An example: individuals with Parkinson-plus syndromes, such as Lewy Body dementia, are susceptible to orthostatic hypotension, which can cause episodes of fainting and falls.

3. This is, of course, a future technology, though as I write this, self-driving cars are already in existence and have begun road testing in some US states. It is more likely than not that organizations that serve elders (e.g., the American Association of Retired Persons [AARP] and the Alzheimer's Association, to name only two [both of these address issues of driving safety in the elderly]) will be keeping close watch on the development, safety, and availability of self-driving technology.

4. Graafmans, J.A.M., The history and incubation of gerontechnology, in Sunkyo Kwon (Ed.), *Gerontechnology: Research, Practice and Principles in the Field of Technology and Aging* (New York: Springer, 2017), 7.

5. Ibid.

6. The department website is https://www.hhs.gov. For its mission statement see https://www.hhs.gov/about/indexhtml (accessed February 18, 2017).

7. The quotes that follow are taken from the FDA website, accessible at http://www.fda.gov/medicaldevices/deviceregulationandguidance/overview/classifyyourdevice/ucm051512.htm (accessed January 14, 2017).

8. Examples in the field of psychiatry include the use of older antidepressant medications such as amitriptyline for the management of peripheral pain and the use of acetylcholinesterase inhibitors for the treatment of psychosis (visual hallucinations) in the context of Lewy body dementia (with Lewy body dementia individuals become hypersensitive to many medications, especially neuroleptics, so this provides an important alternative with lower risk).

9. Other products related to healthcare for both humans and animals are regulated by the FDA, which also covers "other FDA regulated products such as drugs. Biological products which include blood and blood products, and blood banking equipment are regulated by FDA's Center for Biologics Evaluation and Research (CBER). FDA's Center for Veterinary Medicine (CVM) regulates products used with animals." See the FDA website for details on the activities of these divisions.

10. See FDA website.

11. The issue of cognitive enhancement in the normally aging population, as well as in younger adults and children, touches on this area as well and is likely to be discussed with increasing frequency in the future.

12. Recognizing the rapid growth in use of mobile technologies, the FDA has commented:

> Mobile applications (apps) can help people manage their own health and wellness, promote healthy living, and gain access to useful information when and where they need it. These tools are being adopted almost as quickly as they can be developed. According to industry estimates, 500 million smartphone users worldwide will be using a health care application by 2015, and by 2018, 50 percent of the more than 3.4 billion smartphone and tablet users will have downloaded mobile health applications (http://www.research2guidance.com/500m-people-will-be-using-healthcare-mobile-applications-in-2015/). These users include health care professionals, consumers, and patients.
>
> The FDA encourages the development of mobile medical apps that improve health care and provide consumers and health care professionals with valuable health information. The FDA also has a public health responsibility to oversee the safety and effectiveness of medical devices—including mobile medical apps.
>
> The FDA issued the Mobile Medical Applications Guidance for Industry and Food and Drug Administration Staff (PDF—269KB) on September 25, 2013, which explains the agency's oversight of mobile medical apps as devices and our focus only on the apps that present a greater risk to patients if they don't work as intended and on apps that cause smartphones or other mobile platforms to impact the functionality or performance of traditional medical devices.

13. The agency attempts to make clear distinctions about what does and does not fall under the category of low-risk medical apps, how they will be regulated, and guidance in determining which applications fall under FDA regulation:

> The FDA will apply the same risk-based approach the agency uses to assure safety and effectiveness for other medical devices. The guidance document

(PDF—269KB) provides examples of how the FDA might regulate certain moderate-risk (Class II) and high-risk (Class III) mobile medical apps. The guidance also provides examples of mobile apps that are not medical devices, mobile apps that the FDA intends to exercise enforcement discretion and mobile medical apps that the FDA will regulate in Appendix A, Appendix B and Appendix C. We encourage app developers to contact the FDA—as early as possible—if they have any questions about their mobile app, its level of risk, and whether a premarket application is required.

14. The complete policy is available at http://www.fda.gov/medicaldevices/digitalhealth/mobilemedicalapplications/default.htm (accessed January 14, 2017).
15. This information is available at the FTC website, https://www.ftc.gov, under https://www.ftc.gov/about-ftc/what-we-do (accessed January 14, 2017).
16. Federal Trade Commission, https://www.ftc.gov/about-ftc/what-we-do
17. Federal Trade Commission, https://www.ftc.gov/news-events/press-releases/2016/01/lumosity-pay-2-million-settle-ftc-deceptive-advertising-charges
18. FTC, "Lumosity to Pay $2 Million to Settle FTC Deceptive Advertising Charges for Its "Brain Training" Program Company Claimed Program Would Sharpen Performance in Everyday Life and Protect Against Cognitive Decline. https://www.ftc.gov/news-events/press-releases/2016/01/lumosity-pay-2-million-settle-ftc-deceptive-advertising-charges
19. The announcement of the settlement, which reviews the history of the FTC's assessment of Lumosity, can be found at https://www.ftc.gov/news-events/press-releases/2016/01/lumosity-pay-2-million-settle-ftc-deceptive-advertising-charges (accessed January 14, 2017).
20. This issue also arises in the many products, classified as herbal products, medical foods, or vitamins, marketed as adjunct treatments for dementia. Many of them were started in FDA clinical drug trials, which were then stopped by the manufacturer due to concerns about lack of demonstrable efficacy in rigorous testing, and instead were marketed as items such as medical foods, herbal products, or vitamins, not regulated in the same way by the FDA. These include coconut oil, vitamin E, Prevagen, coral calcium, and so forth. A review of the various adjunct products, including potential interactions with prescription drugs, can be found through the search engine of the Alzheimer's Association website, alz.org. In clinical practice, when patients ask about these products, it is important to encourage them to speak with their prescribers about any adjunct treatments they are considering (most older patients are unaware, for example, that vitamin E can lower the efficacy of statin drugs used to treat hypercholesterol, and that gingko can cause visual hallucinations) and to seek out reliable information about the product through the Alzheimer's Association.
21. The complete document is available at the GAO website, http://www.gao.gov/assets/100/95747.pdf. Quotes are taken from this document. See Figure 15.1 for the complete listing of critical infrastructures and information about the applicability of federal regulations (accessed February 18, 2017).
22. http://www.gao.gov/assets/100/95747.pdf
23. http://www.gao.gov/assets/100/95747.pdf
24. http://www.gao.gov/assets/100/95747.pdf

25. See GAO, *Progress Coordinating Government and Private Sector Efforts Varies by Sectors' Characteristics,* GAO-07-39 (Washington, DC: October 16, 2006).

26. http://www.gao.gov/assets/100/95747.pdf. See the section Results: Objective 2: Enforcement Mechanisms.

27. Note that these are all under the aegis of the HHS. I have considered them separately from the general overview of the HHS earlier and as a group because they are all *health insurance entities* that will be direct payers for dementia technology and thus exert a direct influence on which dementia technologies come into widespread use and which do not through decisions by these agencies on what specific technologies will and will not be reimbursed.

28. Information about Medicare and dementia care is available at https://www.medicare.gov/site-search/search-results.html?q=dementia.

29. The federal website for Medicaid is https://www.medicaid.gov. For an overview of the program, see https://www.medicaid.gov/about-us/index.html (accessed January 14, 2017).

30. Information about the VA system is available at http://www.va.gov/. The VA provides services to all veterans, including younger ones who have served in the military; our focus here though will be on those over 65, which already includes individuals who fought in World War II, the Korean War, and the Vietnam War, and which will eventually include military personnel who served in the Middle East from the 1990s, and so forth. One example of the changes in medical care needs the VA will deal with is the incidence of chronic traumatic encephalopathy (CTE), no longer seen only in professional athletes (e.g., boxing, football, and hockey, as well as other professional sports) but also in members of the military who served over the past two decades in the Middle East due to exposure to improvised explosive devices (IEDs). The common causal denominator to CTE is repeated concussions, and the condition, which causes dementia as well as behavioral and movement symptoms, can have a delay of symptom onset of one to two decades.

31. As I write this in mid-2017, legislation to repeal the ACA, known as Obama Care, was passed by the House of Representatives and sent to the Senate, where it will likely undergo changes before a Senate vote. Whatever final form the plan takes, it will need to address access to the technologies of healthcare.

32. For a listing of health insurance companies in the United States with the largest market share, see https://health.usnews.com/health-news/health-insurance.

33. Available for use across healthcare professions, the Montreal Cognitive Assessment (MoCA) is a highly useful, brief, valid, and reliable screening for cognitive functioning that has been shown to be better than other widely used screening instruments (e.g., Mini Mental Status Exam, St. Louis University Mental Status exam) at detecting early/mild cognitive impairment, enabling earlier diagnosis and intervention.

Bibliography

Alzheimer, A. Über eigenartige Krankheitsfalle der späteren Alters. *Zeitschrift für die Gesamte Neurologie und Psychiatrie,* 4 (1911): 356–385.

Bengtson, V.L., and R.A. Settersten Jr. *Handbook of Theories of Aging,* Third Edition. New York: Springer, 2016.

Berridge, C., P.I. Furseth, R. Cuthbertson, and S. Demello. Technology-based innovation for independent living: Policy and innovation in the United Kingdom, Scandinavia, and the United States. *Journal of Aging and Social Policy*, 26 (2014): 213–228.

Bozeat, S., C.A. Gregory, M.A. Ralph, and A.R. Hodges. Which neuropsychiatric features distinguish front-temporal and temporal variants of frontotemporal dementia form Alzheimer's disease? *Journal of Neurology, Neurosurgery and Psychiatry*, 69 (2000): 178–186.

Braak, H., I. Alafuzoff, T. Arzberger, H. Kretzschmar, and K. Del Tredici. Staging of Alzheimer's disease-associated neurofibrillary pathology using paraffin sections and immunocytochemistry. *Acta Neuropathologica*, 112 (2006): 389–404.

Cardarelli, R., A. Kertesz, and J.A. Knebel. Frontotemporal dementia: A review for primary care physicians. *American Family Physician*, 82 (2010): 1372–1377.

Cavanaugh, J.C., and F. Blanchard-Fields. *Adult Development and Aging*, Seventh Edition. Stamford, CT: Cengage, 2015.

Chatterjee, A., and M.J. Farah. *Neuroethics in Practice: Medicine, Mind and Society*. New York: Oxford University Press, 2013.

DeCarli, C. Vascular cognitive impairment. In B. Dickerson and A. Atri (Eds.), *Dementia, Comprehensive Principles and Practice*. New York: Oxford University Press, 2014.

Dickerson, B., and A. Atri. *Dementia: Comprehensive Principles and Practice*. New York: Oxford University Press, 2014.

Farah, M.J. *Neuroethics: An Introduction with Readings*. Cambridge, MA: MIT Press, 2010.

Gitlin, L., H. Kales, and C.G. Lykestos. Nonpharmacologic management of behavioral symptoms in dementia. *Journal of the American Medical Association*, 308 (2012): 2020–2029.

Glannon, W. *Defining Right and Wrong in Brain Science: Essential Readings in Neuroethics*. New York: Dana Press, 2007.

Graafmans, J.A.M. The history and incubation of gerontechnology. In S. Kwon (Ed.), *Gerontechnology: Research, Practice and Principles in the Field of Technology and Aging*. New York: Springer, 2017.

Guardini, R. *Letters from Lake Como: Explorations in Technology and the Human Race*. Grand Rapids, MI: William B. Eerdmans, 1994.

Jotterand, F., and V. Dubljevi. *Cognitive Enhancement: Ethical and Policy Implications in International Perspectives*. New York: Oxford University Press, 2016.

Kwon, S. *Gerontechnology: Research, Practice and Principles in the Field of Technology and Aging*. New York: Springer, 2017.

Miller, B.L., J.L. Cummings, J. Villaneuva-Meyer, C.M. Mehringer, and I. Mena. Frontal lobe degeneration: Clinical, neuropsychological and SPECT characteristics. *Neurology*, 41 (1991): 1374–1382.

Seshardi, S., and P.A. Wolf. Lifetime risk of stroke and dementia: Current concepts and estimates from the Framingham study. *Lancet Neurology*, 6, 12 (2007): 1106–1114.

Sugar, J.A., R.J. Rieske, H. Holstege, and M.A. Faber. *Introduction to Aging: A Positive, Interdisciplinary Approach*. New York: Springer, 2014.

Vallor, S. *Technology and the Virtues: A Philosophical Guide to a Future Worth Living*. Oxford: Oxford University Press, 2016.

Weiner, J.B. The regulation of technology and the technology of regulation. *Technology in Society* 26 (2004): 483–500.

Wilmoth, J.M., Ferraro, K.F. *Gerontology: Perspectives and Issues*, 4th Ed. New York: Springer Publishing Company, 2013.

Epilogue

Dementia in the Digital Age

Tenzin Wangmo and Marcello Ienca

Alzheimer's disease (AD) and other dementias afflict millions of older adults worldwide. The global prevalence of dementia is placing a high financial and caregiving burden on both individual families and the healthcare systems. Furthermore, it raises the risk of jeopardizing the delivery of care services in both the institutional and home care setting. No less important, dementia has a devastating impact on the lives of the person diagnosed and his or her families, friends, and loved ones. The silent global epidemic of dementia calls for urgent measures to alleviate this global burden and for improving the delivery of effective care services for patients in need and their families.

Achieving this goal will require a coordinated multilevel effort involving (a) advances in basic science aimed at cracking the pathological conundrum of AD and casting light on its etiology, (b) generating innovative pharmacological solutions aimed at mitigating—and possibly reversing—its symptoms, and (c) developing technological solutions that can assist people with dementia and their families, improve their quality of life, and facilitate and ameliorate the delivery of healthcare services.

The digital transformation of medicine is expected to contribute to achieving these aims. Public health is increasingly incorporating data from expanded digital sources including electronic patient records, mobile technology and digital phenotyping, and social media content and other online behavior. This opens the prospect of a "digital epidemiology of dementia," which could improve the bandwidth and scope of current epidemiological models and improve the adaptiveness of existing public health plans. In parallel, healthcare provision will increasingly benefit from the deployment of intelligent assistive technologies and other digital health solutions, especially those reliant on automated artificial intelligence applications such as machine learning.

This book has shown, however, that the future of dementia care in the digital era will be dependent not only on technology development but also on fundamental ethical considerations, unavoidable societal discussions, well-calibrated regulatory interventions, and adaptive governance frameworks.

By bringing together experts from the fields of medicine, public health, computer science, engineering, gerontology, law, social science, and ethics, this volume attempted to outline a first comprehensive and multidisciplinary vision to prepare the terrain for the future of dementia in the digital age. The more technology advances, the more it becomes clear that there should be no easy shortcuts to the digital transformation of dementia care. The 15 chapters compiled in this book give us a glimpse of the multifaceted complexity of digitalizing dementia care through intelligent technology.

This collection stands to show that hard work needs to be done to ensure an effective, safe, and inclusive digital transition and that the big technical, ethical, and policy challenges ahead cannot be avoided. These include identifying concrete strategies to alleviate caregiving burden through intelligent assistive technology (IAT), promoting successful public-private cooperation, transitioning to patient-centered and caregiver-centered approaches to technology design, developing standards for gerontechnology applications, preserving data privacy both by design and through effective data governance frameworks, ensuring informed consent in the ever-evolving digital ecosystem, addressing the complex philosophical and psychological nature of personal identity in light of both the transformative nature of dementia and the intimate interaction with artificially intelligent systems, adequately disseminating information to end-users, sustaining trust in the technology and in data collection, and preventing a technological divide that could aggravate preexisting inequalities.

This volume provided an up-to-date overview of these challenges and an examination of their implications for individual stakeholders, healthcare, and society at large. It thus stands to benefit both the academic and nonacademic community working in the fields of dementia care, digital health, and assistive technology. The timely analyses contained in this collection emphasize that successful IATs require a deeper understanding of the multilevel complexity of dementia, which encompasses a continuum going from single molecules to personal identities, families, healthcare systems, and the global population. Also necessary are policy measures that ensure the evidence-based validation of new technologies and their fair dissemination to all people in need. In a world where digital technology is becoming pervasive and indispensable in all facets of our lives, we should not aim for societal models that create divisions between those with the means to afford it and those without, especially when it comes to vulnerable groups such as people with dementia.

Index